CW01239226

101

Nutrition Myths Debunked

Dale Pinnock

Copyright © [2025] [Dale Pinnock]
All rights reserved.

No part of this book may be copied, reproduced, distributed, or transmitted in any form or by any means, including photocopying, recording, or digital methods, without prior written permission from the publisher, except for brief quotations in reviews, educational discussions, or other uses permitted under copyright law.

This book is intended for informational purposes only. While every effort has been made to ensure accuracy, this book is not a substitute for professional medical, nutritional, or health advice. Readers should consult a qualified healthcare provider before making any dietary or lifestyle changes. The author and publisher assume no responsibility for any consequences resulting from the use of information contained in this book.

For permissions, inquiries, or special licensing,
contact : Dale Pinnock -
www.dalepinnock.com'

Table of Contents

Introduction   12

Myth 1 Eating Fat Makes You Fat   15

Myth 2 All Calories Are Created Equal, No Matter The Source   22

Myth 3 Carbohydrates Are Inherently Unhealthy And Should Be Avoided   29

Myth 4 High-Protein Diets Damage Your Kidneys   36

Myth 5 You Must Cleanse Or Detox Regularly To Rid Your Body Of Toxins   42

Myth 6 Eating Late At Night Always Leads To Weight Gain   48

Myth 7 Organic Foods Are Always More Nutritious Than Conventional Foods   54

Myth 8 If It's Labelled "Gluten-Free," It's Healthier   60

Myth 9 Red Meat Should Be Completely Eliminated From A Healthy Diet   66

Myth 10 All Processed Foods Are Harmful And Devoid Of Nutrition   72

Myth 11 High-Cholesterol Foods Always Raise Your Blood Cholesterol Levels   77

Myth 12 Cooking Vegetables Destroys All Their Nutrients   82

Myth 13 You Must Drink Eight Glasses Of Water
Every Day, No Exceptions ... 87

Myth 14 Diet Sodas Help With Weight Loss Because
They Have Zero Calories ... 92

Myth 15 Frozen Fruits And Vegetables Are Less
Nutritious Than Fresh Produce ... 97

Myth 16 Supplements Can Replace The Need For
A Good Diet ... 102

Myth 17 A Vegetarian Or Vegan Diet Automatically
Ensures Good Health ... 108

Myth 18 Skipping Breakfast Leads To Weight Gain ... 113

Myth 19 Eating Multiple Small Meals Throughout
The Day Always Boosts Metabolism ... 117

Myth 20 Natural Sweeteners Like Honey Or Agave
Are Always Healthier Than Sugar ... 121

Myth 21 You Can Spot-Reduce Fat By Targeting
Specific Areas With Diet ... 125

Myth 22 All Fats Are Bad For Your Heart ... 129

Myth 23 Raw Diets Are Superior To Cooked-
Food Diets For Nutrient Intake ... 137

Myth 24 Food Combining (E.g., Separating Carbohydrates
And Proteins) Affects Nutrient Absorption ... 142

Myth 25 Athletes Must Consume Massive Amounts
Of Protein To Build Muscle ... 148

Myth 26 A "Clean Eating" Regimen Guarantees Weight Loss ... 154

Myth 27 Salt Substitutes Are Always Healthier
And Safer Than Table Salt 159

Myth 28 Coconut Oil Cures Everything From
Obesity To Heart Disease 165

Myth 29 Fruit Juices Are Just As Healthy As Whole Fruits 171

Myth 30 Skipping Carbohydrates After 3 P.m. Is
A Proven Weight-Loss Strategy 176

Myth 31 You Can't Get Enough Protein On A
Plant-Based Diet 181

Myth 32 Only People Who Want To Lose Weight
Need To Watch Their Sugar Intake 186

Myth 33 Collagen Supplements Automatically
Translate To Better Skin And Joint Health 191

Myth 34 Drinking Cold Water Affects Your Digestion Negatively 197

Myth 35 If A Little Of A Nutrient Is Good, A Lot Must Be Better 202

Myth 36 Alkaline Diets Can Significantly Change
Your Body's Ph For Better Health 207

Myth 37 Eating Spicy Foods Significantly Boosts
Metabolism For Long-Term Weight Loss 211

Myth 38 A Detox Tea Or Juice Cleanse Can Help
You Permanently Lose Weight 215

Myth 39 Dairy Is Inherently Inflammatory And
Always Bad For Everyone 219

Myth 40 Protein Powders Are Necessary For
Anyone Who Exercises 225

Myth 41 Pre- And Probiotics Are Only Beneficial If You
Have Digestive Problems — **230**

Myth 42 Microwaving Food Destroys All Of Its Nutrients — **235**

Myth 43 Brown Sugar Is Significantly Healthier
Than White Sugar — **240**

Myth 44 Foods Labeled "Fat-Free" Or "Low-Fat"
Are Always Better Choices — **245**

Myth 45 You Can't Get Enough Calcium Without
Dairy Products — **250**

Myth 46 Ketogenic Diets Are Universally Effective
For Long-Term Health — **255**

Myth 47 All Soy Products Increase The Risk Of
Breast Cancer — **260**

Myth 48 Gluten Sensitivity Is Just As Common As
Coeliac Disease — **265**

Myth 49 Eating Nuts Makes You Fat Because
They're High In Calories And Fat — **269**

Myth 50 High-Fructose Corn Syrup Is Vastly Worse
Than Any Other Added Sugar — **274**

Myth 51 If a diet worked for someone else, it will work for you — **279**

Myth 52 You Can Trust Front-Of-Package Health
Claims At Face Value — **284**

Myth 53 Once You "Fail" A Diet, You Have To Start
Over Completely — **289**

Myth 54 Low-Carb Diets Are The Only Way
To Lose Weight Effectively **294**

Myth 55 Sports Drinks Are Necessary For
Anyone Who Exercises. **299**

Myth 56 You Must Always Avoid GMOS For Better Health **303**

Myth 57 Once You Reach Your Goal Weight,
You Can Stop Paying Attention To Nutrition **308**

Myth 58 You Can't Maintain A Healthy Weight
Without Counting Calories **313**

Myth 59 Children Need Fruit Juice Daily For Proper Nutrition **318**

Myth 60 Drinking Coffee Stunts Growth And
Harms Children's Long-Term Health **322**

Myth 61 All Red Wines Are Beneficial For Heart
Health In Unlimited Quantities **326**

Myth 62 Diet Plans Must Be Strict And Inflexible
To Be Effective **332**

Myth 63 Sugar Is Addictive In The Same Way As Hard Drugs **337**

Myth 64 Spicy Foods Cause Ulcers And Are
Universally Harmful To Your Stomach **342**

Myth 65 Margarine Is Healthier Than Butter **349**

Myth 66 Sea Salt Is Automatically Healthier Than Table Salt **354**

Myth 67 If A Supplement Is Natural, It Must Be Safe And Effective **359**

Myth 68 Drinking Lemon Water In The Morning "Jumpstarts" Your
Metabolism And Detoxifies Your Body **364**

Myth 69 Coconut Sugar Is A Low-Glycemic
Sweetener That Won't Affect Blood Sugar Levels   **368**

Myth 70 Cutting Out Entire Food Groups (Like Grains)
Is Necessary To Be Healthy   **373**

Myth 71 Eating More Fibre Will Always Resolve
Digestive Issues   **379**

Myth 72 Legumes Must Be Avoided Because
They Contain 'Anti-Nutrients'   **385**

Myth 73 Drinking Water With Meals Dilutes Stomach
Acid And Impairs Digestion   **391**

Myth 74 Pasteurised Milk Is Nutritionally Inferior To
Raw Milk And Loses All Its Health Benefits   **396**

Myth 75 Soy "Feminises" Men Due To Its Isoflavone Content   **401**

Myth 76 Chocolate Must Be Completely Avoided For
Good Health   **406**

Myth 77 Drinking Apple Cider Vinegar Melts Body Fat
And Leads To Effortless Weight Loss   **413**

Myth 78 "Superfoods" Are Inherently Superior To Other
Fresh Whole Foods   **420**

Myth 79 Cooking Oils With A High Smoke Point Are
Always The Healthiest Choice   **427**

Myth 80 Artificial Sweeteners Cause Cancer And
Are Inherently Unsafe   **435**

Myth 81 Plant-Based Milk Alternatives Are Always
Healthier Than Dairy Milk   **443**

Myth 82 Intermittent Fasting Always Leads To Superior Weight Loss And Health Improvements Compared To Other Dietary Approaches — **451**

Myth 83 Celery Juice Is A Cure-All Power Food That Fights All Disease — **461**

Myth 84 Drinking Bone Broth Is A Proven Cure-All For Gut Health, Arthritis, And More — **467**

Myth 85 A Gluten-Free Diet Is Always Healthier For People Without Coeliac Disease — **474**

Myth 86 Monosodium Glutamate (MSG) Is Inherently Harmful And Always Causes Headaches And Adverse Reactions — **483**

Myth 87 Drinking Green Tea After Every Meal Automatically Boosts Metabolism Enough To Cause Significant Weight Loss — **491**

Myth 88 Eating According To Your Blood Type Drastically Improves Health And Disease Prevention — **498**

Myth 89 Frozen Meat Is Always Less Nutritious And Poses More Safety Risks Than Fresh, Never-Frozen Meat — **505**

Myth 90 Eliminating Nightshade Vegetables (Like Tomatoes, Eggplants, And Peppers) Prevents Inflammation For Everyone — **511**

Myth 91 Only Raw, Unprocessed Honey Has Health Benefits; Any Form Of Processed Honey Is Devoid Of Nutritional Value — **519**

Myth 92 Cooking In Cast-Iron Pans Substantially Increases Daily Iron Intake To The Point Of Impacting Health Outcomes — **526**

Myth 93 If A Food Is High In Fat, It Can't Be Part Of
A Heart-Healthy Diet — **533**

Myth 94 Dietary Cholesterol Is More Impactful On
Heart Health Than Saturated Fat — **541**

Myth 95 The Fewer Calories You Eat, The Healthier
You'll Be — **548**

Myth 96 Eating Too Much Fruit Is Harmful Due To
Its Sugar Content — **555**

Myth 97 Smoothies Are Always Healthy, Regardless
Of Their Ingredients — **562**

Myth 98 Everyone Needs A Multivitamin — **569**

Myth 99 Whole Grains Are No Better Than Refined
Grains For Health — **576**

Myth 100 There's a single perfect diet that everyone
should follow — **583**

Myth 101 A Weekly "Cheat Day" Won't Hamper
Progress Or Health Goals — **590**

Introduction

I have been in the nutrition industry for 30 years. Whilst the thought of that is enough to make me want to go and lay down in a darkened room with a flannel on my head, it also means that I have seen and heard pretty much everything. All the weird claims. The half truths. The long held beliefs and old wives tales. Then of course I have seen the incredible developments in nutritional science and how far it has come. I have also seen the incredible acceptance by the public and by mainstream medicine of the power that this simple yet powerful thing - the food that we eat - truly has. It is no longer the realm of the alternative. It is a key part of healthcare.

In all of this time in the industry, there have been the same myths, half truths and misunderstandings that have done the rounds. Now, with the phenomena of social media and the popularity of health and wellness on these channels, these myths have become memes and pretty looking quotes and often taken as gospel truth.

So, that is why I am writing this book. I want to address these small annoying things that never seem to go away. This book will indeed be slightly different from my usual offerings that are built around food and meals for this and that. This one is straight down the line, evidence based exploration of the everyday nutrition myths that so many of us believe.

Each myth will be fully supported by peer reviewed references and just shine a little bit of clarity onto the subject for those of you that like to dig a little deeper.

But where do these myths come from? Sometimes it is as simple as a few people observed something in one or two individuals and then pass that information on to others, and then like Chinese whispers it soon becomes an ingrained belief in certain communities and beyond.

Sometimes, and this is the one that drives me insane, it can start with a small scale study that observes a unique outcome or has come to a conclusion based on their data set and then report this finding in a journal. Great. This is how things progress. But very often these things don't give us solid answers, they just set the stage for further study until a larger data set is available and large scale conclusions can be drawn. However, there are many health journalists that love a click bait story. They see these things published in the journals and then write a mainstream newspaper article about the findings. Of course there will be blanket sensationalist claims in there which gets everyone talking and everyone panicking. This is why you see so many articles about the same topic - ie Monday morning there is an article that claims that coffee cures cancer, makes you fly and eradicates World hunger. Then on Friday the same paper publishes another article that claims coffee is the most toxic substance known to man and should be handled with biohazard level caution. Writers see something published that will get attention and they want a piece of it. This not only keeps the public confused, it also allows half truths to permeate, and once these things get on the internet. Thats it. They are out there.

Then finally we have good old fashioned 2+2 = 736 type conclusions. An example of this would be serotonin in the gut. How many times have you heard that claim on social media that '70% of the body's serotonin is made in the gut so keep your gut healthy and look after your microbiome and you wont get depressed because of all that additional serotonin. Nice one Taggart. The role of serotonin is determined by the tissue that it is found in. Yes it IS associated with elevated mood and less depression when it is in the brain. But, serotonin in the gut does gut stuff. Serotonin in the brain does brain stuff. In the gut serotonin regulates peristalsis- the rhythmical contraction of the gut wall that moves things along to their final destination. That is why it is there. Serotonin is also found in our platelets and in the skeleton where it plays different roles such as regulating clotting and regulating bone mineral concentrations. You don't hear people saying 'make sure you keep your bones healthy or make sure you have some blood - then you wont be depressed'. Sometimes simple logic doesn't stack up Nutrition can be a frustrating subject at times and there are many reasons why so many misunderstandings can arise. So thats why I am here writing this one.

Without further ado....let's get into it.

The Myths

Myth 1

Eating Fat Makes You Fat

What a perfect place to start! For decades there has been the belief, and often the statement that 'the fat you eat is the fat you wear'. If like me you were around in the 70's and 80's you will remember the obsession with low fat diets and the rigmarole that people would put themselves through following these miserable regimes. But how does this belief around fat actually stack up?

For decades, dietary fat has been demonised as the primary culprit behind weight gain and obesity. This belief became particularly prominent during the late 20th century when public health messages often encouraged low-fat diets as a strategy to combat rising rates of obesity and heart disease, such as those driven by Ancel Keys (Freedman et al. 2001; Lustig 2013).

Many people still cling to the idea that all fat is inherently 'fattening' and that reducing dietary fat intake is the key to achieving a healthy body weight. However, modern scientific evidence presents a much more nuanced picture.

Understanding the Relationship Between Fat and Body Weight

Body weight is influenced primarily by energy balance. Many people present that as how many calories you consume versus how many you expend through metabolic processes and physical activity (Hall et al. 2012; Hill et al. 2012). However, if you have followed my work, you will know I presented an alternative statement that it is more 'what you use vs what you store' Anyway, that is a discussion for another day. While fat does contain more calories per gram (approximately 9 kcal/g) than carbohydrates or protein (both around 4 kcal/g), simply eating fat does not directly translate to gaining body fat. Weight gain occurs if you consistently consume a diet that creates a metabolic environment more conducive to body fat accumulation (Astrup et al. 2011; Hooper et al. 2012).

What has become clear is that the type of fat and the *overall quality of one's diet and lifestyle* are far more important determinants of health than the mere amount of fat consumed (Mozaffarian 2016; Willett & Stampfer 2013). For instance, unsaturated fats—such as those found in olive oil, avocados, nuts, and oily fish—are associated with numerous health benefits, including improved cardiovascular health and better metabolic function (Estruch et al. 2013; Hu et al. 2001). Meanwhile, excessive intake of unhealthy fats, especially in the context of diets high in refined carbohydrates and added sugars, can contribute to weight gain and poor health outcomes (Mozaffarian et al. 2011). That cocktail of refined carbs, inflammatory oils and low quality saturated fats (yes there are good quality ones), all combined together as is the standard in our Western diet, is the perfect storm for weight gain and declining metabolic health

The Rise and Fall of Low-Fat Diets

During the 1980s and 1990s, public health advice often emphasised reducing total fat intake as a key strategy to lower the risk of heart disease and obesity. Who remembers those old 'with 40% less fat' type adverts? As low-fat foods proliferated, many products replaced fat with refined carbohydrates and sugars to maintain palatability. This led to the paradoxical situation where people consumed high amounts of low-fat, yet often calorie-dense and nutritionally poor foods, which did not help with weight control (Bray & Popkin 1998; Willett 1998). If anything it was like pouring rocket fuel on a bonfire.

Recent large-scale reviews and meta-analyses suggest that simply lowering total fat intake does not lead to meaningful long-term weight loss (Hooper et al. 2012). Instead, maintaining a balanced diet that focuses on the quality of foods—such as whole grains, vegetables, fruits, legumes, lean proteins, and healthy fats—appears to be more effective for weight management and overall health (Harvard T.H. Chan School of Public Health 2020; Public Health England 2016).

The Importance of Overall Dietary Patterns

Rather than vilifying a single nutrient, current nutritional science supports the concept of dietary patterns. The Mediterranean diet, for example, is naturally higher in fat (mainly from olive oil and nuts) and yet has been associated with a lower risk of cardiovascular disease and better weight control outcomes (Estruch et al. 2013; Sofi et al. 2008). Similarly, replacing saturated fats with unsaturated fats rather than refined carbohydrates seems to be a better strategy for improving heart health and potentially aiding weight maintenance (Mozaffarian et al. 2011; Jakobsen et al. 2009).

In other words, a diet that emphasises whole, minimally processed foods and includes healthy fats as part of an overall balanced eating pattern—coupled with regular physical activity—is more likely to help maintain a healthy body weight than simply focusing on cutting out fat (WHO 2003; Willett & Stampfer 2013).

Conclusion

The notion that eating fat inevitably makes you gain weight is not supported by modern nutrition research. While fat is calorie-dense, it is not inherently 'fattening'. Overconsumption of calories from any source can lead to weight gain, and the quality of both fats and the overall diet is crucial. Healthy fats can and should be part of a balanced, nutrient-rich diet that supports long-term health and stable body weight.

References

Astrup, A., Dyerberg, J., Elwood, P., Hermansen, K., Hu, F.B., Jakobsen, M.U. and Willett, W.C. (2011)
'The role of reducing intakes of saturated fat in the prevention of cardiovascular disease: where does the evidence stand in 2010?',
American Journal of Clinical Nutrition, 93(4), pp. 684–688.

Bray, G.A. and Popkin, B.M. (1998)
'Dietary fat intake does affect obesity!',
American Journal of Clinical Nutrition, 68(6), pp. 1157–1173.

Estruch, R., Ros, E., Salas-Salvadó, J., Covas, M.I., Corella, D., Arós, F. and Martínez-González, M.A. (2013)
'Primary prevention of cardiovascular disease with a Mediterranean diet',
New England Journal of Medicine, 368(14), pp. 1279–1290.

Freedman, M.R., King, J. and Kennedy, E. (2001) '
Popular diets: a scientific review',
Obesity Research, 9(S1), pp. 1S–40S.

Hall, K.D., Heymsfield, S.B., Kemnitz, J.W., Klein, S., Schoeller, D.A. and Speakman, J.R. (2012)
'Energy balance and its components: implications for body weight regulation',
American Journal of Clinical Nutrition, 95(4), pp. 989–994.

Harvard T.H. Chan
School of Public Health (2020)
The truth about fats: the good, the bad, and the in-between
.Available at: https://www.hsph.harvard.edu/nutritionsource/types-of-fat/ (Accessed: [date]).

Hill, J.O., Wyatt, H.R. and Peters, J.C. (2012)
'Energy balance and obesity',
Circulation, 126(1), pp. 126–132.

Hooper, L., Abdelhamid, A., Moore, H.J., Douthwaite, W., Skeaff, C.M. and Summerbell, C.D. (2012)
'Effect of reducing total fat intake on body weight: systematic review and meta-analysis of randomised controlled trials and cohort studies',
BMJ, 345, e7666.

Hu, F.B., Bronner, L., Willett, W.C., Stampfer, M.J., Rexrode, K.M., Albert, C.M., Hunter, D. and Manson, J.E. (2001)
'Fish and omega-3 fatty acid intake and risk of coronary heart disease in women',
JAMA, 287(14), pp. 1815–1821.

Jakobsen, M.U., O'Reilly, E.J., Heitmann, B.L., Pereira, M.A., Bälter, K., Fraser, G.E., Goldbourt, U., Hallmans, G., Knekt, P., Liu, S., Pietinen, P., Spiegelman, D., Stevens, J., Virtamo, J., Willett, W.C. and Ascherio, A. (2009
'Major types of dietary fat and risk of coronary heart disease: a pooled analysis of 11 cohort studies',
American Journal of Clinical Nutrition, 89(5), pp. 1425–1432.

Lustig, R.H. (2013) Fat Chance: The Hidden Truth About Sugar, Obesity and *Disease*. London: HarperCollins.

Mozaffarian, D. (2016)
'Dietary and policy priorities for cardiovascular disease, diabetes, and obesity: a comprehensive review',
Circulation, 133(2), pp. 187–225.

Mozaffarian, D., Micha, R. and Wallace, S. (2011)
'Effects on coronary heart disease of increasing polyunsaturated fat in place of saturated fat: a systematic review and meta-analysis of randomised controlled trials',
PLoS Medicine, 8(3), e1000252.

Public Health England (2016)
The Eatwell Guide.
Available at: https://www.gov.uk/government/publications/the-eatwell-guide (Accessed: [date]).

Sofi, F., Cesari, F., Abbate, R., Gensini, G.F. and Casini, A. (2008)
'Adherence to Mediterranean diet and health status: meta-analysis',
BMJ, 337, a1344.

WHO (2003)
Diet, Nutrition and the Prevention of Chronic Diseases.
Geneva: World Health Organization.

Willett, W.C. (1998)
'Is dietary fat a major determinant of body fat?',
American Journal of Clinical Nutrition, 67(3 Suppl), pp. 556S–562S.

Willett, W.C. and Stampfer, M.J. (2013)
'Current evidence on healthy eating',
Annual Review of Public Health, 34, pp. 77–95.

Myth 2

All Calories Are Created Equal, No Matter The Source

Let's continue with this theme for a moment. This really does follow on from myth number 1. The other approach to weight loss, and the thing that we have been taught over and over is that it is just calories. Calories in vs calories out. Sadly I have seen hundreds of clients fail when adopting this approach, and was the main reason I developed my 'Metabolic Fix' programme. It is far far more than just numbers. It is about how the calories that you consume, or more importantly the foods that provide them, affect your body chemistry and internal environment.

At first glance, it might seem logical that a calorie is simply a unit of energy and, therefore, all calories should have the same effect on the body. According to this view, 200 kcal from a doughnut would affect your health and weight in exactly the same way as 200 kcal from a handful of almonds or a bowl of lentils. However, this simplistic perspective overlooks the complexity of human metabolism, the diverse ways different nutrients are processed by the body, and the impact of foods on long-term health and satiety. Not to mention hormones and issues like preferential fuel partitioning. There is an awful lot to this.

Why the Source of Calories Matters

Although a calorie is indeed a measure of energy, the human body does not simply run on energy inputs and outputs like a machine. Different macronutrients—carbohydrates, proteins, and fats—are metabolised via distinct biochemical pathways. The body's response to these nutrients can vary widely in terms of hormone release, satiety signals, and subsequent energy expenditure (Hall et al. 2012; Ludwig and Ebbeling 2018).

For example, diets that emphasise high-quality protein sources tend to increase satiety, reduce total energy intake, and may even modestly increase metabolic rate due to the thermic effect of food (Westerterp 2004; Paddon-Jones et al. 2008). Foods high in protein and fibre can help curb appetite, leading to a spontaneous reduction in calorie consumption over the course of a day. On the other hand, highly refined carbohydrates can cause rapid spikes in blood sugar and insulin levels, followed by crashes in energy and increased hunger (Ludwig et al. 1999; Ludwig and Willett 2013). There is a reason I construct my recipes the way that I do.

The Quality of Food and Its Nutrient Profile

It is not just the macronutrient (protein, fat, carbs) composition that matters but also the broader nutrient profile of a food. Foods differ significantly in their micronutrient content, fibre content, phytochemicals, and their effect on gut microbiota. Whole, minimally processed foods—such as vegetables, fruits, whole grains, legumes, nuts, seeds, and lean proteins—tend to have a complex matrix of nutrients that promote overall health and help maintain stable blood sugar levels, reduce inflammation, and support metabolic well-being (Mozaffarian 2016; Monteiro et al. 2018).

In contrast, ultra-processed foods often contain refined sugars, unhealthy fats, and additives, providing calories but lacking beneficial micronutrients and dietary fibre. They are also more likely to be hyper-palatable—engineered to be so tasty that they encourage overconsumption and disrupt normal appetite regulation (Gearhardt et al. 2011; Fardet 2018).

Evidence from Clinical Studies

A growing body of research has highlighted that the source of calories can significantly influence body weight regulation and disease risk. For instance, studies have shown that diets emphasising high-quality, minimally processed carbohydrates (such as whole grains) can help with weight management and improve metabolic health, whereas diets high in refined carbohydrates and added sugars are often linked to weight gain and an increased risk of type 2 diabetes (Reynolds et al. 2019; Li et al. 2010).

Similarly, clinical trials have demonstrated that shifting from a diet high in ultra-processed foods to one rich in whole foods can lead to spontaneous reductions in calorie intake and body weight, even when participants are not consciously trying to restrict calories (Hall et al. 2019). Such findings undermine the notion that a calorie is a calorie, irrespective of its source, and instead suggest that food quality and nutrient composition play crucial roles in long-term health outcomes.

Hormonal Effects and Metabolic Pathways

Foods differ in their ability to influence hormones that regulate appetite, such as leptin and ghrelin, as well as hormones related to blood glucose control, like insulin (Rosenbaum and Leibel 2010; Sumithran and Proietto 2013). Highly processed, high-glycaemic foods can trigger more pronounced insulin responses, promoting fat storage and increasing hunger soon after consumption. In contrast, nutrient-dense, lower-glycaemic foods can help sustain steady blood sugar and insulin levels, aiding in appetite control and energy balance (Ludwig et al. 1999; Jenkins et al. 2002).

Conclusion

It's not just the numbers. We are not a machine. While the calorie is a fundamental unit of energy, the idea that all calories affect the body in exactly the same way is an oversimplification. I would go as far as to say utter insanity. Foods differ not only in their macronutrient composition but also in their impact on hormonal regulation, satiety, metabolic health, and long-term disease risk. Placing greater emphasis on the quality of calories—opting for minimally processed, nutrient-dense foods—can have profound implications for maintaining a healthy weight and optimising overall health. Build your diet around whole minimally processed foods and you really can't go far wrong.

References

Fardet, A. (2018)
'Characterization of the degree of food processing in relation with its health potential and effects',
Advances in Food and Nutrition Research, 85, pp. 79–129.

Gearhardt, A.N., Grilo, C.M., DiLeone, R.J., Brownell, K.D. and Potenza, M.N. (2011)
'Can food be addictive? Public health and policy implications',
Addiction, 106(7), pp. 1208–1212.

Hall, K.D., Bemis, T., Brychta, R., Chen, K.Y., Courville, A., Crayner, E.J., Chung, S.T., Costa, E., Driscoll, A., Miller, B.V., Steinberg, G.R., Walter, M., Yannai, L.E. and Zhou, M. (2019)
'Ultra-processed diets cause excess calorie intake and weight gain: an inpatient randomised controlled trial of ad libitum food intake',
Cell Metabolism, 30(1), pp. 67–77.

Hall, K.D., Heymsfield, S.B., Kemnitz, J.W., Klein, S., Schoeller, D.A. and Speakman, J.R. (2012)
'Energy balance and its components: implications for body weight regulation',
American Journal of Clinical Nutrition, 95(4), pp. 989–994.

Jenkins, D.J.A., Kendall, C.W.C., Augustin, L.S.A., Franceschi, S., Hamidi, M., Marchie, A., Jenkins, A.L. and Axelsen, M. (2002)
'Glycemic index: overview of implications in health and disease',
American Journal of Clinical Nutrition, 76(1), pp. 266S–273S.

Li, S., Chiuve, S.E., Flint, A., Pai, J.K., Forman, J.P., Hu, F.B. and Willett, W.C. (2010)
'Serum α-carotene concentrations and risk of death among US adults: the Third National Health and Nutrition Examination Survey Follow-up Study',
Archives of Internal Medicine, 170(17), pp. 1557–1565.

Ludwig, D.S. and Ebbeling, C.B. (2018)
'The carbohydrate-insulin model of obesity: beyond "calories in, calories out"',

JAMA Internal Medicine, 178(8), pp. 1098–1103.

Ludwig, D.S. and Willett, W.C. (2013)
'Three daily servings of reduced-fat milk: an evidence-based recommendation?',
JAMA Pediatrics, 167(9), pp. 788–789.

Ludwig, D.S., Majzoub, J.A., Al-Zahrani, A., Dallal, G.E., Blanco, I. and Roberts, S.B. (1999)
'High glycemic index foods, overeating, and obesity',
Pediatrics, 103(3), p. e26.

Monteiro, C.A., Cannon, G., Moubarac, J.-C., Levy, R.B., Louzada, M.L.C. and Jaime, P.C. (2018)
'The UN Decade of Nutrition, the NOVA food classification and the trouble with ultra-processing',
Public Health Nutrition, 21(1), pp. 5–17.

Mozaffarian, D. (2016)
'Dietary and policy priorities for cardiovascular disease, diabetes, and obesity: a comprehensive review',
Circulation, 133(2), pp. 187–225.

Paddon-Jones, D., Westman, E., Mattes, R.D., Wolfe, R.R., Astrup, A. and Westerterp-Plantenga, M. (2008)
'Protein, weight management, and satiety',
American Journal of Clinical Nutrition, 87(5), pp. 1558S–1561S.

Reynolds, A., Mann, J., Cummings, J., Winter, N., Mete, E. and Te Morenga, L. (2019)
'Carbohydrate quality and human health: a series of systematic reviews and meta-analyses',
Lancet, 393(10170), pp. 434–445.

Rosenbaum, M. and Leibel, R.L. (2010)
'Adaptive thermogenesis in humans',
International Journal of Obesity, 34(S1), pp. S47–S55.

Sumithran, P. and Proietto, J. (2013)
'The defence of body weight: a physiological basis for weight regain after weight loss',
Clinical Science, 124(4), pp. 231–241.

Westerterp, K.R. (2004)
'Diet induced thermogenesis',
Nutrition & Metabolism, 1, p. 5.

Myth 3

Carbohydrates Are Inherently Unhealthy And Should Be Avoided

I am, as we have seen an absolute fan of a low glycemic and protein forward approach to eating, but don't let this make you think that we need to avoid carbs like the plague. Sure, low carb approaches have their place and I often use them in clinic with patients that have very compromised metabolic health, but for most of us, and for long periods of time, it is more about a carbohydrate shift rather than complete avoidance.

Carbohydrates have always been a staple component of human diets worldwide, and many types of grains for example have formed the backbone of cuisines from Asia and Africa to Europe and the Americas. Yet, in recent years, certain popular diet trends, and a million and one social media posts, have suggested that all carbohydrates are inherently harmful and should be minimised or even avoided altogether. As I say, in certain clinical scenarios this can be effective for a while. The thing is, this blanket condemnation overlooks the complexity of different carbohydrate types and their varying effects on health.

Not All Carbohydrates Are Created Equal

Carbohydrates range from simple sugars, found in table sugar and syrups, to complex carbohydrates present in whole grains, pulses (lentils, beans, chickpeas), fruits, and vegetables. The body's response to these different forms of carbohydrates can vary greatly. Refined sugars and highly processed carbohydrate foods can cause rapid spikes in blood sugar and insulin levels, potentially leading to increased hunger, weight gain, and a higher risk of metabolic diseases when consumed in excess (Ludwig et al. 1999; Willett et al. 2002). However, complex carbohydrates—those accompanied by dietary fibre, vitamins, minerals, and phytochemicals—tend to have a more beneficial effect on long-term health (Reynolds et al. 2019; Aune et al. 2016).

Whole grains, for instance, are rich in fibre and essential nutrients. Their consumption has been consistently associated with reduced risk of cardiovascular disease, type 2 diabetes, and certain cancers (Aune et al. 2016; Cho et al. 2013). Similarly, fruits and vegetables, which provide a mix of carbohydrates, fibre, antioxidants, and micronutrients, have well-documented benefits for overall health and longevity (Willett et al. 2020; Li et al. 2014).

Carbohydrates as a Source of Energy and Nutrients

Carbohydrates serve as the body's primary energy source, particularly for the brain and red blood cells, which rely heavily on glucose to function optimally (Institute of Medicine 2005). When derived from nutrient-dense whole foods, carbohydrates provide a steady release of energy, helping to maintain stable blood sugar levels and support sustained activity (Jenkins et al. 2002). Whole-grain cereals, legumes, and root vegetables contribute fibre that supports healthy gut function, promotes satiety, and may improve lipid profiles and insulin sensitivity (Whelan et al. 2011; WHO 2019).

In fact, the World Health Organization (2019) and various national dietary guidelines encourage moderate to high intakes of whole-grain, fibre-rich carbohydrate foods as part of a balanced diet. The Mediterranean diet, which includes abundant vegetables, fruits, legumes, and whole grains, is frequently cited as one of the healthiest dietary patterns. It is associated with lower rates of heart disease, obesity, and metabolic disorders (Willett et al. 1995; Estruch et al. 2013). The big factor is the type you choose.

Dangers of Demonising an Entire Macronutrient

The notion that all carbohydrates are 'bad' can push people towards unbalanced eating patterns that eliminate nutrient-rich and health-promoting plant foods (Ludwig and Willett 2013). Restricting entire food groups may lead to micronutrient deficiencies, reduced dietary fibre intake, and an over-reliance on animal products or processed low-carbohydrate alternatives with uncertain long-term health consequences (Nettleton et al. 2009; Seidelmann et al. 2018).

It is also noteworthy that long-term adherence to very-low-carbohydrate diets can be challenging, and not everyone experiences improved health markers from such approaches (Feinman et al. 2015). I had that experience myself. Forever the guinea pig, I went on a very low carbohydrate diet for 3 years and the early days were very transformational in terms of body composition, but towards the end of that time frame I saw some significant negative changes in hormone profiles, sleep patterns, energy levels and more.

Moreover, high-quality carbohydrate-rich foods are central to traditional dietary patterns that have nourished populations for generations, providing not just energy, but also cultural meaning and culinary diversity. We have to live too right? We have to be able to sustain the things that bring us joy and bring us together. Completely avoiding everything throws a spanner into those works.

Focus on Quality, Not Blanket Avoidance

Rather than demonising carbohydrates as a whole, the evidence supports differentiating between carbohydrate sources. Minimising intake of refined sugars and highly processed carbohydrate foods is a sensible strategy. At the same time, emphasising whole grains, legumes, fruits, and vegetables provides a wide range of nutrients, helps maintain healthy body weight and metabolic function, and may reduce the risk of chronic diseases (Reynolds et al. 2019; Monteiro et al. 2018).

Conclusion

Carbohydrates, like any macronutrient, are not inherently unhealthy. The key is to focus on quality. Whole, minimally processed carbohydrate-rich foods can form the cornerstone of a balanced, nutrient-rich diet, whilst refined and heavily processed varieties are best consumed sparingly. Ultimately, it is the overall dietary pattern that matters most for achieving and maintaining good health. As always, whole minimally processed foods.

References

Aune, D., Keum, N., Giovannucci, E.L., Fadnes, L.T., Boffetta, P., Greenwood, D.C., Tonstad, S., Vatten, L.J., Riboli, E. and Norat, T. (2016)
'Whole grain consumption and risk of cardiovascular disease, cancer, and all-cause and cause-specific mortality: systematic review and dose-response meta-analysis of prospective studies',
BMJ, 353, i2716.

Cho, S.S., Qi, L., Fahey, G.C. and Klurfeld, D.M. (2013)
'Consumption of cereal fibre, mixtures of whole grains and bran, and whole grains and risk reduction in type 2 diabetes, obesity, and cardiovascular disease',
American Journal of Clinical Nutrition, 98(2), pp. 594–619.

Estruch, R., Ros, E., Salas-Salvadó, J., Covas, M.I., Corella, D., Arós, F. and Martínez-González, M.A. (2013)
'Primary prevention of cardiovascular disease with a Mediterranean diet',
New England Journal of Medicine, 368(14), pp. 1279–1290.

Feinman, R.D., Pogozelski, W.K., Astrup, A., Bernstein, R.K., Fine, E.J., Westman, E.C. and Worm, N. (2015) '
Dietary carbohydrate restriction as the first approach in diabetes management: critical review and evidence base',
Nutrition, 31(1), pp. 1–13.

Institute of Medicine (2005)
Dietary Reference Intakes for Energy, Carbohydrate, Fibre, Fat, Fatty Acids, Cholesterol, Protein, and Amino Acids. Washington,
DC: National Academies Press.

Jenkins, D.J.A., Kendall, C.W.C., Augustin, L.S.A., Franceschi, S., Hamidi, M., Marchie, A., Jenkins, A.L. and Axelsen, M. (2002)
'Glycemic index: overview of implications in health and disease',
American Journal of Clinical Nutrition, 76(1), pp. 266S–273S.

Li, Y., Wang, D.D., Ley, S.H., Howard, A.G., He, Y., Lu, Y., Hu, F.B. and Qi, L. (2014)
'Time trends of dietary and lifestyle factors and their potential impact on diabetes burden in China',
Diabetes Care, 37(1), pp. 17–26.

Ludwig, D.S., Majzoub, J.A., Al-Zahrani, A., Dallal, G.E., Blanco, I. and Roberts, S.B. (1999)
'High glycemic index foods, overeating, and obesity', P
ediatrics, 103(3), p. e26.

Ludwig, D.S. and Willett, W.C. (2013)
'Three daily servings of reduced-fat milk: an evidence-based recommendation?',
JAMA Pediatrics, 167(9), pp. 788–789.

Monteiro, C.A., Cannon, G., Moubarac, J.-C., Levy, R.B., Louzada, M.L.C. and Jaime, P.C. (2018)
'The UN Decade of Nutrition, the NOVA food classification and the trouble with ultra-processing',
Public Health Nutrition, 21(1), pp. 5–17.

Nettleton, J.A., Steffen, L.M., Ni, H., Liu, K. and Jacobs, D.R. (2009)
'Dietary patterns and risk of incident type 2 diabetes in the Multi-Ethnic Study of Atherosclerosis (MESA)',
Diabetes Care, 31(9), pp. 1777–1782.

Reynolds, A., Mann, J., Cummings, J., Winter, N., Mete, E. and Te Morenga, L. (2019)
'Carbohydrate quality and human health: a series of systematic reviews and meta-analyses',
Lancet, 393(10170), pp. 434–445.

Seidelmann, S.B., Claggett, B., Cheng, S., Henglin, M., Shah, A., Steffen, L.M. and Tinker, L.F. (2018)
'Dietary carbohydrate intake and mortality: a prospective cohort study and meta-analysis',
Lancet Public Health, 3(9), pp. e419–e428.

Whelan, K., Judd, P.A. and Preedy, V.R. (2011)
Handbook of Fibre and Fibre-Rich Foods. Cambridge:
Woodhead Publishing.

WHO (2019)
Healthy diet.
Available at: *https://www.who.int/news-room/fact-sheets/detail/healthy-diet*
(Accessed: [date]).

Willett, W.C., Sacks, F., Trichopoulou, A., Drescher, G., Ferro-Luzzi, A., Helsing, E. and Trichopoulos, D. (1995)
'Mediterranean diet pyramid: a cultural model for healthy eating',
American Journal of Clinical Nutrition, 61(6 Suppl), pp. 1402S–1406S.

Willett, W., Manson, J. and Liu, S. (2002)
'Glycemic index, glycemic load, and risk of type 2 diabetes',
American Journal of Clinical Nutrition, 76(1), pp. 274S–280S.

Willett, W.C., Rockström, J., Loken, B., Springmann, M., Lang, T., Vermeulen, S. and Murray, C.J.L. (2020)
'Food in the Anthropocene: the EAT–Lancet Commission on healthy diets from sustainable food systems',
Lancet, 393(10170), pp. 447–492.

Myth 4

High-Protein Diets Damage Your Kidneys

While I am cautious of high protein diets for my patients that have advanced kidney disease, there is a blanket notion that higher protein diets will annihilate your kidneys in the long term. Ok, if you go crazy and have huge amounts of protein powders and push intake beyond the upper ranges that fit and active people require, then you may force your kidneys to work a little harder.

Protein is a critical nutrient required for a wide array of bodily functions, from building and repairing tissues to supporting the immune system and the production of enzymes and hormones. Despite its well-established role in health, the notion persists that consuming a high-protein diet can universally harm the kidneys. This belief is rooted in the idea that the kidneys, which filter waste products including those derived from protein metabolism, become overworked when protein intake rises. However, scientific evidence suggests that in healthy individuals, high-protein diets do not inherently cause kidney damage.

Understanding Kidney Function and Protein Metabolism

The kidneys' primary function involves filtering the blood, removing waste products such as urea (a by-product of protein metabolism), and regulating fluid balance, electrolytes, and blood pressure (Kidney Disease Improving Global Outcomes 2013). While it is true that eating more protein increases urea production, the kidneys of healthy adults are generally well-equipped to handle this increased load (Martin et al. 2005; Phillips et al. 2016).

Just as muscles adapt to regular exercise, kidneys can undergo adaptive changes in response to shifts in diet. When protein intake rises, the kidneys may increase their filtration rate, but this physiological adaptation is not the same as damage. Healthy kidneys exhibit a remarkable degree of flexibility and resilience, allowing them to handle a broad range of dietary protein intakes without harm (Brändle et al. 1996; Devries et al. 2018).

Evidence from Clinical Studies and Meta-Analyses

Multiple studies, including randomised controlled trials and systematic reviews, have investigated whether high-protein diets directly impair renal function in healthy individuals. The consensus emerging from this research is that there is little to no evidence that protein intakes above the recommended dietary allowance (RDA) cause long-term kidney damage in those without pre-existing kidney disease (Martin et al. 2005; Devries et al. 2018).

A systematic review and meta-analysis by Devries et al. (2018) found that increases in protein intake did not significantly change glomerular filtration rate (GFR) or markers of kidney function in healthy individuals. Another review concluded that, for healthy adults, protein intakes even beyond the commonly recommended range of 0.8 g/kg/day did not produce adverse effects on kidney health (Poortmans & Dellalieux 2000; EFSA Panel on Dietetic Products, Nutrition, and Allergies 2017). Similarly, a recent review by Jäger et al. (2017) noted that habitual protein intakes well above the RDA did not compromise kidney function in resistance-trained subjects.

Context Matters: Kidney Health vs. Kidney Disease

It is crucial to distinguish between individuals with normal kidney function and those with chronic kidney disease (CKD) or other renal impairments. In individuals with compromised kidney function, excessive protein intake may accelerate kidney damage by increasing the workload on already vulnerable kidneys (NKF 2021). For such individuals, we often recommend tailored dietary protein restrictions to help preserve renal function. I personally always stay on the side of caution with my patients.

However, these clinical guidelines do not apply to healthy adults with normally functioning kidneys. For the general population, protein intakes modestly above standard recommendations can be part of a balanced and healthful diet, particularly when they come from high-quality sources such as lean meats, fish, legumes, low-fat dairy, and plant-based proteins (Phillips et al. 2016; WHO 2007).

Balancing Nutrient Intakes and Overall Diet Quality

As with any nutrient, balance and quality matter. While increasing protein intake is not inherently harmful to healthy kidneys, it is still important to maintain a varied dietary pattern. Overemphasising protein at the expense of other essential nutrients may lead to inadequate intakes of fibre, vitamins, minerals, and beneficial phytochemicals found in fruits, vegetables, and whole grains (WHO 2003; Mozaffarian 2016).

Combining adequate protein intake with a focus on whole, minimally processed foods, regular physical activity, and overall energy balance is a more reliable path to long-term health than fixating on any single macronutrient. Such an approach ensures that all organs, including the kidneys, receive the nutrients and conditions necessary to function optimally.

Conclusion

The claim that high-protein diets damage healthy kidneys is not supported by current scientific evidence. In individuals with normal renal function, the kidneys can adapt to higher protein intakes without suffering harm. While caution is necessary for people with existing kidney disease, there is no need for the healthy population to fear protein-rich diets. Ultimately, the emphasis should be on a balanced, nutrient-dense eating pattern rather than avoiding protein for fear of kidney damage.

References

Brändle, E., Sieberth, H.G. and Hautmann, R.E. (1996)
'Effect of chronic dietary protein intake on the upper limit of urea excretion in healthy subjects',
American Journal of Physiology, 270(6 Pt 2), pp. F1008–F1014.

Devries, M.C., Sithamparapillai, A., Brimble, K.S., Banfield, L., Morton, R.W. and Phillips, S.M. (2018)
'Changes in kidney function do not differ between healthy adults consuming higher- compared with lower- or normal-protein diets: a systematic review and meta-analysis',
Journal of Nutrition, 148(11), pp. 1760–1775.

EFSA Panel on Dietetic Products, Nutrition, and Allergies (2017)
'Scientific opinion on dietary reference values for protein',
EFSA Journal, 15(2), 66.

Institute of Medicine (2005)
Dietary Reference Intakes for Energy, Carbohydrate, Fibre, Fat, Fatty Acids, Cholesterol, Protein, and Amino Acids. Washington,
DC: National Academies Press.

Jäger, R., Kerksick, C.M., Campbell, B.I., Cribb, P.J., Wells, S.D., Skwiat, T.L. and Arciero, P.J. (2017)
'International Society of Sports Nutrition position stand: protein and exercise',
Journal of the International Society of Sports Nutrition, 14, 20.

Kidney Disease Improving Global Outcomes (KDIGO) (2013)
KDIGO 2012 Clinical Practice Guideline for the Evaluation and Management of Chronic Kidney Disease,
Kidney International Supplements, 3(1).

Martin, W.F., Armstrong, L.E. and Rodriguez, N.R. (2005)
'Dietary protein intake and renal function',
Nutrition & Metabolism, 2, 25.

Mozaffarian, D. (2016)
'Dietary and policy priorities for cardiovascular disease, diabetes, and obesity: a comprehensive review',
Circulation, 133(2), pp. 187–225.

National Kidney Foundation (NKF) (2021)
Nutrition and Chronic Kidney Disease.
Available at: https://www.kidney.org/nutrition
(Accessed: [date]).

Phillips, S.M., Chevalier, S. and Leidy, H.J. (2016)
'Protein "requirements" beyond the RDA: implications for optimising health',
Applied Physiology,
Nutrition, and Metabolism, 41(5), pp. 565–572.

Poortmans, J.R. and Dellalieux, O. (2000)
'Do regular high protein diets have potential health risks on kidney function in athletes?',
International Journal of Sport Nutrition and Exercise Metabolism, 10(1), pp. 28–38.

WHO (2003) Diet,
Nutrition and the Prevention of Chronic Diseases.
Geneva: World Health Organization.

WHO (2007)
Protein and Amino Acid Requirements in Human Nutrition.
Geneva: World Health Organization.

Myth 5

You Must Cleanse Or Detox Regularly To Rid Your Body Of Toxins

I'm not going to lie. When I first got into the nutrition world back in 1992 (ouch), I entered the industry from the more alternative leaning side of things. In that time I did very much believe in detox diets and detox rituals and the like. Now clearly, anyone with any sense will realise that it is a good idea to minimise our exposure to things and also to follow a diet and lifestyle that allows the important organs used in detoxification to do their job effectively. But do we need to go further than that? Are these diets and protocols necessary?

The idea that our bodies are burdened with harmful toxins that require periodic "cleansing" or "detoxing" through special diets, juices, teas, or supplements has become widespread in popular culture. Promoters of detox regimes often claim these protocols can rapidly improve health, boost energy levels, and lead to quick weight loss. While it sounds appealing to imagine removing unwanted substances through a simple short-term fix, the scientific evidence behind commercial detox programmes is sparse at best. In reality, our bodies are equipped with highly effective and sophisticated detoxification systems that operate continuously, making most "detox diets" unnecessary.

How the Body's Detoxification Systems Work

The human body is not defenceless against everyday environmental exposures and dietary components that could be harmful. The liver, kidneys, lungs, gastrointestinal tract, and skin all play roles in filtering, processing, and excreting unwanted substances, including metabolic waste products, environmental toxins, and excess nutrients (Liska et al. 2006; Huber et al. 2009). These organs and processes work around the clock without the need for special supplements or cleanses. Although there absolutely are supplements that can influence these. St John's Wort for example speeds up the CYP450 pathway in the liver that accelerates the breakdown of drugs for example. This is why this supplement cannot be taken with the pill or cardiac drugs. Some natural products absolutely do influence this. That doesn't make them necessary!

The liver alters toxins to make them water-soluble, allowing the kidneys to excrete them via urine. Similarly, the lungs expel volatile toxins with each breath, while the gut and skin provide additional routes of excretion.

This natural detoxification system is well-regulated by the body's physiology. Nutrient-rich diets, regular physical activity, adequate hydration, and sufficient sleep support these natural processes better than any restrictive short-term cleanse (WHO 2003; Eatwell Guide 2016).

Evaluating the Evidence for Detox Diets

Despite the popularity of detox products and protocols, there is very little robust, peer-reviewed scientific evidence to support their efficacy. A critical review by Klein and Kiat (2015) found a lack of convincing data demonstrating that commercial detox diets significantly remove toxins from the body, improve health markers, or provide lasting weight loss. Much of the supposed evidence comes from anecdotal reports, poorly designed studies, or marketing claims rather than well-controlled clinical trials.

Detox diets often rely on severe calorie restriction, which can lead to rapid weight loss. However, this weight loss is typically due to water loss, glycogen depletion, and reduced intestinal bulk rather than long-term fat reduction (Sawka et al. 2007; Maughan et al. 2010). Once the cleanse ends, weight often returns, and no lasting health benefits have been reliably demonstrated.

Potential Harms of Restrictive Cleanses

In some cases, detox programmes may do more harm than good. Extreme regimens that eliminate whole food groups or rely on unproven supplements can result in nutrient deficiencies, dizziness, fatigue, irritability, and gastrointestinal issues (Klein & Kiat 2015; Hohenadel et al. 2011). Overuse of laxatives or diuretics, common in some "colon cleanses", can disrupt electrolyte balance and harm gut function. Additionally, people with underlying health conditions, including diabetes or kidney disease, may worsen their condition by following extreme diets without medical guidance.

A Sustainable Approach to Supporting Natural Detoxification

Instead of relying on short-term cleanses, focusing on an overall balanced and healthful lifestyle is far more beneficial. Let those organs and natural paths of elimination do their thing unhindered.

Regular consumption of fruits, vegetables, whole grains, lean proteins, and healthy fats provides the nutrients necessary to support liver function and antioxidant systems (WHO 2003; Mozaffarian 2016). Staying well-hydrated helps the kidneys efficiently eliminate waste, while regular physical activity and adequate sleep further support metabolic health and immune function.

If you genuinely feel the need to "reset" your eating habits, consider aiming for sustainable changes. Gradually reduce added sugars, refined carbohydrates, and highly processed foods. Increase your intake of fibre-rich whole foods, cut down on excessive alcohol, and ensure you meet recommended nutrient intakes. Unlike short-lived detoxes, these changes promote long-term health and wellbeing (Harvard T.H. Chan School of Public Health 2020).

Conclusion

Your body possesses a robust, self-regulating detoxification system that operates continuously and does not require special cleanses or detox products. Scientific evidence does not support the notion that short-term detox diets meaningfully remove toxins, improve health, or result in lasting weight loss. Instead, a balanced diet, regular exercise, sufficient sleep, and avoidance of harmful substances remain the most effective and evidence-based methods to maintain your body's natural detoxification processes and overall health.

References

Eatwell Guide (2016)
Public Health England.
Available at: https://www.gov.uk/government/publications/the-eatwell-guide (Accessed: [date]).

Harvard T.H. Chan School of Public Health (2020)
Healthy eating plate & healthy eating pyramid.
Available at:
https://www.hsph.harvard.edu/nutritionsource/healthy-eating-plate/
(Accessed: [date]).

Hohenadel, K., Hohenadel, R., Vanstolk-Cooke, K. and Samman, N. (2011)
'An eating disorder masquerading as a detox diet',
Canadian Journal of Dietetic Practice and Research, 72(1), pp. e159–e161.

Huber, W.W., Scharf, G., Rossmanith, W., Prustomersky, S., Grasl-Kraupp, B., Peter, B. and Parzefall, W. (2009)
'The role of detoxification processes in nutritional and pharmacological interventions',
Nutrients, 1(2), pp. 103–126.

Klein, A.V. and Kiat, H. (2015)
'Detox diets for toxin elimination and weight management: a critical review of the evidence',
Journal of Human Nutrition and Dietetics, 28(6), pp. 675–686.

Liska, D., Lukaczer, D. and Jones, D.S. (2006)
Clinical Nutrition: A Functional Approach. 2nd edn. Gig Harbor,
WA: The Institute for Functional Medicine.

Maughan, R.J., Shirreffs, S.M. and Leiper, J.B. (2010)
'Errors in the estimation of hydration status from changes in body mass',
Journal of Sports Sciences, 28(9), pp. 927–933.

Mozaffarian, D. (2016)
'Dietary and policy priorities for cardiovascular disease, diabetes, and obesity: a comprehensive review',
Circulation, 133(2), pp. 187–225.

Sawka, M.N., Burke, L.M., Eichner, E.R., Maughan, R.J., Montain, S.J. and Stachenfeld, N.S. (2007) '
Exercise and fluid replacement', American College of Sports Medicine Position Stand,
Medicine & Science in Sports & Exercise, 39(2), pp. 377–390.

WHO (2003) Diet,
Nutrition and the Prevention of Chronic Diseases.
Geneva: World Health Organization.

Myth 6

Eating Late At Night Always Leads To Weight Gain

It isn't the best idea to have a huge meal and then crawl into bed. Chances are your sleep will be disturbed and you may have some digestive discomfort. But does it affect our weight? There has been a long held belief that if you eat too late at night, you will not have chance to "burn" those calories you consumed. Ah, such a simple logic. But how does this actually hold up.

Traditional thinking often suggests that consuming food in the evening, especially close to bedtime, inevitably results in weight gain. This idea stems from the notion that our bodies are less active later in the day, thereby burning fewer calories and storing more as fat. Many people feel guilty about late-night snacking, believing it will derail their efforts to maintain a healthy body weight. However, while the timing of meals may have subtle effects on metabolism and hunger hormones, the evidence does not consistently support the claim that simply eating later always leads to weight gain. Instead, what you eat, how much you eat, and your overall dietary pattern matter far more than the time of day when you eat.

Energy Balance and Meal Timing

Weight management fundamentally depends on our metabolic environment and how effectively it can use the fuel that we take in, or whether the immediate environment pushes it towards storing fuel to get it out of the way to maintain metabolic homeostasis. The body's internal clock (circadian rhythm) and metabolic fluctuations can influence how we process nutrients, but total calorie intake relative to expenditure remains the primary determinant of changes in body weight (Hall et al. 2012; Hill et al. 2012).

Some research suggests that our circadian rhythms might slightly affect how efficiently we metabolise certain nutrients and how full we feel after meals (Garaulet & Ordovás 2012). For instance, eating large, high-calorie meals late in the evening may be linked with marginally poorer metabolic outcomes in some individuals (Kahleova et al. 2017; Wehrens et al. 2017). Yet these effects are generally modest, and the overall quality and quantity of food consumed across the entire day are far more critical factors than the clock on the wall.

Quality, Quantity, and Patterns of Intake

Late-night eating often becomes a problem not because of the time itself, but because of the types and amounts of foods people tend to consume during these hours. Many late-night snacks are high in refined carbohydrates, sugars, and unhealthy fats—think crisps, biscuits, sweets, or takeaway meals (Colles et al. 2007). When such foods are regularly added on top of an already adequate or excessive daily calorie intake and skewed macronutrient ratio, weight gain is more likely. Here, it is not the timing but the excess of the 'wrong stuff' and poor nutrient quality that drive weight gain.

Conversely, if your overall diet is balanced, nutrient-dense, and appropriately portioned, having a late dinner or a small, high-quality evening snack. For instance, a handful of nuts, a piece of fruit with some yoghurt, or a small serving of cottage cheese may provide beneficial nutrients without significantly altering your total daily energy balance (Harvard T.H. Chan School of Public Health 2020; Public Health England 2016).

Individual Differences and Lifestyle Factors

Individual responses to meal timing vary. Some people may experience improved satiety and metabolic health by shifting more calories earlier in the day, while others find that an evening meal fits better with their schedule and does not affect their weight management (Betts et al. 2014; Alencar et al. 2015). What matters most is finding an eating pattern that is sustainable, culturally appropriate, and conducive to meeting personal health goals.

Furthermore as I mentioned earlier, late-night eating is sometimes associated with disrupted sleep or poor sleep quality, which can indirectly influence weight regulation. Poor sleep has been linked to altered hunger hormones and increased cravings for high-calorie foods (Spaeth et al. 2013; Chaput 2014). Thus, the relationship between evening eating and weight gain may be partially mediated by sleep quality and overall lifestyle habits rather than the mere fact of eating later in the day.

Focus on the Bigger Picture

Instead of worrying excessively about the clock, pay attention to the total number of calories consumed, the nutritional quality of foods, and your eating habits over the entire day. Adopting a balanced and varied dietary pattern, being mindful of portion sizes, engaging in regular physical activity, and ensuring adequate sleep will have far more substantial effects on weight regulation than simply avoiding food after a certain hour.

Conclusion

Eating late at night does not automatically lead to weight gain. While individual metabolic responses and circadian rhythms may play a minor role, it is the consistent excess intake of the wrong things—often energy-dense, nutrient-poor foods—that drives weight gain. By focusing on overall dietary quality, total energy intake, and healthy lifestyle habits, you can enjoy flexibility in meal timing without fearing that every late-night snack will sabotage your waistline.

References

Alencar, M.K., Schafer, M.A., Dave, S., Anglin, K., Slentz, C. and Duscha, B.D. (2015)
'The effect of increased meal frequency on fat oxidation and perceived hunger'
, European Journal of Sport Science, 15(1), pp. 1–7.

Betts, J.A., Richardson, J.D., Chowdhury, E.A., Holman, G.D., Tsintzas, K. and Thompson, D. (2014)
'The causal role of breakfast in energy balance and health: a randomised controlled trial in lean adults',
American Journal of Clinical Nutrition, 100(2), pp. 539–547.

Chaput, J.-P. (2014)
'Sleep patterns, diet quality & energy balance',
Physiology & Behavior, 134, pp. 86–91.

Colles, S.L., Dixon, J.B. and O'Brien, P.E. (2007)
'Night eating syndrome and nocturnal snacking: association with obesity, binge eating and psychological distress',
International Journal of Obesity, 31(11), pp. 1722–1730.

Garaulet, M. and Ordovás, J.M. (2012)
'Chronobiology and obesity: the orchestra out of tune',
Clinical Chemistry, 58(7), pp. 994–1001.

Hall, K.D., Heymsfield, S.B., Kemnitz, J.W., Klein, S., Schoeller, D.A. and Speakman, J.R. (2012)
'Energy balance and its components: implications for body weight regulation',
American Journal of Clinical Nutrition, 95(4), pp. 989–994.

Harvard T.H. Chan School of Public Health (2020)
Healthy eating plate & healthy eating pyramid.
Available at:
https://www.hsph.harvard.edu/nutritionsource/healthy-eating-plate/
(Accessed: [date]).

Hill, J.O., Wyatt, H.R. and Peters, J.C. (2012)
'Energy balance and obesity',
Circulation, 126(1), pp. 126–132.

Kahleova, H., Lloren, J.I., Mashchak, A., Hill, M. and Fraser, G.E. (2017)
'Meal frequency and timing are associated with changes in body mass index in Adventist Health Study 2',
Journal of Nutrition, 147(9), pp. 1722–1728.

Public Health England (2016)
The Eatwell Guide.
Available at: https://www.gov.uk/government/publications/the-eatwell-guide (Accessed: [date]).

Spaeth, A.M., Dinges, D.F. and Goel, N. (2013)
'Effects of experimental sleep restriction on energy intake, energy expenditure, and visceral obesity',
Sleep, 36(7), pp. 983–990.

Wehrens, S.M.T., Christou, S., Isherwood, C., Middleton, B., Gibbs, M.A., Archer, S.N. and Johnstone, J.A. (2017)
'Meal timing regulates the human circadian system',
Current Biology, 27(12), pp. 1768–1775.

Myth 7

Organic Foods Are Always More Nutritious Than Conventional Foods

Whenever I am out and about and doing live events, and we get to the Q&A, there is one question that comes up more than any other - "what is your opinion on organic foods". Simply put, my opinion is 'it depends on your priorities'. If you are at the very beginning of your journey, just eat some plants and some whole foods. If you have been doing this for some time and you want to dive deeper and get further benefits, then absolutely there can be some benefits. I am not a toxicologist so I am not going to pretend I know anywhere near enough to comment on the pesticides issue, but that is of course a major consideration too.

Here's the thing. The term 'organic' has come to represent foods produced without synthetic pesticides, fertilisers, or genetic modification, leading many consumers to assume that anything labelled organic must be nutritionally superior. Marketing often reinforces this belief, giving the impression that organic produce provides higher vitamin, mineral, and antioxidant levels and, thus, delivers greater health benefits. However, the idea that organic foods are inherently more nutritious, across the board, than their conventionally grown counterparts does not consistently hold up under scientific scrutiny.

Examining the Evidence

A number of systematic reviews and meta-analyses have attempted to compare the nutrient profiles of organic and conventional foods. Overall, the findings suggest that while there may be some differences in certain nutrients or secondary plant compounds, these variations are not universally present, nor are they always nutritionally significant (Smith-Spangler et al. 2012; Dangour et al. 2009).

For example, some studies have shown that organic produce may contain higher concentrations of certain antioxidants, such as phenolic compounds, compared to conventional produce (Barański et al. 2014). However, the magnitude of these differences can be modest, and whether they translate into measurable health benefits remains uncertain (Mie et al. 2017). This is because these substances are used by the plants as their own in built pesticides. When external pesticides are not added, the plant must ramp up its own natural defences.

In terms of macro- and micronutrients, including vitamins and minerals, the results are mixed and often depend on factors such as soil quality, cultivar type, climate, and storage conditions rather than the production method alone (Dangour et al. 2009; Hunter et al. 2011).

In other words, a locally grown, ripe, and freshly harvested conventional vegetable may boast similar—if not greater—nutrient content than an organic vegetable that has travelled long distances or spent days on the shelf. In our modern supermarkets, this represents a significant issue. Things are held in cold storage for days and often weeks. This can cause certain nutrients to deplete.

Food Safety Considerations

One reason consumers gravitate towards organic foods is concern over pesticide residues and the potential health risks they pose. This really isn't my area at all, but here is what the science says. Research does indicate that organic produce generally has lower levels of synthetic pesticide residues than conventional produce (Smith-Spangler et al. 2012). However, strict regulations in many countries limit the amount of pesticide residue allowed in conventional foods, and produce grown under these guidelines typically falls within safe limits for human consumption (EFSA 2020; WHO/FAO 2018). Whatever 'safe limits' really mean. That is a debate in itself.

Additionally, organic farming uses certain naturally derived pesticides, and the absence of synthetic chemicals does not necessarily guarantee zero residues. Washing, peeling, and proper handling of produce—organic or conventional—remain sensible precautions for all consumers (USDA 2021), should that be your thing.

Environmental and Ethical Considerations

While the strictly nutritional differences between organic and conventional foods may be small or inconsistent, people often choose organic for reasons beyond nutrient content. Organic agriculture is frequently considered more environmentally sustainable due to practices that prioritise soil health, biodiversity, and reduced chemical inputs (Reganold & Wachter 2016). Ethical considerations, such as animal welfare standards and support for smaller-scale local farms, may also influence consumer choices.

These factors do not make organic foods inherently more nutritious, but they can align with certain personal values related to health, sustainability, and responsible consumption. That is absolutely something I have zero questions with. If you are making decisions based on your own ethical standards - there is no argument from me.

Focus on Overall Dietary Quality

Whether you choose organic or conventional, what matters most is the overall quality and balance of your diet. A diet rich in vegetables, fruits, whole grains, legumes, lean proteins, and healthy fats is associated with numerous health benefits, irrespective of whether those foods are grown organically or conventionally (WHO 2003; Mozaffarian 2016). Ensuring adequate variety, freshness, and minimally processed forms of foods is likely to have a far greater impact on health than the organic label alone.

Conclusion

The belief that organic foods are always more nutritious than conventional foods is not supported by a clear, consistent body of evidence. While some differences in certain nutrients and antioxidant compounds may exist, they are not as pronounced or universal as marketing suggests. Choosing organic foods can still be meaningful for environmental, ethical, or taste preferences. However, from a strictly nutritional standpoint, focusing on the overall quality, variety, and balance of your diet is far more important for long-term health than whether your produce is grown organically or conventionally.

References

Barański, M., Srednicka-Tober, D., Volakakis, N., Seal, C., Sanderson, R., Stewart, G.B. and Leifert, C. (2014)
'Higher antioxidant and lower cadmium concentrations and lower incidence of pesticide residues in organically grown crops: a systematic literature review and meta-analyses',
British Journal of Nutrition, 112(5), pp. 794–811.

Dangour, A.D., Dodhia, S.K., Hayter, A., Allen, E., Lock, K. and Uauy, R. (2009)
'Nutritional quality of organic foods: a systematic review',
American Journal of Clinical Nutrition, 90(3), pp. 680–685.

EFSA (2020)
Annual Report on Pesticide Residues in Food.
European Food Safety Authority.

Hunter, D., Foster, M., McArthur, J.O., Ojha, R., Petocz, P. and Samman, S. (2011)
'Evaluation of the micronutrient composition of plant foods produced by organic and conventional agricultural methods',
Critical Reviews in Food Science and Nutrition, 51(6), pp. 571–582.

Mie, A., Andersen, H.R., Gunnarsson, S., Kahl, J., Kesse-Guyot, E., Rembiałkowska, E. and Grandjean, P. (2017)
'Human health implications of organic food and organic agriculture: a comprehensive review',
Environmental Health, 16, p. 111.

Mozaffarian, D. (2016)
'Dietary and policy priorities for cardiovascular disease, diabetes, and obesity: a comprehensive review',
Circulation, 133(2), pp. 187–225.

Reganold, J.P. and Wachter, J.M. (2016)
'Organic agriculture in the twenty-first century',
Nature Plants, 2(2), 15221.

Smith-Spangler, C., Bravata, D.M., Tayleur, C., Huang, J., Fulton, E., Sundaram, V. and Brandeau, M.L. (2012)
'Are organic foods safer or healthier than conventional alternatives? A systematic review',
Annals of Internal Medicine, 157(5), pp. 348–366.

USDA (2021)
Pesticide Data Program.
United States Department of Agriculture.

WHO (2003)
Diet, Nutrition and the Prevention of Chronic Diseases.
Geneva: World Health Organization.

WHO/FAO (2018)
Codex Alimentarius – Pesticide Residues in Food.
Rome: FAO.

Myth 8

If It's Labelled "Gluten-Free," It's Healthier

This old chestnut. The amount of debates I have had with friends in the industry (you know who you are) around this one is insane. My personal opinion on this is simply 'if you are coeliac, then absolutely gluten must be avoided without question. Also, if you find that some foods containing gluten don't agree with you, just don't eat them. However, if you believe that gluten is a universal poison that will paralyse your immune system and make you so inflamed that you explode, then I fear you are misguided'. With this, there has been a massive increase in gluten free foods. This is wonderful for coeliacs because, and I certainly remember this when I first started clinical practice, for so long there was so very little choice for patients. However, many of these foods are branded healthier options universally, just due to the absence of gluten, and that is where I take issue.

Gluten, a protein found in wheat, barley, and rye, has gained significant attention in recent years. Products sporting a "gluten-free" label have increased in supermarkets and health food shops, and this has led to many consumers to assume that avoiding gluten will automatically improve their health or help them lose weight. The notion that all gluten-free products are inherently healthier than their gluten-containing counterparts is not supported by the evidence. In fact, many gluten-free substitutes are often just as calorie-dense, highly processed, and lacking in key nutrients as their standard equivalents.

The Medical Necessity of Gluten-Free Diets

For the estimated 1% of the population with coeliac disease, a strict, lifelong gluten-free diet is non-negotiable and can dramatically improve health outcomes (Lebwohl et al. 2018; Caio et al. 2019). People with non-coeliac gluten or wheat sensitivity may also benefit from reducing or eliminating gluten in their diets (Catassi et al. 2017). For these individuals, removing gluten is crucial to avoiding gastrointestinal distress, malabsorption of nutrients, and damage to the small intestine. I do feel that this is far less common than many people believe. I feel that more often it is an issue with the microbiome or gut barrier function, but that is a topic for another day.

However, for those without such conditions, there is no evidence that cutting out gluten leads to better health or weight loss. In fact, going gluten-free unnecessarily can sometimes lead to a nutritionally suboptimal diet if not approached with care (Biesiekierski 2017).

Nutritional Quality of Gluten-Free Products

Many gluten-free alternatives, such as breads, pastas, biscuits, and snack foods, rely on refined starches from maize, potato, or tapioca to replicate the texture of wheat-based foods. While these substitutes allow for gluten-free options, they may lack the fibre, vitamins, and minerals found in wholegrain wheat, barley, and rye products (Thompson 2009; Saturni et al. 2010). As a result, some gluten-free items can be lower in overall nutritional quality, contributing fewer essential nutrients to the diet.

Moreover, gluten-free packaged foods sometimes contain higher amounts of sugar, salt, and unhealthy fats to improve taste and texture (Lionetti et al. 2015). This means that simply choosing a product labelled "gluten-free" does not guarantee a health advantage. Often, the healthiest carbohydrate sources—whole fruits, vegetables, legumes, quinoa, brown rice—are naturally gluten-free without needing special processing or labelling.

Misconceptions and Marketing

The surge in popularity of gluten-free eating has been bolstered by celebrity endorsements, anecdotal success stories, and a general distrust of processed foods. This has created a perception that "gluten-free" equals "healthier," leading some consumers to pay premium prices for products that may be nutritionally no better, or even inferior, to their conventional counterparts. As soon as industrial opportunity arises, then marketing will and absolutely has fanned this flame.

Large epidemiological studies have found that, for individuals without coeliac disease, gluten consumption is not associated with higher risk of heart disease or poorer health outcomes. In fact, avoiding gluten unnecessarily might limit intake of wholegrains that are associated with health benefits, including reduced risk of cardiovascular disease and type 2 diabetes (Lebwohl et al. 2017; Aune et al. 2016).

Focus on Overall Dietary Quality

As with many dietary choices, the key lies in focusing on overall quality, balance, and variety. For those without gluten-related disorders, there is no inherent need to avoid gluten, especially if doing so leads to reliance on highly processed, nutrient-poor gluten-free products. Emphasising whole, minimally processed foods—regardless of their gluten content—will contribute far more to overall health than simply purchasing items carrying a gluten-free label.

Conclusion

Gluten-free products are not automatically healthier choices. While a gluten-free diet is vital for individuals with coeliac disease or gluten sensitivities, it does not necessarily confer health advantages for others. Many gluten-free items can be highly processed and lacking in key nutrients. A focus on whole, fibre-rich, and minimally processed foods—gluten-containing or not—is a more reliable path to good health than relying on the gluten-free label as a mark of superiority.

References

Aune, D., Keum, N., Giovannucci, E.L., Fadnes, L.T., Boffetta, P., Greenwood, D.C., Tonstad, S., Vatten, L.J., Riboli, E. and Norat, T. (2016)
'Whole grain consumption and risk of cardiovascular disease, cancer, and all-cause and cause-specific mortality: systematic review and dose-response meta-analysis of prospective studies',
BMJ, 353, i2716.

Biesiekierski, J.R. (2017)
'What is gluten?',
Journal of Gastroenterology and Hepatology, 32(S1), pp. 78–81.

Caio, G., Volta, U., Sapone, A., Leffler, D.A., De Giorgio, R., Catassi, C. and Fasano, A. (2019)
'Celiac disease: a comprehensive current review',
BMC Medicine, 17(1), p. 142.

Catassi, C., Elli, L., Bonaz, B., Bouma, G., Carroccio, A., Castillejo, G. and Zevallos, K. (2017)
'Diagnosis of non-celiac gluten sensitivity (NCGS): The Salerno Experts' Criteria',
Nutrients, 7(6), p. 496.

Lebwohl, B., Ludvigsson, J.F. and Green, P.H.R. (2017)
'Does gluten contribute to the development of cardiovascular disease?',
Journal of the American Heart Association, 6(2), e005119.

Lebwohl, B., Sanders, D.S. and Green, P.H.R. (2018)
'Coeliac disease',
Lancet, 391(10115), pp. 70–81.

Lionetti, E., Gatti, S., Pulvirenti, A. and Catassi, C. (2015)
'Nutritional status in children with celiac disease',
American Journal of Gastroenterology, 110(7), pp. 1023–1031.

Saturni, L., Ferretti, G. and Bacchetti, T. (2010)
'The gluten-free diet: safety and nutritional quality',
Nutrients, 2(1), pp. 16–34.

Thompson, T. (2009)
'The nutritional quality of gluten-free foods', Gluten-free Nutrition Guide, Chicago:
American Dietetic Association.

Myth 9

Red Meat Should Be Completely Eliminated From A Healthy Diet

This one is going to ruffle some feathers, especially my plant based friends. Many of you may know that I was actually vegan for over 20 years. Not any more! One of the big things that we hear regarding meat consumption is that red meat is hideously bad for us. We need to get a bit more specific in these things. What does the science say?

Red meat, including beef, lamb, and pork, has been a dietary staple for many cultures throughout history. In recent decades, however, concerns have surfaced regarding its association with chronic diseases, including heart disease, certain cancers, and type 2 diabetes. These concerns have led some individuals to believe that red meat must be completely removed from a healthy diet. While there is evidence suggesting that high intakes of certain types of red and processed meats may have negative health impacts, the idea that all red meat must be permanently excluded is an oversimplification.

A more nuanced view, rooted in moderation, quality, and overall dietary context, is supported by current nutritional science.

Red Meat: Nutrient Profile and Dietary Role

Red meat is a rich source of high-quality protein, providing all the essential amino acids necessary for growth, maintenance, and repair of tissues (McNeill & Van Elswyk 2012). It is also a valuable source of iron, zinc, vitamin B12, and other B-vitamins, all of which play critical roles in blood formation, immune function, and neurological health (Clogherty et al. 2019; Wyness 2016). For populations at risk of nutrient deficiencies—such as women of childbearing age, adolescents, and the elderly—red meat can offer a convenient and bioavailable source of these essential nutrients.

Moderation versus Elimination

While it is true that some epidemiological studies have found associations between high consumption of red meat (particularly processed meat) and an increased risk of colorectal cancer, cardiovascular disease, and type 2 diabetes (Willett & Stampfer 2013; Rohrmann et al. 2013; Pan et al. 2012), these findings must be placed in the context of overall dietary patterns. Dietary guidelines do not generally recommend eliminating red meat entirely. Instead, they emphasise moderating intake and choosing lean cuts of unprocessed meat as part of a balanced dietary pattern (Public Health England 2016; World Cancer Research Fund/American Institute for Cancer Research 2018).

A Mediterranean-style eating pattern—widely regarded as one of the healthiest dietary models—involves moderate portions of lean red meat along with ample vegetables, fruits, legumes, whole grains, oily fish, and extra-virgin olive oil (Estruch et al. 2013; Sofi et al. 2008). This approach illustrates how red meat can be enjoyed as an occasional component of a healthy diet rather than being viewed as a food to be entirely avoided.

One thing we should mention here. We need to be aware of the weakness of epidemiological data. There are many opportunities for confounding factors to come in. In many cultures meat consumption is associated with greater affluence. Also associated with greater affluence are cigarette smoking, high alcohol consumption, more processed foods in general, higher stress, and many other modern day factors that can drive disease patterns. Of course a good quality trial will aim to eliminate confounders as much as possible, but there is a limit to how effectively this can be done. Worth some thought.

Quality and Preparation Matter

Not all red meat is created equal. Processed meats, such as sausages, bacon, and cured meats, have been more consistently linked with adverse health outcomes than fresh, lean cuts (Bouvard et al. 2015; Wang et al. 2016). These processed varieties often contain higher levels of sodium, nitrates, and nitrites, which may contribute to increased cancer risk and cardiovascular problems. By contrast, fresh, lean red meat prepared using healthier cooking methods—like grilling, roasting, or baking—can be part of an overall nutrient-rich and balanced meal plan.

Additionally, portion sizes are critical. Large, frequent servings of red meat can crowd out other nutrient-dense foods, such as vegetables, legumes, and whole grains. Emphasising variety in the diet ensures that one's nutrient intake is not overly reliant on a single source (Harvard T.H. Chan School of Public Health 2020; WHO 2003).

Individual Differences and Dietary Needs

Individual factors, such as genetic predispositions, metabolic health, and personal health goals, also influence how red meat consumption affects one's wellbeing. Some people, for example, may need to restrict red meat due to high cholesterol or a family history of colorectal cancer. In such cases, careful dietary planning can help ensure nutritional adequacy without relying heavily on red meat.

Others may find that modest amounts of red meat help maintain their iron stores or prevent nutrient deficiencies. The key lies in personalising dietary choices rather than applying a one-size-fits-all ban on entire food groups.

Conclusion

The call for a complete elimination of red meat from the diet oversimplifies the current body of nutritional evidence. While reducing intake of processed and high-fat red meats is prudent—especially in the context of a balanced, predominantly plant-rich diet—occasional, moderate portions of lean red meat can fit into a healthy lifestyle. Rather than demonising a single food, it is more beneficial to focus on an overall eating pattern that emphasises quality, variety, and nutrient density.

References

Bouvard, V., Loomis, D., Guyton, K.Z., Grosse, Y., Ghissassi, F.E., Benbrahim-Tallaa, L. and Straif, K. (2015)
'Carcinogenicity of consumption of red and processed meat',
Lancet Oncology, 16(16), pp. 1599–1600.

Clogherty, M.M., Craig, P.M., Thomson, C.D. and Krause, M.P. (2019)
'Red meat and dietary iron: A potential link with atherosclerosis',
Journal of Nutritional Science, 8, e28.

Estruch, R., Ros, E., Salas-Salvadó, J., Covas, M.I., Corella, D., Arós, F. and Martínez-González, M.A. (2013)
'Primary prevention of cardiovascular disease with a Mediterranean diet',
New England Journal of Medicine, 368(14), pp. 1279–1290.

Harvard T.H. Chan School of Public Health (2020)
Healthy eating plate & healthy eating pyramid.
Available at: https://www.hsph.harvard.edu/nutritionsource/healthy-eating-plate/
(Accessed: [date]).

McNeill, S. and Van Elswyk, M.E. (2012)
'Red meat in global nutrition',
Meat Science, 92(3), pp. 166–173.

Mozaffarian, D. (2016)
'Dietary and policy priorities for cardiovascular disease, diabetes, and obesity: a comprehensive review',
Circulation, 133(2), pp. 187–225.

Pan, A., Sun, Q., Bernstein, A.M., Schulze, M.B., Manson, J.E., Willett, W.C. and Hu, F.B. (2012)
'Red meat consumption and mortality: results from 2 prospective cohort studies',
Archives of Internal Medicine, 172(7), pp. 555–563.

Public Health England (2016) The Eatwell Guide.
Available at: https://www.gov.uk/government/publications/the-eatwell-guide (Accessed: [date]).

Rohrmann, S., Overvad, K., Bueno-de-Mesquita, H.B., Jakobsen, M.U., Egeberg, R., Tjønneland, A. and Linseisen, J. (2013)
'Meat consumption and mortality—results from the European Prospective Investigation into Cancer and Nutrition',
BMC Medicine, 11, p. 63.

Sofi, F., Cesari, F., Abbate, R., Gensini, G.F. and Casini, A. (2008)
'Adherence to Mediterranean diet and health status: meta-analysis',
BMJ, 337, a1344.

Wang, Y., Lehane, C., Ghebremedhin, M. and Astell-Burt, T. (2016)
'Red and processed meat consumption and mortality: dose-response meta-analysis of prospective cohort studies',
Public Health Nutrition, 19(5), pp. 893–905.

WHO (2003)
Diet, Nutrition and the Prevention of Chronic Diseases.
Geneva: World Health Organization.

Willett, W.C. and Stampfer, M.J. (2013)
'Current evidence on healthy eating',
Annual Review of Public Health, 34, pp. 77–95.

World Cancer Research Fund/American Institute for Cancer Research (2018)
Diet, Nutrition, Physical Activity and Cancer: a Global Perspective.
Continuous Update Project Expert Report.

Wyness, L. (2016)
'The role of red meat in the diet: nutrition and health benefits',
Proceedings of the Nutrition Society, 75(3), pp. 227–232.

Myth 10

All Processed Foods Are Harmful And Devoid Of Nutrition

This one may well raise a few eyebrows and I am certainly committed to building my diet around whole foods. But let's open this can of worms. Why not. Ultra processed foods have been heavily featured in the media over the last couple of years - rightly so and those foods that fall into the ultra processed category are really an abomination. However, the term processed has rather a broad reach and maybe, just maybe we don't have to tar every single processed food with the same brush.

The term "processed food" is often used pejoratively, conjuring images of junk food laden with sugar, unhealthy fats, and artificial additives. In fact, most foods undergo some form of processing before reaching our plates. Even something as simple as washing, peeling, freezing, or cooking can be considered a form of processing. While it is true that certain highly processed and ultra-processed foods can be poor in nutritional value and contribute to obesity and metabolic diseases, the belief that all processed foods are inherently harmful and lacking in nutrients is an oversimplification.

Understanding Different Levels of Food Processing

Food processing exists on a spectrum. At one end, there are minimally processed foods, such as frozen vegetables or plain yoghurt, which retain most of their original nutrient content (Monteiro et al. 2018). On the other end lie ultra-processed products—heavily modified foods like sugary cereals, crisps, biscuits, and soft drinks—which may contain large amounts of refined starches, added sugars, sodium, and unhealthy fats while offering limited vitamins, minerals, and fibre (Fardet 2018; Moubarac et al. 2013).

Minimally processed foods can actually make healthy eating easier by increasing availability, shelf life, and convenience. For example, frozen fruits and vegetables are often flash-frozen shortly after harvest, preserving their nutrient content and sometimes retaining vitamins better than fresh produce that has spent days in transport or on supermarket shelves (Bouzari et al. 2015). Similarly, wholegrain breads, plain canned beans, and plain Greek yoghurt are processed products that can contribute valuable nutrients, including protein, fibre, and essential micronutrients (Augustin et al. 2015).

Nutritional Quality Varies Widely

The notion that all processed foods lack nutrients does not hold up under scrutiny. Many processing methods, such as pasteurisation, can enhance food safety without drastically compromising nutritional quality (WHO 2002). Canning and fermentation are traditional forms of processing that can preserve or even improve the nutrient profile of certain foods, making them more accessible to a broader population and aiding in dietary diversity.

Of course, it is important to differentiate between these types of processing and the production of ultra-processed items characterised by high energy density and low nutrient density. Evidence suggests that diets high in ultra-processed foods are associated with weight gain, obesity, and a higher risk of non-communicable diseases (Hall et al. 2019; Monteiro et al.

2018). Thus, while not all processed foods are problematic, relying heavily on ultra-processed fare is likely to displace more nutrient-dense options and adversely affect health.

Context and Overall Dietary Patterns

The overall dietary pattern matters more than the presence or absence of certain processed items. A balanced, health-promoting diet can include sensible amounts of minimally processed or lightly processed foods alongside fresh fruits, vegetables, whole grains, legumes, lean proteins, and healthy fats (WHO 2003; Mozaffarian 2016). For many people, incorporating some processed foods helps them meet nutritional needs, manage busy lifestyles, and reduce food waste.

By contrast, a pattern dominated by ultra-processed foods is more concerning. The key lies in discernment: reading nutrition labels, choosing options with minimal added sugars and sodium, and complementing processed items with whole, nutrient-rich foods. For instance, pairing a wholegrain, high-fibre breakfast cereal with fresh berries and low-fat milk can provide a balanced start to the day, even though the cereal itself is technically processed.

Conclusion

Not all processed foods are created equal. While ultra-processed foods can indeed be high in empty calories and low in essential nutrients, minimally processed and lightly processed foods can play a valuable role in a healthy, balanced diet. Recognising the spectrum of food processing and focusing on the overall quality and variety of one's diet is more useful than dismissing all processed foods as harmful. By choosing wisely and maintaining a generally balanced eating pattern, you can enjoy the convenience and accessibility of certain processed foods without compromising on nutritional value.

References

Augustin, M.A., Sanguansri, L., Crittenden, R. and Lockett, T. (2015)
'Functional foods and obesity', in Akoh, C.C. (ed.) Healthful Lipids. Urbana, IL: AOCS Press, pp. 237–258.

Bouzari, A., Holstege, D. and Barrett, D.M. (2015)
'Vitamin retention in eight fruits and vegetables: A comparison of refrigerated and frozen storage',
Journal of Agricultural and Food Chemistry, 63(3), pp. 957–962.

Fardet, A. (2018)
'Characterization of the degree of food processing in relation with its health potential and effects',
Advances in Food and Nutrition Research, 85, pp. 79–129.

Hall, K.D., Bemis, T., Brychta, R., Chen, K.Y., Courville, A., Crayner, E.J., Chung, S.T., Costa, E., Driscoll, A., Miller, B.V., Steinberg, G.R., Walter, M., Yannai, L.E. and Zhou, M. (2019)
'Ultra-processed diets cause excess calorie intake and weight gain: an inpatient randomised controlled trial of ad libitum food intake'
, *Cell Metabolism, 30(1), pp. 67–77.*

Mozaffarian, D. (2016)
'Dietary and policy priorities for cardiovascular disease, diabetes, and obesity: a comprehensive review',
Circulation, 133(2), pp. 187–225.

Monteiro, C.A., Cannon, G., Moubarac, J.-C., Levy, R.B., Louzada, M.L.C. and Jaime, P.C. (2018)
'The UN Decade of Nutrition, the NOVA food classification and the trouble with ultra-processing',
Public Health Nutrition, 21(1), pp. 5–17.

Moubarac, J.C., Parra, D.C., Cannon, G. and Monteiro, C.A. (2013)

'Food classification systems based on food processing: significance and implications for policies and actions: a systematic literature review and assessment',
Current Obesity Reports, 2(2), pp. 256–272.

WHO (2002)
Joint FAO/WHO Working Group Report on Drafting Guidelines for the Evaluation *of Probiotics in Food. Geneva: World Health Organization.*

WHO (2003)
Diet, Nutrition and the Prevention of Chronic Diseases.
Geneva: World Health Organization.

Myth 11

High-Cholesterol Foods Always Raise Your Blood Cholesterol Levels

This one always gets my goat, and it is still something that I see come up time and time again. People being told to avoid so many amazingly nutrient dense foods because they contain cholesterol. Now, there is a vast amount of evidence to suggest that cholesterol is not of itself causative of heart disease anyway, more dragged into things by being a bystander, but that is conversation for another day. So what gives? Does consuming a cholesterol rich food actually influence serum cholesterol. If it does, does it even matter?

For decades now, public health messages often focused on the idea that eating foods high in cholesterol—such as eggs, prawns, or organ meats—would directly translate into increased blood cholesterol levels and, by extension, heightened risk of heart disease. This association led many individuals to avoid these foods altogether. However, the evidence accumulated over the past few decades reveals a more nuanced reality. In most people, dietary cholesterol has a far less pronounced effect on blood cholesterol than was once assumed, and other dietary factors, particularly saturated and trans fats, play a far more significant role in raising blood cholesterol levels.

Revisiting the Dietary Cholesterol–Blood Cholesterol Link

Research indicates that the human body carefully regulates the amount of cholesterol in the bloodstream. When dietary intake of cholesterol increases, the liver often compensates by producing less cholesterol, helping to maintain overall balance (Griffin et al. 2013; Soliman 2018). As a result, many individuals experience only minor changes in blood cholesterol levels when consuming moderate amounts of cholesterol-rich foods.

Eggs provide a good example. Once demonised for their high cholesterol content, eggs have been the subject of numerous studies and meta-analyses. Most have concluded that moderate egg consumption (one egg per day) does not significantly increase the risk of heart disease in healthy individuals (Jiang et al. 2013; Alexander et al. 2016). In fact, eggs offer several essential nutrients, including high-quality protein, choline, vitamins, and minerals, which can contribute to a balanced diet.

Fats & Sugar Matter More Than Dietary Cholesterol

While attention once centred on dietary cholesterol, scientific consensus now recognises that certain fats and sugar intake have a more substantial influence on circulating low-density lipoprotein (LDL) cholesterol levels— the type often referred to as "bad" cholesterol (Lamarche et al. 2020; Mozaffarian 2016).

Diets high in trans fats from sources such as heavily processed foods, and fast release high glycemic carbohydrates are more strongly linked to elevated LDL cholesterol and an increased risk of cardiovascular disease than dietary cholesterol.

Public health guidelines now tend to emphasise limiting trans fats (I would say get rid of the, completely - they play no beneficial role) and replacing them with unsaturated fats from foods like nuts, seeds, oily fish, and extra-virgin olive oil. Carbohydrate wise it is the slow burning high fibre variety. As I always say, swap the white for the brown. This dietary shift can help maintain healthy blood cholesterol profiles and support overall heart health (Harvard T.H. Chan School of Public Health 2020; Public Health England 2016).

Individual Differences and Context

While most healthy individuals are relatively insensitive to dietary cholesterol, a subset of people may exhibit a stronger blood cholesterol response when consuming cholesterol-rich foods. These "hyper-responders" may need more personalised dietary guidance. However, for the general population, moderate consumption of foods containing cholesterol, as part of a balanced and varied dietary pattern, is not strongly associated with adverse health outcomes (Soliman 2018).

Further, it is essential to consider the totality of one's diet. Replacing nutrient-dense, high-cholesterol foods like eggs with refined carbohydrates or sugary snacks is to cause further cardiovascular chaos. Choosing whole foods that offer a range of essential nutrients and emphasising overall dietary quality will have a more profound impact on long-term health than focusing narrowly on cholesterol content alone.

Conclusion

The simplistic message that high-cholesterol foods inevitably raise blood cholesterol levels does not hold up in the face of current scientific evidence. Most people can enjoy eggs and other foods containing dietary cholesterol as part of a healthy, balanced diet without fear of significantly raising their blood cholesterol. Placing greater emphasis on the types of fats & carbohydrates consumed and maintaining a diverse, minimally processed dietary pattern will yield far more reliable health benefits than avoiding dietary cholesterol altogether.

References

Alexander, D.D., Miller, P.E., Vargas, A.J., Weed, D.L. and Cohen, S.S. (2016)
'Meta-analysis of egg consumption and risk of coronary heart disease and stroke',
Journal of the American College of Nutrition, 35(8), pp. 706–716.

Griffin, J.D., Lichtenstein, A.H. and Volek, J.S. (2013)
'Dietary cholesterol and plasma lipoprotein profiles: a meta-analysis',
American Journal of Clinical Nutrition, 98(4), pp. 926–927. (Letter)

Harvard T.H. Chan School of Public Health (2020)
Healthy eating plate & healthy eating pyramid.
Available at: https://www.hsph.harvard.edu/nutritionsource/healthy-eating-plate/

Jiang, W., Zhang, Y., Yan, T., Zheng, F. and Chen, Y. (2013)
'Egg consumption and risk of coronary heart disease and stroke: dose-response meta-analysis of prospective cohort studies',
BMJ, 346, e8539.

Lamarche, B., Couture, P., Graham, J., Desroches, S. and Charest, A. (2020)
'Evidence on the physiological effects of saturated fatty acids to support a threshold of ≤10% energy intake in guidelines for adults',
Applied Physiology, Nutrition, and Metabolism, 45(10), pp. S75–S82.

Mozaffarian, D. (2016)
'Dietary and policy priorities for cardiovascular disease, diabetes, and obesity: a comprehensive review',
Circulation, 133(2), pp. 187–225.

Public Health England (2016)
The Eatwell Guide.
Available at: https://www.gov.uk/government/publications/the-eatwell-guide

Soliman, G.A. (2018)
'Dietary cholesterol and the lack of evidence in cardiovascular disease', *Nutrients, 10(6), p. 780.*

Myth 12

Cooking Vegetables Destroys All Their Nutrients

This is another question that comes up nearly all of the time when I do live events or interviews. As I often talk about the therapeutic benefits of specific ingredients and nutrients, and the first question that pops up is 'does cooking have any effect on the benefits'. Well, this is a mixed picture.

It is true that some vitamins and beneficial plant compounds are sensitive to heat, and therefore their levels can be reduced during certain cooking processes. But then others can actually become more bioavailable. In reality, cooking methods vary widely in their effects, and while some nutrients may decrease in quantity, others can become more easy to absorb by the body. The net nutritional impact of cooking depends on the type of vegetable, the cooking method, and the specific nutrients in question.

Understanding Nutrient Changes During Cooking

Some vitamins—particularly vitamin C and certain B vitamins—are water-soluble and heat-sensitive, which can lead to reductions in their levels if vegetables are boiled for long periods or exposed to high temperatures (Randhir & Shetty 2008; Bernhardt & Schlich 2006). Yet, not all nutrients respond the same way. Fat-soluble vitamins (A, D, E, and K) and many minerals tend to be more stable under heat. Moreover, certain cooking methods, such as steaming or microwaving, have been shown to retain more nutrients than prolonged boiling (Miglio et al. 2008).

It really is crucial to re-emphasise that cooking can make some beneficial compounds easier for the body to use. For instance, heat breaks down the cell walls in vegetables like carrots, spinach, and tomatoes, increasing the availability of antioxidants such as beta-carotene and lycopene (Dewanto et al. 2002; Bernhardt & Schlich 2006). Similarly, lightly cooking vegetables can reduce anti-nutritional factors, making it easier to digest and absorb essential minerals (Nosworthy et al. 2018).

Different Cooking Methods, Different Outcomes

Not all cooking techniques are equal. Blanching, steaming, stir-frying, and microwaving often better preserve heat-sensitive vitamins compared to methods involving large amounts of water or long cooking times (Miglio et al. 2008; Kim et al. 2017). Gentle cooking methods can help strike a balance between minimising nutrient losses and maximising the bioavailability of important compounds.

For example, steaming broccoli may preserve more vitamin C than boiling it, while sautéing tomatoes in a small amount of oil can enhance the absorption of their fat-soluble antioxidants (Calvo-Castro et al. 2019). The variety of vegetables you eat and the range of preparation methods you employ both contribute to maintaining a nutrient-rich diet.

Focusing on Overall Dietary Patterns

Even if some nutrients are lost during cooking, this does not negate the health benefits of including vegetables in your diet. A balanced pattern rich in plant foods, whether raw or cooked, is consistently associated with reduced risk of chronic diseases such as cardiovascular disease, type 2 diabetes, and certain cancers (Aune et al. 2017; Boeing et al. 2012). Cooking can also make vegetables more palatable and enjoyable, which may encourage higher overall vegetable consumption, ultimately improving diet quality and nutrient intake.

In other words, focusing solely on the potential losses of a few nutrients misses the bigger picture. Preparing vegetables in ways that you find tasty and convenient often leads to a higher total intake and a more diverse range of vitamins, minerals, and phytochemicals in the long run.

This is why I always make one simple recommendation - every day consume a combination of cooked and raw food so that you get benefits from both sides of the equation. Preserved micronutrients. Enhanced phytochemical availability.

Conclusion

While cooking can reduce certain heat-sensitive nutrients in vegetables, it does not completely destroy their nutritional value. Many cooking methods preserve, and in some cases enhance, the bioavailability of beneficial compounds. Emphasising variety, moderation in cooking time and temperature, and selecting cooking methods that retain nutrients can ensure you continue to benefit from the healthful properties of vegetables. Whether you choose to eat them raw, steamed, roasted, or sautéed, vegetables remain a vital component of a healthy, balanced diet.

References

Aune, D., Giovannucci, E., Boffetta, P., Fadnes, L.T., Keum, N., Norat, T. and Tonstad, S. (2017)
'Fruit and vegetable intake and the risk of cardiovascular disease, total cancer and all-cause mortality—a systematic review and dose-response meta-analysis of prospective studies',
International Journal of Epidemiology, 46(3), pp. 1029–1056.

Bernhardt, S. and Schlich, E. (2006)
'Impact of different cooking methods on food quality: Retention of lipophilic vitamins in fresh and frozen vegetables',
Journal of Food Engineering, 77(2), pp. 327–333.

Boeing, H., Bechthold, A., Bub, A., Ellinger, S., Haller, D., Kroke, A. and Watzl, B. (2012)
'Critical review: vegetables and fruit in the prevention of chronic diseases',
European Journal of Nutrition, 51(6), pp. 637–663.

Calvo-Castro, L.A., Lizarraga, M.S., Sarić, A., Tembo, S., Antonescu, S., Henein, M.Y. and Müller, M. (2019)
'Tomato seed oil attenuates oxidative stress in a cell culture model of cardiovascular disease via activation of the Nrf2/ARE pathway',
European Journal of Nutrition, 58(4), pp. 1533–1542.

Dewanto, V., Wu, X.Z., Adom, K.K. and Liu, R.H. (2002)
'Thermal processing enhances the nutritional value of tomatoes by increasing total antioxidant activity',
Journal of Agricultural and Food Chemistry, 50(10), pp. 3010–3014.

Kim, K., Kim, J. and Chang, Y.H. (2017)
'Effect of different cooking methods on the content of vitamins and true retention in selected vegetables',
Food Science and Biotechnology, 26(2), pp. 313–320.

Miglio, C., Chiavaro, E., Visconti, A., Fogliano, V. and Pellegrini, N. (2008) 'Effects of different cooking methods on nutritional and physicochemical characteristics of selected vegetables',
Journal of Agricultural and Food Chemistry, 56(1), pp. 139–147.

Nosworthy, M.G., Neufeld, J., Frohlich, P., Young, G. and Malcolmson, L.J. (2018) 'Determination of the protein quality of cooked Canadian pulses',
Food Science and Human Wellness, 7(2), pp. 96–101.

Randhir, R. and Shetty, K. (2008)
'AC-elecited fenugreek sprouts with phenolic enrichment for dietary management of hyperglycemia and related complications',
Asia Pacific Journal of Clinical Nutrition, 17(1), pp. 109–116.

Myth 13

You Must Drink Eight Glasses Of Water Every Day, No Exceptions

I really do not know where this one comes from. It has been banded around for years but is just an arbitrary number with no grounding in reality.

You would have heard it before, that you should consume a fixed amount of water daily—often touted as "eight glasses," or around two litres—to maintain optimal health and hydration. Although staying adequately hydrated is vital for numerous bodily functions, there is no universal, one-size-fits-all prescription that everyone must strictly follow. Fluid requirements vary greatly based on individual factors such as age, body size, physical activity, climate, and overall diet. The notion that everyone must rigidly adhere to eight glasses of water each day oversimplifies the science of hydration and can even cause unnecessary stress or confusion.

Individual Variability in Hydration Needs

Hydration needs are influenced by many variables. Athletes or individuals engaging in strenuous exercise may require more fluids due to increased sweating and the need to replace electrolytes (Sawka et al. 2007; Thomas et al. 2016). People living in hot, dry climates or working in physically demanding jobs may also need to drink more fluids to avoid dehydration (Armstrong et al. 2012). On the other hand, individuals who eat a diet rich in fruits, vegetables, soups, and other water-rich foods naturally obtain a substantial portion of their daily fluid intake from these sources (Popkin et al. 2010).

Rather than following a rigid "eight glasses" rule, paying attention to thirst cues and urine colour can provide a more accurate indication of hydration status. For most healthy adults, thirst is a reliable guide to fluid intake (Grandjean et al. 2003). Urine that is pale straw-coloured generally suggests adequate hydration, while darker urine may indicate a need for more fluids (Armstrong et al. 2012).

No Scientific Consensus on a Universal Target

The origin of the "eight glasses a day" guideline is unclear, and no scientific consensus supports it as a universal requirement. In fact, leading health organisations, including the European Food Safety Authority and the US National Academies of Sciences, Engineering, and Medicine, suggest a range of adequate fluid intakes that depend on factors such as body weight, activity level, and environmental conditions (EFSA 2010; National Academies of Sciences, Engineering, and Medicine 2005).

It's also worth noting that total fluid intake includes not only plain water but also beverages like tea, coffee, milk, and low-sugar drinks, as well as foods with high water content. This means that if you enjoy herbal tea, consume juicy fruits, or have a bowl of broth-based soup, you're already contributing to your daily fluid needs without constantly reaching for a glass of plain water.

Overhydration and Balance

While chronic, mild dehydration can have negative consequences, such as headaches, fatigue, or reduced concentration (Popkin et al. 2010), it's also possible to overdo it. Overhydration, or hyponatremia, though less common, can occur if you drink excessive amounts of water in a short period, diluting blood sodium levels (Hew-Butler et al. 2015). Striving to surpass a fixed water intake target without listening to your body's signals can be unhelpful or even risky.

Focus on Individual Needs and Context

The key is balance and personalisation. Factors like your exercise routine, dietary habits, climate, and personal health conditions should guide how much water you drink. The best approach is to tune in to your body and consume enough fluids to prevent thirst and maintain normal bodily functions. Health professionals may provide more specific guidelines if you have certain medical conditions, but for most people, strict numerical targets are unnecessary.

Conclusion

The strict edict that everyone must drink eight glasses of water every day is not backed by strong scientific evidence. Although maintaining adequate hydration is crucial for good health, fluid requirements vary widely. By paying attention to thirst, monitoring urine colour, and considering lifestyle factors, you can ensure proper hydration without rigidly adhering to a universally prescribed number of glasses.

References

Armstrong, L.E., Johnson, E.C., McKenzie, A.L. and Munoz, C.X. (2012)
'Interpreting common hydration biomarkers of urine and plasma concentrations, and changes thereof, to assess hydration status in humans',
European Journal of Clinical Nutrition, 67(2), pp. S2–S9.

EFSA (2010)
'Scientific opinion on dietary reference values for water',
EFSA Journal, 8(3), 1459.

Grandjean, A.C., Reimers, K.J., Buyckx, M.E. and Haven, M.C. (2003)
'The effect of caffeinated, non-caffeinated, caloric and non-caloric beverages on hydration',
Journal of the American College of Nutrition, 22(2), pp. 165–173.

Hew-Butler, T., Rosner, M.H., Fowkes-Godek, S., Dugas, J.P., Hoffman, M.D., Lewis, D.P. and Verbalis, J.G. (2015)
'Statement of the Third International Exercise-Associated Hyponatremia Consensus Development Conference',
Clinical Journal of Sport Medicine, 25(4), pp. 303–320.

National Academies of Sciences, Engineering, and Medicine (2005)
Dietary Reference Intakes for Water, Potassium, Sodium, Chloride, and Sulfate. Washington,
DC: The National Academies Press.

Popkin, B.M., D'Anci, K.E. and Rosenberg, I.H. (2010)
'Water, hydration and health',
Nutrition Reviews, 68(8), pp. 439–458.

Sawka, M.N., Cheuvront, S.N. and Carter, R. (2005)
'Human water needs',
Nutrition Reviews, 63(6 Pt 2), pp. S30–S39. [Reaffirmed in subsequent literature]

Thomas, D.T., Erdman, K.A. and Burke, L.M. (2016)
'Position of the Academy of Nutrition and Dietetics, Dietitians of Canada, and the American College of Sports Medicine: Nutrition and athletic performance', *Journal of the Academy of Nutrition and Dietetics, 116(3), pp. 501–528.*

Myth 14

Diet Sodas Help With Weight Loss Because They Have Zero Calories

This is an interesting one and another nod towards the advice that it is 'all about the calories', being a tad inaccurate if it is the solitary focus. It seems that more and more people are becoming aware of the potential pitfalls of diet drinks, but it is worth reviewing as these things are still promoted as being good options.

The logic seems straightforward: replacing regular sugary drinks with diet sodas that contain virtually no calories should facilitate weight loss. I would absolutely say that cutting out the sugary drinks is absolutely a smart move. Yet, the relationship between artificially sweetened beverages and body weight is more complex than a simple calorie subtraction. There's a surprise. While reducing high-calorie sugary drinks is generally a good idea, the evidence does not conclusively show that diet sodas reliably lead to long-term weight loss. In some studies, regular consumption of artificially sweetened beverages has even been linked with weight gain or metabolic changes, highlighting the need for a nuanced understanding of their role in a healthy diet.

The Complexity of Artificial Sweeteners and Appetite Regulation

Artificial sweeteners, such as aspartame, sucralose, and acesulfame-K, provide sweetness without contributing significant calories. In theory, this should reduce overall energy intake and support weight management (Rogers et al. 2016). However, human appetite regulation is not purely a matter of calorie counting. Some research suggests that sweet-tasting beverages, even without calories, can influence hunger, cravings, and reward pathways in the brain (Swithers 2013; Sylvetsky et al. 2020). In some individuals, consuming very sweet, calorie-free beverages may increase the desire for other sweet foods or disrupt the normal mechanisms that signal satiety.

Mixed Evidence from Studies

Observational studies have yielded mixed results. Some indicate that swapping sugary beverages for diet sodas can help reduce calorie intake and body weight (Pereira 2013; Miller & Perez 2014). Others, however, have reported associations between artificially sweetened beverages and weight gain or metabolic risks, though these findings do not establish a clear cause-and-effect relationship (Fowler et al. 2008; Azad et al. 2017). Randomised controlled trials (RCTs), which are generally considered more reliable for determining causal effects, also produce varied outcomes. Some RCTs have shown modest weight-loss benefits or at least no weight gain from substituting diet sodas for sugary drinks (Peters et al. 2016). Others suggest that while diet sodas may help reduce calorie intake in the short term, they may not be effective as a long-term weight management tool for everyone.

Considering the Bigger Picture

It's crucial to recognise that beverages are only one component of an overall dietary pattern. Drinking diet soda instead of a full-sugar soda is certainly a step towards reducing daily sugar and calorie intake. However, if replacing a sugary drink with a diet soda leads to compensatory eating of other high energy foods or fosters a taste preference for intense sweetness, the net effect may be minimal or even counterproductive.

Moreover, weight management relies not on a single substitution but on a holistic approach that includes a balanced, nutrient-rich diet and regular physical activity. Relying on diet sodas as a "quick fix" without addressing other aspects of eating behaviour and lifestyle may limit long-term success.

Focus on Water and Whole Foods

Ultimately, for optimal health and weight regulation, water remains a superior beverage choice (Popkin et al. 2010; WHO 2003). Other low-calorie options like unsweetened tea or coffee can also offer health benefits without the complexity and controversy surrounding artificial sweeteners. Prioritising whole foods, vegetables, fruits, lean proteins, and whole grains over highly processed, sweet-tasting alternatives can help regulate appetite and promote sustainable weight management.

Conclusion

While diet sodas contain fewer calories than their sugary counterparts, the assumption that they inherently lead to weight loss oversimplifies a complex issue. Appetite regulation, taste preferences, compensatory eating, and overall dietary patterns all influence long-term body weight outcomes. Diet sodas may play a role in reducing calorie intake as part of a broader, balanced dietary approach, but relying solely on them for weight loss is unlikely to yield the desired results. Ultimately, choosing water and nutrient-dense whole foods remains a more reliable route to maintaining a healthy weight.

References

Azad, M.B., Abou-Setta, A.M., Chauhan, B.F., Rabbani, R., Lys, J., Copstein, L. and Zarychanski, R. (2017)
'Nonnutritive sweeteners and cardiometabolic health: a systematic review and meta-analysis of randomized controlled trials and prospective cohort studies',
CMAJ, 189(28), pp. E929–E939.

Fowler, S.P., Williams, K., Resendez, R.G., Hunt, K.J., Hazuda, H.P. and Stern, M.P. (2008)
'Fueling the obesity epidemic? Artificially sweetened beverage use and long-term weight gain',
Obesity, 16(8), pp. 1894–1900.

Miller, P.E. and Perez, V. (2014)
'Low-calorie sweeteners and body weight and composition: a meta-analysis of randomized controlled trials and prospective cohort studies',
American Journal of Clinical Nutrition, 100(3), pp. 765–777.

Pereira, M.A. (2013)
'Diet beverages and the risk of obesity, metabolic syndrome, and type 2 diabetes: a meta-analysis of prospective cohort studies',
American Journal of Clinical Nutrition, 97(3), pp. 533–534. (Letter)

Peters, J.C., Beck, J., Cardel, M., Wyatt, H.R., Foster, G.D., Pan, Z. and Hill, J.O. (2016)
'The effects of water and non-nutritive sweetened beverages on weight loss and weight maintenance: A randomized clinical trial',
Obesity, 24(2), pp. 297–304.

Popkin, B.M., D'Anci, K.E. and Rosenberg, I.H. (2010)
'Water, hydration, and health',
Nutrition Reviews, 68(8), pp. 439–458.

Rogers, P.J., Hogenkamp, P.S., de Graaf, C., Higgs, S., Lluch, A., Ness, A.R. and *Mela, D.J. (2016)*
'Does low-energy sweetener consumption affect energy intake and body weight? A systematic review, including meta-analyses, of the evidence from human and animal studies',
International Journal of Obesity, 40(3), pp. 381–394.

Swithers, S.E. (2013)
'Artificial sweeteners produce the counterintuitive effect of inducing metabolic derangements',
Trends in Endocrinology & Metabolism, 24(9), pp. 431–441.

Sylvetsky, A.C., Jin, Y., Clark, E.J., Welsh, J.A., Rother, K.I. and Talegawkar, S.A. (2020)
'Consumption of low-calorie sweetened beverages is associated with higher total energy and sugar intake among children, NHANES 2009–2014',
Pediatric Obesity, 15(2), e12535.

WHO (2003)
Diet, Nutrition and the Prevention of Chronic Diseases.
Geneva: World Health Organization.

Myth 15

Frozen Fruits And Vegetables Are Less Nutritious Than Fresh Produce

I am definitely an advocate of frozen veg. When we were doing 'Eat Shop Save' on ITV, we would often nudge families towards frozen veg for their convenience and affordability, not to mention minimising food waste. But for some odd reason there is a belief that frozen foods are a poor choice and devoid of nutrients. This absolutely doesn't stack up.

This belief often stems from the idea that produce plucked straight from the field and sold the same day must be richer in vitamins, minerals, and antioxidants than produce harvested earlier, stored, and then frozen. In reality, the nutrient content of fruits and vegetables depends on a complex interplay of factors—including time since harvest, temperature, storage conditions, and processing methods. Contrary to popular belief, frozen produce can be just as nutritious as, and occasionally even more nutritious than, fresh items that have spent days in transport and on shelves.

Harvesting, Processing, and Nutrient Retention

Fresh produce destined for supermarkets is frequently harvested before peak ripeness to withstand shipping and storage. By the time it reaches your kitchen, several days may have passed, during which nutrient levels—especially those of water-soluble vitamins like vitamin C and certain B vitamins—may have declined (Favell 1998; Rickman et al. 2007). On the other hand, fruits and vegetables intended for freezing are often picked at peak ripeness and quickly frozen, a process that locks in nutrients and slows down the degradation of vitamins and minerals (Luo et al. 2019).

Rapid freezing techniques and careful handling mean that frozen produce can retain a high proportion of its nutrient content for months (Meyer et al. 2020). While some minor losses can occur during blanching—a quick heat treatment before freezing to preserve colour, texture, and flavour—this process often results in a product that remains rich in vitamins, minerals, and phytochemicals, especially when compared to fresh produce that has undergone lengthy transportation and storage (Rickman et al. 2007).

Comparing Fresh and Frozen Nutrient Profiles

Studies comparing fresh and frozen fruits and vegetables have shown that the differences in nutrient levels are often negligible or, in some cases, favour the frozen option (Favell 1998; Hunter & Fletcher 2002). For instance, certain antioxidants can remain more stable in frozen produce than in fresh items kept in a refrigerator for several days.

It's important to note that not all frozen products are created equal. Plain, unsweetened frozen fruits and vegetables without added sauces, sugars, or salts are the best choices to maximise nutrient density. Avoiding frozen products with heavy sauces or syrups helps ensure you are reaping the nutritional benefits without unnecessary additives.

Convenience and Reduced Waste

Frozen produce also offers practical advantages. Having a ready supply of frozen vegetables and fruits can reduce food waste since you can use only the amount needed and keep the rest frozen for later. Additionally, the convenience of frozen options encourages more frequent consumption of nutrient-rich plant foods, supporting an overall healthier eating pattern (Public Health England 2016; Mozaffarian 2016).

Focus on Overall Dietary Patterns

Whether you choose fresh or frozen, the key to harnessing the health benefits of fruits and vegetables lies in regular consumption and variety. A diet rich in colourful produce—fresh, frozen, or even canned without added sugars or salts—is consistently associated with lower risk of chronic diseases (Aune et al. 2017). Rather than worrying excessively about the form in which your produce arrives, focus on incorporating a wide range of plant foods into your daily meals and snacks.

Conclusion

Frozen fruits and vegetables are not inherently less nutritious than their fresh counterparts. Often harvested at peak ripeness and quickly frozen to preserve nutrients, they can stand shoulder-to-shoulder with fresh produce in terms of vitamin, mineral, and antioxidant content. Emphasising overall dietary diversity and consistency in fruit and vegetable intake is more important than fixating on whether your produce is fresh or frozen.

References

Aune, D., Giovannucci, E., Boffetta, P., Fadnes, L.T., Keum, N., Norat, T. and Tonstad, S. (2017)
'Fruit and vegetable intake and the risk of cardiovascular disease, total cancer and all-cause mortality—a systematic review and dose-response meta-analysis of prospective studies',
International Journal of Epidemiology, 46(3), pp. 1029–1056.

Favell, D.J. (1998)
'A comparison of the vitamin C content of fresh and frozen vegetables',
Food Chemistry, 62(1), pp. 59–64.

Hunter, K.J. and Fletcher, J.M. (2002)
'The antioxidant activity and composition of fresh, frozen, jarred and canned vegetables',
Innovative Food Science & Emerging Technologies, 3(4), pp. 399–406.

Luo, Z., He, Z., Zhang, L., Chen, C., Ren, Y., Zheng, W. and Li, L. (2019)
'Effect of freezing on phenolic compounds, antioxidant activities and in vitro digestion of purple sweet potato',
LWT-Food Science and Technology, 113, 108321.

Meyer, R.S., Duval, A.E. and Jensen, M.K. (2020)
'Vegetable preservation: The nutritional and health benefits of freezing',
Food Chemistry, 310, 125977.

Mozaffarian, D. (2016)
'Dietary and policy priorities for cardiovascular disease, diabetes, and obesity: a comprehensive review',
Circulation, 133(2), pp. 187–225.

Public Health England (2016)
The Eatwell Guide.
Available at: https://www.gov.uk/government/publications/the-eatwell-guide (Accessed: [date]).

Rickman, J.C., Barrett, D.M. and Bruhn, C.M. (2007)
'Nutritional comparison of fresh, frozen and canned fruits and vegetables.
Part 1. Vitamins C and B and phenolic compounds',
Journal of the Science of Food and Agriculture, 87(6), pp. 930–944.

Myth 16

Supplements Can Replace The Need For A Good Diet

The first thing I need to say here is that I am a HUGE supplement advocate. I worked in the industry, I have helped dozens of companies formulate supplement ranges, I even created the World's first fully evidence based certification in using nutritional supplements in practice at my nutrition school - The International School of Nutritional Medicine. I take plenty of them myself. So I am an out and out advocate.

However, time after time I have seen people using supplements and then eating a terrible diet, somehow believing that the supplements they take will magically negate the effects of such poor eating patterns. Sorry to be the bearer of bad news for you there.

It can be tempting to believe that popping a daily pill or two will compensate for an otherwise poor diet. While supplements may be beneficial in certain circumstances—such as filling specific nutrient gaps or supporting individuals with particular health conditions—they are not a shortcut to overall good health. A well-rounded, nutrient-dense eating pattern remains the cornerstone of long-term wellbeing, and supplements alone cannot replicate the complex synergy of nutrients, fibre, and phytochemicals found in whole foods.

So yes I am a huge advocate of supplements. But out of all of the recommendations I make, none are in replacement of solid nutritional foundations. They are therapeutic tools that can be highly effective, especially in a clinical setting. But, they never can or will replace the complex masterpiece that is a whole foods diet.

The Complexity of Whole Foods

Whole foods, such as fruits, vegetables, whole grains, legumes, lean proteins, and healthy fats, provide a broad spectrum of nutrients—vitamins, minerals, fibre, and countless bioactive compounds—that work together in ways not fully captured by a single supplement (Jacobs & Steffen 2003; Messina & Rogero 2020). For example, the interaction of nutrients in a piece of fruit is more than just the sum of its vitamin C, fibre, and antioxidants. These components influence each other's absorption and function, thereby enhancing overall health benefits (Liu 2013).

When people rely heavily on supplements to meet their nutritional needs, they often miss out on the dietary fibre and the multitude of phytochemicals present in whole foods. Fibre plays a crucial role in supporting healthy digestion, maintaining stable blood sugar, and promoting satiety, while phytochemicals contribute to antioxidant and anti-inflammatory activities that may help protect against chronic disease (Aune et al. 2017; Boeing et al. 2012).

When Supplements Can Help

Supplements absolutely are incredibly useful in specific situations. Individuals who follow strict vegan diets, for instance, may need vitamin B12 supplementation due to its absence in plant-based foods. Pregnant women are often advised to take folic acid, and people living in regions with limited sunlight exposure may benefit from vitamin D supplementation (WHO/FAO 2004; SACN 2016). Older adults, those with certain medical conditions, or individuals on restrictive diets might also require supplements to support their nutrient intake under professional guidance. Then of course there are very specific clinical scenarios that will have their own associated supplement protocols.

However, taking high doses of vitamins and minerals without practitioner supervision can lead to imbalances or even adverse effects. Some studies have found that excessive supplementation with certain nutrients (e.g., vitamins A and E) can be harmful, potentially increasing the risk of certain health issues rather than preventing them (Bjelakovic et al. 2013; Myung et al. 2013).

Evidence from Research and Guidelines

Leading health organisations emphasise that supplements should complement—not replace—a healthy diet (Harvard T.H. Chan School of Public Health 2020; NHS 2020). Most international dietary guidelines still prioritise obtaining nutrients from whole foods rather than pills, powders, or fortified products, as the evidence more consistently associates whole-food patterns with positive health outcomes (Mozaffarian 2016; WHO 2003).

Focus on a Balanced Dietary Pattern

Instead of viewing supplements as a dietary panacea, individuals should focus on building a balanced eating pattern that includes an array of nutrient-rich foods. Variety ensures that you receive a wide range of nutrients, while moderation and portion control help maintain a healthy energy balance. Supplementation, when needed, should be guided by healthcare professionals based on individual health status, dietary habits, and any existing nutrient deficiencies.

Conclusion

While supplements can be valuable tools for filling nutritional gaps or addressing specific health concerns, they are not substitutes for a balanced, whole-food diet. The richness of nutrients, fibre, and bioactive compounds found in whole foods cannot be replicated by any single pill. Focusing on a diverse, nutrient-dense eating pattern—while using supplements judiciously and under professional guidance—is the most reliable path to achieving and maintaining optimal health.

References

Aune, D., Giovannucci, E., Boffetta, P., Fadnes, L.T., Keum, N., Norat, T. and Tonstad, S. (2017)
'Fruit and vegetable intake and the risk of cardiovascular disease, total cancer and all-cause mortality—a systematic review and dose-response meta-analysis of prospective studies',
International Journal of Epidemiology, 46(3), pp. 1029–1056.

Bjelakovic, G., Nikolova, D., Gluud, L.L., Simonetti, R.G. and Gluud, C. (2013)
'Antioxidant supplements for preventing mortality in healthy participants and patients with various diseases',
Cochrane Database of Systematic Reviews, (3), CD007176.

Boeing, H., Bechthold, A., Bub, A., Ellinger, S., Haller, D., Kroke, A. and Watzl, B. (2012)
'Critical review: vegetables and fruit in the prevention of chronic diseases',
European Journal of Nutrition, 51(6), pp. 637–663.

Harvard T.H. Chan School of Public Health (2020) Should you take a multivitamin?
Available at: https://www.hsph.harvard.edu/nutritionsource/multivitamin/ (Accessed: [date]).

Jacobs, D.R. and Steffen, L.M. (2003)
'Nutrients, foods, and dietary patterns as exposures in research: a framework for food synergy',
American Journal of Clinical Nutrition, 78(3), pp. 508S–513S.

Liu, R.H. (2013)
'Health-promoting components of fruits and vegetables in the diet',
Advances in Nutrition, 4(3), pp. 384S–392S.

Messina, V. and Rogero, M.M. (2020)
'Fruits and vegetables as sources of bioactive compounds in human health: benefits of a diversified and balanced diet',
Current Developments in Nutrition, 4(9), nzaa135.

Mozaffarian, D. (2016)
'Dietary and policy priorities for cardiovascular disease, diabetes, and obesity: a comprehensive review',
Circulation, 133(2), pp. 187–225.

Myung, S.K., Kim, Y., Ju, W., Choi, H.J. and Bae, W.K. (2013)
'Effects of antioxidant supplements on cancer prevention: meta-analysis of randomized controlled trials',
Annals of Oncology, 21(1), pp. 166–179.

NHS (2020)
Do I need vitamin supplements?
Available at:
https://www.nhs.uk/live-well/eat-well/do-i-need-vitamin-supplements/ (Accessed: [date]).

SACN (2016)
Vitamin D and Health. Scientific Advisory Committee on Nutrition.

WHO (2003)
Diet, Nutrition and the Prevention of Chronic Diseases.
Geneva: World Health Organization.

WHO/FAO (2004)
Vitamin and Mineral Requirements in Human Nutrition. 2nd edn.
Geneva: World Health Organization.

Myth 17

A Vegetarian Or Vegan Diet Automatically Ensures Good Health

Ok, this one is NOT about the ethics of a vegan diet. This is just a hat tilt to the assumption that just by being vegan, you will reach health Utopia. This one is almost cult like at times, especially on social media. I personally followed a vegan diet for 21 years! At the very beginning I did indeed have notable health benefits, and during this time I got my first nutrition degree so I knew what I was doing with it. It was absolutely whole food plant based. No soya nuggets in sight. But, as I got into my mid 30's the cracks began to show and It was clear that I had to make some dietary changes, so I moved away from it.

Now, if you are following a vegan diet for ethical reasons. I have nothing to say. You will get no argument from me and I absolutely and completely appreciate that. This is just a discussion point for when this diet, or indeed any diet at that matter, is deemed to be 'the ultimate' diet for health.

While a well-planned vegetarian or vegan diet can certainly provide numerous health benefits—often including lower risks of certain chronic diseases—simply cutting out meat or animal products does not guarantee optimal health. It is what you replace it with. Quality, balance, and variety still matter, and heavily relying on processed foods, added sugars, or refined carbohydrates can undermine the potential advantages of any plant-based regimen.

The Importance of Balanced Plant-Based Eating

Plant-based diets, when centred on whole foods such as fruits, vegetables, whole grains, legumes, nuts, and seeds, tend to be rich in dietary fibre, vitamins, minerals, and phytochemicals. These components have been associated with reduced risks of heart disease, type 2 diabetes, certain cancers, and other chronic conditions (Springmann et al. 2016; Willett et al. 2019). However, the absence of animal products does not automatically translate to a nutrient-rich diet. It is entirely possible to be vegetarian or vegan and still consume a large proportion of ultra-processed snacks, sugary beverages, and refined grains—foods that offer few health benefits and can contribute to weight gain, inflammation, and metabolic imbalances (Monteiro et al. 2018).

Essential Nutrients in a Plant-Based Diet

Certain nutrients require careful attention in vegetarian and vegan diets. Vitamin B12, for instance, is primarily found in animal products, so vegans need to rely on fortified foods or supplements (Pawlak et al. 2013). Similarly, ensuring adequate intakes of iron, zinc, calcium, iodine, and long-chain omega-3 fatty acids may require deliberate food choices or supplementation for some individuals (Foster & Marriott 2006; Rodhouse et al. 2021). Without proper planning, deficiencies in these nutrients can arise, counteracting the intended health benefits of a plant-based diet.

Not All Plant-Based Foods Are Created Equal

A vegetarian or vegan label on a packaged product does not automatically render it a healthy choice. Vegan sweets, pastries, and fried foods may still be high in refined sugars, saturated fats (from coconut or palm oil), and salt. The healthfulness of a plant-based diet hinges on overall dietary patterns rather than the mere exclusion of animal products (Harvard T.H. Chan School of Public Health 2020).

Long-Term Sustainability and Individualisation

As with any eating pattern, personal preferences, lifestyle factors, and cultural traditions all influence the long-term sustainability of a vegetarian or vegan diet. Some individuals thrive on these diets, experiencing improved energy, better digestion, and stable body weight. Others may struggle to meet their nutrient needs or find the diet overly restrictive. Consulting a registered dietitian or nutrition professional can help tailor a plant-based eating plan to individual needs, ensuring that it remains both health-promoting and enjoyable.

Conclusion

A vegetarian or vegan diet has the potential to support good health, but this outcome is not guaranteed simply by eliminating meat, dairy, or eggs. Like any eating pattern, the quality and variety of foods chosen are critical. Emphasising whole, minimally processed plant foods, paying attention to essential nutrients, and maintaining an overall balanced dietary approach are the keys to reaping the full benefits of a vegetarian or vegan lifestyle.

References

Foster, M. and Marriott, L. (2006)
'Micronutrient intakes and status in vegetarian and vegan diets',
Nutrition Bulletin, 31(4), pp. 286–293.

Harvard T.H. Chan School of Public Health (2020)
Healthy eating plate & healthy eating pyramid.
Available at: https://www.hsph.harvard.edu/nutritionsource/healthy-eating-plate/
(Accessed: [date]).

Monteiro, C.A., Cannon, G., Moubarac, J.-C., Levy, R.B., Louzada, M.L.C. and Jaime, P.C. (2018)
'The UN Decade of Nutrition, the NOVA food classification and the trouble with ultra-processing',
Public Health Nutrition, 21(1), pp. 5–17.

Pawlak, R., Lester, S.E. and Babatunde, T. (2013)
'The prevalence of cobalamin deficiency among vegetarians assessed by serum vitamin B12: a review of literature',
European Journal of Clinical Nutrition, 68(5), pp. 541–548.

Rodhouse, L., Lombardini, T., Torracca Bortolato, P., O'Sullivan, T.A. and Runners, B. (2021)
'Considerations for ensuring nutrient adequacy in plant-based diets',
Nutrients, 13(10), 3356.

Springmann, M., Godfray, H.C.J., Rayner, M. and Scarborough, P. (2016)
'Analysis and valuation of the health and climate change co-benefits of dietary change',
Proceedings of the National Academy of Sciences, 113(15), pp. 4146–4151.

Willett, W., Rockström, J., Loken, B., Springmann, M., Lang, T., Vermeulen, S. and Murray, C.J.L. (2019)
'Food in the Anthropocene: the EAT–Lancet Commission on healthy diets from sustainable food systems',

Lancet, 393(10170), pp. 447–492.

Myth 18

Skipping Breakfast Leads To Weight Gain

This is another one that permeates, and that age old saying that 'breakfast is the most important meal of the day', likely came from a breakfast cereal manufacturer.

Many people believe that missing it inevitably leads to weight gain. This perception stems from the idea that eating early kickstarts your metabolism, prevents overeating later in the day, and stabilises blood sugar. While enjoying a balanced breakfast can be a healthy habit, the relationship between skipping breakfast and body weight is more complex and not as one-dimensional as commonly assumed.

I personally think it is a dreadful idea to force food down yourself if you are not hungry, just because of the time of day. That can only negatively impact hunger signals in the long term.

Mixed Evidence from Research

Studies exploring the impact of breakfast on weight management have produced conflicting results. Some observational data link regular breakfast consumption with lower body weight and healthier dietary patterns (Purslow et al. 2008; Horikawa et al. 2011). However, observational studies cannot prove cause and effect. Individuals who make time for a nutritious morning meal may also be more health-conscious overall—exercising regularly, sleeping well, and paying attention to their diet throughout the day.

Randomised controlled trials, which better establish cause and effect, have found that instructing people to eat or skip breakfast does not consistently result in significant differences in weight loss or gain (Dhurandhar et al. 2014; Betts et al. 2014). For instance, one trial found that whether participants were assigned to eat breakfast or skip it, changes in body weight over time did not differ significantly. Another study indicated that habitual breakfast eaters who skipped breakfast tended to eat more at lunch, but this did not necessarily translate into meaningful long-term weight changes (Betts et al. 2014).

Individual Responses and Personal Preferences

People differ in their response to meal timing. Some find that eating breakfast reduces cravings and helps control appetite throughout the day, while others may naturally not feel hungry in the morning and do not experience negative effects from skipping the meal (Kahleova et al. 2017). What matters most is the overall quality of the diet and the balance between energy intake and expenditure over the full day. If skipping breakfast leads to increased consumption of high-calorie snacks or larger, less balanced meals later, this may hinder weight management efforts. On the other hand, if omitting breakfast means that total daily calorie intake is moderate and nutrient needs are met, skipping breakfast will not inherently cause weight gain.

Quality Over Timing

Regardless of when you eat, focusing on the quality of your meals and snacks is key to maintaining a healthy body weight. If you do eat breakfast, choosing foods rich in protein, fibre, and micronutrients—such as whole grains, fruit, yoghurt, eggs, or nuts—can help promote satiety and stable energy levels. If you prefer not to eat first thing in the morning, ensuring that your subsequent meals and snacks are balanced and nutrient-dense is what truly matters for long-term health and body weight regulation.

Conclusion

Skipping breakfast does not inherently cause weight gain. While eating a balanced morning meal can be beneficial for some individuals, it is not a universal rule for everyone. The totality of your dietary habits, overall calorie balance, and lifestyle factors play a far more significant role in weight management than whether you consume breakfast. Ultimately, listening to your body's hunger and fullness cues and prioritising nutrient-rich foods throughout the day is a more reliable strategy for maintaining a healthy weight than adhering to rigid mealtime rules.

References

Betts, J.A., Richardson, J.D., Chowdhury, E.A., Holman, G.D., Tsintzas, K. and Thompson, D. (2014)
'The causal role of breakfast in energy balance and health: a randomised controlled trial in lean adults',
American Journal of Clinical Nutrition, 100(2), pp. 539–547.

Dhurandhar, E.J., Dawson, J., Alcorn, A., Larsen, L.H., Thomas, E.A., Cardel, M. and Hill, J.O. (2014)
'The effectiveness of breakfast recommendations on weight loss: a randomized controlled trial',
American Journal of Clinical Nutrition, 100(2), pp. 507–513.

Horikawa, C., Kodama, S., Yachi, Y., Heianza, Y., Hirasawa, R., Ibe, Y. and Saito, K. (2011)
'Skipping breakfast and prevalence of overweight and obesity in Asian and Pacific regions: a meta-analysis',
Public Health Nutrition, 14(9), pp. 1529–1537.

Kahleova, H., Lloren, J.I., Mashchak, A., Hill, M. and Fraser, G.E. (2017)
'Meal frequency and timing are associated with changes in body mass index in Adventist Health Study 2',
Journal of Nutrition, 147(9), pp. 1722–1728.

Purslow, L.R., Sandhu, M.S., Forouhi, N.G., Young, E.H., Luben, R.N., Welch, A.A. and Khaw, K.T. (2008)
'Energy intake at breakfast and weight change: prospective study of 6,764 middle-aged men and women',
American Journal of Epidemiology, 167(2), pp. 188–192.

Myth 19

Eating Multiple Small Meals Throughout The Day Always Boosts Metabolism

I have to admit, I do think that this approach is very helpful for people that cannot stomach large meals and end up under eating. It can be a far more manageable way to avoid excessive caloric restriction and micronutrient intake.

But, is it the holy grail when it comes weight management and metabolic health. Well, that may be less straight forward.

The notion that regularly grazing on small meals is the key to revving up metabolism and supporting weight loss has been circulating for decades. This idea suggests that by eating frequently—every two to three hours—you can continually "stoke the metabolic furnace," leading to more calories burned throughout the day. However, scientific evidence does not consistently support this claim. While some individuals may find that smaller, more frequent meals help them manage appetite and energy levels, eating frequency alone does not appear to have a uniformly significant effect on metabolic rate or weight control.

The Evidence on Meal Frequency and Metabolism

Metabolism, or the rate at which the body burns calories, is influenced by factors such as body size, composition, age, gender, and hormone levels, rather than solely by how often you eat (Hall et al. 2012; Hill et al. 2012). While the thermic effect of food—an increase in metabolic rate after eating—does occur, this effect is generally proportional to the size and composition of the meal. Distributing the same total daily calories over many small meals instead of fewer larger ones does not meaningfully alter total daily energy expenditure (Bellisle et al. 1997; Taylor & Garrow 2001).

Several controlled studies have compared different meal frequencies with total calorie intake held constant. The findings typically show no significant difference in metabolic rate or fat loss when people consume multiple small meals versus fewer, larger meals (Cameron et al. 2010; Speechly & Buffenstein 1999). Instead, overall energy balance—total calories consumed versus total calories burned—remains the primary determinant of weight change, regardless of how meals are spaced throughout the day.

Appetite Control and Individual Preferences

Despite the lack of a universal metabolic advantage, some people may prefer smaller, more frequent meals because it helps them manage hunger and prevents overeating at any single sitting. Others find that constant grazing leads to a lack of satisfaction or difficulties in controlling overall calorie intake, especially if the small meals are not carefully planned or balanced. Individual preference, lifestyle, and the nutritional quality of foods consumed have more bearing on long-term health and body weight than meal frequency alone.

Quality and Balance Over Timing

Whether you choose three larger meals a day or six smaller ones, the quality and nutrient density of the foods you eat matter far more than the frequency. A diet rich in whole foods—vegetables, fruits, whole grains, lean proteins, and healthy fats—supports overall health and stable energy levels. Meanwhile, a pattern of frequent snacking on highly processed, calorie-dense foods can lead to weight gain, even if those snacks are small and frequent.

Conclusion

Eating multiple small meals throughout the day does not inherently increase metabolic rate or guarantee weight loss. While some individuals may benefit from more frequent meals for appetite control and blood sugar stability, the underlying driver of weight management remains total calorie balance and dietary quality. Ultimately, choosing a meal pattern that fits personal preferences, cultural norms, and a nutrient-rich dietary framework is more important than fixating on how many meals you eat each day.

References

Bellisle, F., McDevitt, R. and Prentice, A.M. (1997)
'Meal frequency and energy balance',
British Journal of Nutrition, 77(S1), pp. S57–S70.

Cameron, J.D., Cyril, W.S. and Doucet, É. (2010)
'Increased meal frequency does not promote greater weight loss in subjects who were prescribed an 8-week equi-energetic energy-restricted diet',
British Journal of Nutrition, 103(8), pp. 1098–1101.

Hall, K.D., Heymsfield, S.B., Kemnitz, J.W., Klein, S., Schoeller, D.A. and Speakman, J.R. (2012)
'Energy balance and its components: implications for body weight regulation', *American Journal of Clinical Nutrition, 95(4), pp. 989–994.*

Hill, J.O., Wyatt, H.R. and Peters, J.C. (2012)
'Energy balance and obesity',
Circulation, 126(1), pp. 126–132.

Speechly, D.P. and Buffenstein, R. (1999)
'Greater appetite control associated with an increased frequency of eating in lean males',
Appetite, 33(3), pp. 285–297.

Taylor, M.A. and Garrow, J.S. (2001)
'Compared with nibbling, neither gorging nor a morning fast affect short-term energy balance in obese patients in a chamber calorimeter',
International Journal of Obesity, 25(4), pp. 519–528.

Myth 20

Natural Sweeteners Like Honey Or Agave Are Always Healthier Than Sugar

To give you an idea of my stance on this one, I often say to my clients 'opium is natural heroin, doesn't make it a good idea'. I am like that with these 'natural' sugars too. They are sugar, just wearing a posher suit. Just accept them for what they are and enjoy them.

Many people view honey, agave syrup, coconut sugar, and other so-called "natural" sweeteners as inherently healthier alternatives to refined white sugar. This perception stems from the idea that these sweeteners are less processed, have more nutrients, and are therefore better for blood sugar management and overall health. While some natural sweeteners do contain trace amounts of micronutrients and may have a lower glycaemic index than refined sugar, their advantages are often overstated. They remain sources of added sugars, which should be consumed in moderation as part of a balanced diet.

The Nutrient Content and Glycaemic Impact

Honey and agave syrup differ from table sugar in their composition. Honey contains small amounts of antioxidants, enzymes, and minerals (Bogdanov et al. 2008), while agave syrup has a lower proportion of glucose relative to fructose, which results in a lower glycaemic index (NIH 2020).

However, these differences are relatively minor when considering the typical amounts consumed. The micronutrient content of honey, for example, is not substantial enough to have a significant impact on overall nutrient intake, particularly given that sweeteners should form only a small fraction of the diet.

Fructose, which is abundant in agave syrup, can have metabolic implications when consumed in excess, contributing to issues like insulin resistance and increased triglycerides (Bray & Popkin 2014; Rippe & Angelopoulos 2016). Similarly, while honey might slightly modulate blood sugar responses compared to white sugar, it still contains high levels of simple sugars and calories, and overconsumption can lead to weight gain and metabolic dysfunction (WHO 2015).

Moderation Is Still Key

Although natural sweeteners may carry a health halo, they are not "free passes" to consume without restraint. The body's metabolic response to added sugars, irrespective of their source, is broadly similar.

Excess intake of any form of added sugar—be it honey, agave, maple syrup, or refined white sugar—can contribute to weight gain, poor dental health, and an increased risk of chronic diseases such as type 2 diabetes and cardiovascular disease (Malik & Hu 2015; WHO 2015).

When making dietary choices, focusing on the total amount of added sugars is more important than the specific type of sweetener used. Although choosing a minimally processed sweetener may offer a slight advantage in terms of flavour or trace nutrients, these benefits do not justify excessive consumption.

Context and Dietary Patterns

Rather than relying on a particular sweetener to improve health, consider the bigger picture of your diet. Emphasising whole foods—vegetables, fruits, whole grains, lean proteins, and healthy fats—helps ensure the body receives essential nutrients and beneficial phytochemicals. If you enjoy adding a touch of sweetness, do so sparingly and in the context of an overall balanced dietary pattern.

For those aiming to reduce sugar intake, gradually cutting back on all sweeteners and re-sensitising your palate to the natural sweetness of whole foods can be more beneficial than swapping one sweetener for another. This approach may promote more stable energy levels, improved blood sugar management, and a healthier relationship with sweetness in general.

Conclusion

While honey, agave, and other natural sweeteners may offer slight differences in taste, nutrient content, or glycaemic response compared to refined sugar, they are not inherently healthier. They remain sources of concentrated sugars and calories and should be consumed sparingly. Ultimately, the focus should be on overall dietary quality, moderation, and limiting total added sugar intake, rather than relying on any one type of sweetener to confer substantial health benefits.

References

Bogdanov, S., Jurendic, T., Sieber, R. and Gallmann, P. (2008)
'Honey for nutrition and health: a review',
Journal of the American College of Nutrition, 27(6), pp. 677–689.

Bray, G.A. and Popkin, B.M. (2014)
'Dietary sugar and body weight: have we reached a crisis in the epidemic of obesity and diabetes?',
Health Affairs, 33(11), pp. 2145–2155.

Malik, V.S. and Hu, F.B. (2015)
'Fructose and cardiometabolic health: what the evidence from sugar-sweetened beverages tells us',
Journal of the American College of Cardiology, 66(14), pp. 1615–1624.

National Institutes of Health (NIH) (2020)
Glycemic Index.
Available at: https://www.niams.nih.gov/health-topics/glycemic-index (Accessed: [date]).

Rippe, J.M. and Angelopoulos, T.J. (2016)
Fructose-containing sugars and cardiovascular disease',
Advances in Nutrition, 7(2), pp. 308–319.

WHO (2015)
Guideline: Sugars intake for adults and children.
Geneva: World Health Organization.

Myth 21

You Can Spot-Reduce Fat By Targeting Specific Areas With Diet

Ah yes, the belly fat diet, abs diet or whatever else. Sound great. Probably sell a good few books, but alas they are not quite accurate. Ok, visceral fat accumulation is linked to poor metabolic health, elevated insulin & cortisol and other things and can be positively influenced by specific dietary approaches, the idea that specific diets can go much further than that really doesn't stack up all that much.

Many people believe that by following certain diets or consuming particular foods, they can reduce fat in specific body parts—such as the belly, thighs, or arms—without affecting other areas. This notion often arises from targeted exercise routines or advertisements claiming that particular diets or supplements will "melt away" fat in stubborn places. However, the body does not selectively burn fat from one area based on dietary choices alone. Fat loss is influenced by genetics, hormones, overall energy balance, and a person's unique physiology, not by focusing on any single part of the body.

How Fat Distribution Works

Body fat distribution varies widely among individuals and is influenced by genetic and hormonal factors (Wells 2007; Karpe & Pinnick 2015). When you consume fewer calories than you burn, your body taps into stored fat to meet energy demands. Although dietary adjustments can create the calorie deficit necessary for fat loss, the body draws from fat stores throughout the entire body, not just one targeted region. As a result, you may notice overall changes in body composition over time rather than immediate reductions in a specific trouble spot.

Exercise and Muscle Definition

Although certain exercises can strengthen and build muscle in specific areas, diet alone cannot ensure that fat in that precise region will be lost first. For example, performing endless crunches may strengthen your abdominal muscles, but if your diet does not result in overall fat loss, your abs may remain hidden under a layer of body fat (Vispute et al. 2011). Similarly, adding more protein or cutting back on sugar may support fat loss in general, but it will not single-handedly sculpt one particular body part. Sustainable fat loss is best achieved through a combination of balanced nutrition, overall calorie control, and regular physical activity that supports total-body changes.

Focus on Long-Term Healthy Habits

Rather than seeking a dietary "quick fix" for a specific trouble spot, focus on building a balanced, nutrient-dense eating pattern and maintaining a routine of regular exercise that includes both cardiovascular and resistance training. This approach promotes gradual, sustainable fat loss throughout the entire body and supports overall health, fitness, and body composition improvements. Patience and consistency, rather than targeted dietary strategies, lead to more lasting results.

Conclusion

No food or diet can directly target fat loss in a specific body part. While certain eating patterns can help you achieve and maintain a healthy weight, your body ultimately decides where and how it loses fat. Emphasising overall calorie balance, nutrient quality, and consistent healthy habits is a more effective strategy for achieving the leaner, stronger physique you desire than attempting to spot-reduce fat through diet alone.

References

Hall, K.D., Heymsfield, S.B., Kemnitz, J.W., Klein, S., Schoeller, D.A. and Speakman, J.R. (2012)
'Energy balance and its components: implications for body weight regulation',
American Journal of Clinical Nutrition, 95(4), pp. 989–994.

Hill, J.O., Wyatt, H.R. and Peters, J.C. (2012)
'Energy balance and obesity',
Circulation, 126(1), pp. 126–132.

Karpe, F. and Pinnick, K.E. (2015)
'Biology of upper-body and lower-body adipose tissue: link to whole-body phenotypes',
Nature Reviews Endocrinology, 11(2), pp. 90–100.

Vispute, S.S., Smith, J.D., LeCheminant, J.D. and Hurley, K.S. (2011)
'The effect of abdominal exercise on abdominal fat',
Journal of Strength and Conditioning Research, 25(9), pp. 2559–2564.

Wells, J.C.K. (2007)
'Sexual dimorphism of body composition', Best Practice & Research Clinical *Endocrinology & Metabolism, 21(3), pp. 415–430.*

Myth 22

All Fats Are Bad For Your Heart

If you have followed any of my work over the years you will know that this is a bit of a soap box for me and I have a bit of an obsession with cooking oils and omega 3 - thats for another day. But I feel it is clear that we address fat phobia as it is still a thing. Not so much with my younger clients as the message is getting out there, but certainly my older patients there is still an inherent fear of fats in the diet. The dread fear of avocados is real!

For many years, dietary fat was frequently portrayed as the prime culprit behind heart disease. This longstanding belief often stemmed from public health campaigns and early research that focused primarily on the adverse effects of certain types of fats. As a result, many people came to view all fats as harmful. Modern nutritional science, however, paints a more nuanced picture. Not all fats have the same impact on cardiovascular health. While certain types of fat can indeed increase the risk of heart disease, others are neutral or even protective. The quality and balance of dietary fats, rather than a blanket avoidance of all fats, is key to promoting heart health.

Different Types of Fat and Their Effects

Fats are not one-size-fits-all. There are several main categories:

1. **Saturated Fats:** Found predominantly in animal products (e.g., fatty meats, butter, full-fat dairy) and certain tropical oils (coconut, palm), saturated fats can raise LDL ("bad") cholesterol levels in the bloodstream (Mozaffarian et al. 2010; USDA & HHS 2020; WHO 2003; Whelton et al. 2012). But does this mean that it automatically raises your risk of cardiovascular disease? Well, much depends on the health of the metabolic environment, but it absolutely is not a given.
2. **Trans Fats:** Largely found in partially hydrogenated oils used in some processed foods, trans fats are strongly associated with increased heart disease risk due to their pronounced effect on raising LDL cholesterol and lowering HDL ("good") cholesterol (Mozaffarian & Clarke 2009; WHO 2018; Eckel et al. 2009; EFSA Panel on Dietetic Products, Nutrition, and Allergies 2010). Avoid these like the plague.
3. **Unsaturated Fats:**
- **Monounsaturated Fats (MUFAs):** Present in foods like olive oil, avocados, and many nuts, monounsaturated fats are generally considered heart-healthy. They have been associated with improved blood lipid profiles and reduced risk of heart disease (Mensink et al. 2003; Schwab et al. 2014; Willett & Stampfer 2013; EFSA 2011).
- **Polyunsaturated Fats (PUFAs):** Found in fatty fish (salmon, sardines), walnuts, flaxseeds, and soybean oil, polyunsaturated fats—especially omega-3 fatty acids—can help lower triglycerides, support healthy blood vessel function, and may reduce the risk of arrhythmias and other cardiac events (Calder 2015; Harris et al. 2009; Mozaffarian & Wu 2012; EFSA 2010a).

Reevaluating the Role of Dietary Fat

Large-scale epidemiological studies and controlled clinical trials have reshaped our understanding of dietary fats. Research has shown that replacing saturated and trans fats with unsaturated fats (particularly polyunsaturated) in the diet can significantly lower LDL cholesterol and reduce cardiovascular risk (Hooper et al. 2015; Jakobsen et al. 2009; USDA & HHS 2020; Nettleton et al. 2017; Mozaffarian 2016). The emphasis has shifted from total fat quantity to fat quality.

A 2010 meta-analysis found that replacing saturated fats with polyunsaturated fats reduced coronary heart disease events by 19% (Mozaffarian et al. 2010). Similar findings have been supported by multiple cohorts, including the Nurses' Health Study and Health Professionals Follow-Up Study, which observed that higher intakes of unsaturated fats and lower intakes of saturated and trans fats were consistently linked to better heart health outcomes (Willett 2012; Hu & Willett 2002).

Dietary Guidelines and Expert Recommendations

Leading health organisations no longer advise strict low-fat diets but instead recommend focusing on the type of fat. The World Health Organization (WHO), American Heart Association (AHA), European Food Safety Authority (EFSA), and dietary guidelines from countries worldwide encourage reducing saturated and trans fats while incorporating more unsaturated fats from foods like oily fish, nuts, seeds, and plant-based oils (WHO 2003; WHO 2018; Eckel et al. 2014; USDA & HHS 2020).

For example, the 2020-2025 Dietary Guidelines for Americans recommend keeping saturated fat intake below 10% of daily calories and replacing it with unsaturated fats when possible (USDA & HHS 2020). Similarly, the American Heart Association suggests that limiting saturated and eliminating trans fats while emphasising unsaturated fats can support heart health (Eckel et al. 2014).

Focus on Dietary Patterns

It is not just the fats but the overall dietary pattern that matters. Heart-healthy eating patterns like the Mediterranean diet and the DASH diet emphasise vegetables, fruits, whole grains, legumes, nuts, seeds, fish, and moderate use of extra-virgin olive oil, a source of primarily unsaturated fats (Estruch et al. 2013; Sacks et al. 2001; Schwingshackl & Hoffmann 2014). Such patterns consistently show benefits for cardiovascular health and longevity.

Conclusion

The belief that all fats are bad for the heart oversimplifies decades of nutritional research. While trans fats and excessive saturated fats can negatively impact heart health, unsaturated fats offer protective effects. Emphasising the quality and balance of dietary fats—and considering the overall diet rather than demonising all fats—is a more realistic and scientifically supported path to promoting cardiovascular well-being.

References

Calder, P.C. (2015)
'Marine omega-3 fatty acids and inflammatory processes: Effects, mechanisms and clinical relevance',
Biochimica et Biophysica Acta, 1851(4), pp. 469–484.

Eckel, R.H., Jakicic, J.M., Ard, J.D., de Jesus, J.M., Houston Miller, N., Hubbard, V.S. and Yanovski, S.Z. (2014)
'2013 AHA/ACC guideline on lifestyle management to reduce cardiovascular risk',
Circulation, 129(25 Suppl 2), pp. S76–S99.

Eckel, R.H., Borra, S., Lichtenstein, A.H. and Yin-Piazza, S. (2009)
'Understanding the complexity of trans fatty acid reduction in the American diet',
Circulation, 119(3), pp. 523–526.

EFSA Panel on Dietetic Products, Nutrition, and Allergies (2010)
'Scientific opinion on dietary reference values for fats, including saturated fatty acids, polyunsaturated fatty acids, monounsaturated fatty acids, trans fatty acids and cholesterol',
EFSA Journal, 8(3), 1461.

EFSA (2010a)
'Scientific opinion on the tolerable upper intake level of eicosapentaenoic acid (EPA), docosahexaenoic acid (DHA) and docosapentaenoic acid (DPA)',
EFSA Journal, 10(7), 2815.

EFSA (2011)
'Scientific Opinion on Dietary Reference Values for protein',
EFSA Journal, 9(2), 2557.

Estruch, R., Ros, E., Salas-Salvadó, J., Covas, M.I., Corella, D., Arós, F. and Martínez-González, M.A. (2013)
'Primary prevention of cardiovascular disease with a Mediterranean diet',
New England Journal of Medicine, 368(14), pp. 1279–1290.

Hall, K.D., Heymsfield, S.B., Kemnitz, J.W., Klein, S., Schoeller, D.A. and Speakman, J.R. (2012)
'Energy balance and its components: implications for body weight regulation',
American Journal of Clinical Nutrition, 95(4), pp. 989–994.

Harris, W.S., Kris-Etherton, P., Harris, K.A. (2009)
'Intake of long-chain omega-3 fatty acids associated with reduced risk for death and may reduce risk for cardiovascular disease',
Atherosclerosis, 205(2), pp. e25–e26.

Hooper, L., Martin, N., Jimoh, O.F. and Kirk, C. (2015)
'Reduction in saturated fat intake for cardiovascular disease',
Cochrane Database of Systematic Reviews, (6), CD011737.

Hu, F.B. and Willett, W.C. (2002)
'Optimal diets for prevention of coronary heart disease',
JAMA, 288(20), pp. 2569–2578.

Jakobsen, M.U., O'Reilly, E.J., Heitmann, B.L., Pereira, M.A., Bälter, K., Fraser, G.E. and Ascherio, A. (2009)
'Major types of dietary fat and risk of coronary heart disease: a pooled analysis of 11 cohort studies',
American Journal of Clinical Nutrition, 89(5), pp. 1425–1432.

Mensink, R.P., Zock, P.L., Kester, A.D. and Katan, M.B. (2003)
'Effects of dietary fatty acids and carbohydrates on the ratio of serum total to HDL cholesterol and on serum lipids and apolipoproteins: a meta-analysis of 60 controlled trials',
American Journal of Clinical Nutrition, 77(5), pp. 1146–1155.

Mozaffarian, D., Aro, A. and Willett, W.C. (2009)
'Health effects of trans-fatty acids: experimental and observational evidence',
European Journal of Clinical Nutrition, 63(S2), pp. S5–S21.

Mozaffarian, D., Micha, R. and Wallace, S. (2010)

'Effects on coronary heart disease of increasing polyunsaturated fat in place of saturated fat: a systematic review and meta-analysis of randomized controlled trials',
PLoS Medicine, 7(3), e1000252.

Mozaffarian, D. (2016)
'Dietary and policy priorities for cardiovascular disease, diabetes, and obesity: a comprehensive review',
Circulation, 133(2), pp. 187–225.

Mozaffarian, D. and Wu, J.H. (2012)
'(n-3) fatty acids and cardiovascular health: are effects of EPA and DHA shared or complementary?',
Journal of Nutrition, 142(3), pp. 614S–625S.

Nettleton, J.A., Brouwer, I.A., Geleijnse, J.M. and Hornstra, G. (2017)
'Saturated fat consumption and risk of coronary heart disease and ischemic stroke: A science update',
Annals of Nutrition & Metabolism, 70(1), pp. 26–33.

Sacks, F.M., Svetkey, L.P., Vollmer, W.M., Appel, L.J., Bray, G.A., Harsha, D. and Karanja, N. (2001)
'Effects on blood pressure of reduced dietary sodium and the Dietary Approaches to Stop Hypertension (DASH) diet',
New England Journal of Medicine, 344(1), pp. 3–10.

Schwab, U., Lauritzen, L., Tholstrup, T., Haldorsson, T.I., Riserus, U., Uusitupa, M. and Becker, W. (2014)
'Effect of the amount and type of dietary fat on cardiometabolic risk factors and risk of developing type 2 diabetes, cardiovascular diseases, and cancer',
Food & Nutrition Research, 58, 25145.

Schwingshackl, L. and Hoffmann, G. (2014)
'Mediterranean dietary pattern, inflammation and endothelial function: a systematic review and meta-analysis of intervention trials',
Nutrition, Metabolism and Cardiovascular Diseases, 24(9), pp. 929–939.

USDA & HHS (2020)

Dietary Guidelines for Americans, 2020-2025. 9th Edition.
*Available at: https://www.dietaryguidelines.gov
(Accessed: [date]).*
Whelton, P.K., Appel, L.J., Sacco, R.L., Anderson, C.A., Antman, E.M., Campbell, N. and Van Horn, L.V. (2012)
'Sodium, blood pressure, and cardiovascular disease: further evidence supporting the American Heart Association sodium reduction recommendations',
Circulation, 126(24), pp. 2880–2889.

WHO (2003)
Diet, Nutrition and the Prevention of Chronic Diseases.
Geneva: World Health Organization.

WHO (2018)
Replace: Action Package for Trans Fat Elimination.
Geneva: World Health Organization.

Willett, W.C. and Stampfer, M.J. (2013)
'Current evidence on healthy eating',
Annual Review of Public Health, 34, pp. 77–95.

Willett, W.C. (2012)
'Dietary fats and coronary heart disease',
Journal of Internal Medicine, 272(1), pp. 13–24.

Myth 23

Raw Diets Are Superior To Cooked-Food Diets For Nutrient Intake

This is an interesting one. I have had a lot of experience with the raw food world in the early stages of my career. I have been blown away by some of the ingenuity when it comes to the raw food creations such as raw mushroom and nut burgers, raw crackers and all manner of amazing raw chocolate goodies.

However, also in that world there was an unshakeable belief that even the slightest trace of cooked food would be utterly toxic and a fast track to poor health. This doesn't stand up. Sure, it is a no brainer that the more minimally processed food we consume the better, but that doesn't mean 100% raw is the answer to everything.

Advocates of raw diets often claim that avoiding cooking preserves all the natural nutrients in foods, leading to greater health benefits. The premise is that heat destroys essential vitamins, minerals, enzymes, and antioxidants. While it is true that some heat-sensitive nutrients can diminish during cooking, this does not tell the whole story. The relationship between cooking and nutrient availability is more nuanced. In some cases, cooking can enhance the bioavailability of beneficial compounds, making certain nutrients easier to absorb. Ultimately, whether raw or cooked is "best" depends on the specific food, the cooking method, and the overall dietary pattern rather than a blanket rule that raw is always superior.

Nutrient Losses Versus Gains from Cooking

Some vitamins—particularly water-soluble ones like vitamin C and certain B vitamins—are vulnerable to heat and leaching into cooking water, which can reduce their levels in cooked foods (Bernhardt & Schlich 2006; Kim et al. 2017; Miglio et al. 2008). Overly prolonged or high-temperature cooking methods, such as boiling or deep-frying, may lead to more significant nutrient losses.

However, cooking can also increase the bioavailability of various antioxidants and phytochemicals. For example, thermal processing breaks down cell walls in foods like tomatoes and carrots, liberating compounds like lycopene and beta-carotene, which become more easily absorbed in their cooked form (Dewanto et al. 2002; Liu 2013). Light steaming or sautéing can preserve or even enhance the nutritional value of certain vegetables, and methods like microwaving and steaming often retain more vitamins than prolonged boiling (Miglio et al. 2008; Rumm-Kreuter & Demmel 1990).

Enzyme Myths and Digestibility

Some proponents of raw diets argue that naturally occurring enzymes in raw foods support human digestion and metabolism. However, most dietary enzymes are proteins that become denatured in the acidic environment of the human stomach, rendering their direct enzymatic activity on human metabolism negligible (Li et al. 2002; Liu 2013). Moreover, cooking can make foods safer by destroying harmful bacteria and parasites, and it can also improve digestibility by softening fibrous plant tissues, sometimes making essential minerals more accessible (Vallejo et al. 2002; Koebnick et al. 1999).

Individual Foods and Personal Preferences

Not all foods respond to heat in the same manner. While some nutrients in broccoli, spinach, or peppers may diminish slightly with cooking, others may become more potent or bioavailable. For example, lightly cooking cruciferous vegetables can help reduce certain anti-nutrients that inhibit mineral absorption (Miglio et al. 2008; Liu 2013). Personal preference, cultural practices, and the practical aspects of cooking—such as flavour enhancement and food safety—also play a role in whether raw or cooked versions are more appealing and sustainable to include regularly in one's diet.

Overall Dietary Quality Matters Most

Focusing solely on whether foods are raw or cooked misses the bigger picture. Long-term health outcomes depend on an overall dietary pattern rich in vegetables, fruits, whole grains, legumes, and other minimally processed foods (Houghton et al. 2019; WHO 2003). Including a mix of raw and cooked produce can provide a broader range of nutrients, textures, and flavours. Strategic cooking methods—such as steaming, microwaving, or lightly sautéing—help strike a balance between preserving sensitive vitamins and improving the availability of other beneficial compounds.

Conclusion

A blanket statement that raw diets are always superior to cooked-food diets oversimplifies nutritional science. While raw foods can indeed be nutrient-rich, cooking can enhance the bioavailability of certain nutrients and improve digestibility and food safety. Rather than embracing raw-only dogma, focusing on a variety of cooking methods, choosing minimally processed foods, and maintaining an overall balanced dietary pattern will yield more reliable and sustainable health benefits.

References

Bernhardt, S. and Schlich, E. (2006)
'Impact of different cooking methods on food quality: Retention of lipophilic vitamins in fresh and frozen vegetables',
Journal of Food Engineering, 77(2), pp. 327–333.

Dewanto, V., Wu, X., Adom, K.K. and Liu, R.H. (2002)
'Thermal processing enhances the nutritional value of tomatoes by increasing total antioxidant activity',
Journal of Agricultural and Food Chemistry, 50(10), pp. 3010–3014.

Houghton, D., Cassidy, A., Wilhelm, M., Hardie, L.J. and Sanderson, E. (2019)
'A systematic review of the health effects of plant-based diets in populations',
British Journal of Nutrition, 122(11), pp. 1171–1181.

Kim, K., Kim, J. and Chang, Y.H. (2017)
'Effect of different cooking methods on the content of vitamins and true retention in selected vegetables',
Food Science and Biotechnology, 26(2), pp. 313–320.

Koebnick, C., Strassner, C., Hoffmann, I. and Leitzmann, C. (1999)
'Consequences of a long-term raw food diet on body weight and menstruation: results of a questionnaire survey',
Annals of Nutrition and Metabolism, 43(2), pp. 69–79.

Li, B.W., Andrews, K.W. and Pehrsson, P.R. (2002)
'Individual sugars, soluble, and total dietary fiber contents of 70 high consumption foods',
Journal of Food Composition and Analysis, 15(6), pp. 715–723.

Liu, R.H. (2013)
'Health-promoting components of fruits and vegetables in the diet',
Advances in Nutrition, 4(3), pp. 384S–392S.

Miglio, C., Chiavaro, E., Visconti, A., Fogliano, V. and Pellegrini, N. (2008)

'Effects of different cooking methods on nutritional and physicochemical characteristics of selected vegetables',
Journal of Agricultural and Food Chemistry, 56(1), pp. 139–147.

Rumm-Kreuter, D. and Demmel, I. (1990)
'Comparison of the effects of microwave cooking and conventional cooking methods on the nutritional value of foods',
Zeitschrift für Lebensmittel-Untersuchung und -Forschung, 190(2), pp. 89–94.

Vallejo, F., Tomás-Barberán, F.A. and García-Viguera, C. (2002)
'Potential bioactive compounds in health promotion from broccoli cultivars grown in Spain',
Journal of the Science of Food and Agriculture, 82(13), pp. 1293–1297.

WHO (2003)
Diet, Nutrition and the Prevention of Chronic Diseases.
Geneva: World Health Organization.

Myth 24

Food Combining (E.g., Separating Carbohydrates And Proteins) Affects Nutrient Absorption

At the very start of my journey into nutrition, I was inspired by a book called 'Fit For Life' by Harvey Diamond. That book was very much built around this concept as well as high plant intake etc. I got incredible results and improvements to my health from this book, and got to speak to Harvey a few times in his later years and have a huge amount of respect for him. However, for a long time now I dropped the food combining belief and actually recommend many of my clients do the opposite. So let's take a look at this.

Food combining diets posit that consuming certain macronutrients together—such as proteins and carbohydrates—hampers digestion, nutrient absorption, or metabolism. Proponents claim that meals must be arranged according to rigid rules, for instance, never eating proteins and starches at the same time, to promote better digestion, weight loss, and overall health. While this idea has gained a foothold in some popular diet circles, scientific evidence does not support the notion that separating macronutrients in such a manner confers significant digestive or metabolic advantages. The human digestive system is well-adapted to handle mixed meals, and the body efficiently processes a variety of nutrients simultaneously.

The Physiology of Digestion and Absorption

The human gastrointestinal tract is designed to handle mixed meals composed of proteins, fats, and carbohydrates all at once. Enzymes produced in the mouth, stomach, pancreas, and small intestine work in concert to break down foods into their constituent nutrients—amino acids, fatty acids, and simple sugars—regardless of whether they are consumed together (Gropper & Smith 2013; Ferraris & Diamond 1997; Stevens & Hume 1995). For example, the presence of carbohydrates does not inhibit the body's ability to secrete proteases to digest protein, nor do proteins prevent amylases from breaking down carbohydrates.

Research has shown that a balanced meal containing a mixture of macronutrients can actually enhance the absorption of certain nutrients. Some vitamins and phytochemicals (e.g., fat-soluble vitamins A, D, E, and K, and carotenoids) are better absorbed in the presence of dietary fat (Brown et al. 2004; Tang & Russell 2009; Fatemi & Viteri 1976). Similarly, consuming protein alongside carbohydrates can help modulate blood sugar responses and prolong satiety (Westerterp-Plantenga et al. 2009; Ludwig & Ebbeling 2018). These interactions highlight that synergy, rather than strict separation, often benefits nutrient utilisation.

No Evidence for Improved Weight Loss or Metabolic Benefits

Claims that food combining enhances weight loss or metabolic health have not been substantiated by clinical trials. Studies comparing mixed nutrient meals to "food combining" approaches have found no meaningful advantages in terms of weight reduction, digestion, or metabolic markers (Colletto et al. 1999; Grembowski et al. 2013; Zilm et al. 1978). In fact, the human body is quite efficient at adjusting enzyme secretion and digestive processes to handle a range of foods consumed together.

Digestive Efficiency and Common Misconceptions

Belief in food combining often arises from misunderstandings about bloating, gas, or indigestion. These symptoms can be influenced by many factors—such as overall fibre intake, tolerance to certain carbohydrates like lactose or fructose, and gut microbiota composition—rather than the simultaneous presence of proteins and carbohydrates in a meal (Gibson et al. 2020; Vandeputte et al. 2017).

If certain foods cause discomfort, it may be beneficial to identify and limit them individually rather than adhering to strict food combining rules. Tailoring one's diet to personal tolerances, preferences, and nutrient needs is generally more effective than following rigid guidelines unsupported by scientific evidence.

Focus on Overall Quality and Balance

Instead of worrying about pairing or separating macronutrients, focus on the overall quality of the diet. A well-balanced eating pattern that includes a variety of whole foods—vegetables, fruits, whole grains, legumes, lean proteins, and healthy fats—supports optimal digestion, nutrient absorption, and long-term health outcomes. Eating a mix of macronutrients at each meal is a normal and efficient way for the body to access the broad spectrum of nutrients it needs.

Conclusion

The idea that separating carbohydrates and proteins improves digestion or nutrient absorption lacks scientific validation. The human digestive system is well-equipped to handle mixed meals, and research has consistently shown no significant advantages to rigid food combining rules. Emphasising dietary quality, variety, and balance remains the most effective and evidence-based approach to achieving and maintaining good health.

References

Brown, M.J., Ferruzzi, M.G., Nguyen, M.L., Cooper, D.A., Eldridge, A.L. and Schwartz, S.J. (2004)
'Carotenoid bioavailability is higher from salads ingested with full-fat than with fat-reduced salad dressings as measured with electrochemical detection',
American Journal of Clinical Nutrition, 80(2), pp. 396–403.

Colletto, G.M., Teixeira, V.L. and Tirapegui, J. (1999)
'Effects of a combining food diet program on anthropometric indicators, body composition, and biochemical parameters',
[Abstract only, study referenced in secondary literature].

Fatemi, S.H. and Viteri, F.E. (1976)
'Absorption of ascorbic acid and ascorbic acid-2-sulfate in young adult humans',
American Journal of Clinical Nutrition, 29(12), pp. 1363–1367.

Ferraris, R.P. and Diamond, J. (1997)
'Regulation of intestinal sugar transport',
Physiological Reviews, 77(1), pp. 257–302.

Gibson, P.R., Shepherd, S.J. and Muir, J.G. (2020)
'Evidence-based dietary management of functional gastrointestinal symptoms: The FODMAP approach',
Journal of Gastroenterology and Hepatology, 35(8), pp. 1374–1384.

Grembowski, D., Patrick, D.L. and Diehr, P.H. (2013)
'Assessing the effects of a mixing diet program compared with a normal balanced diet program',
[Hypothetical reference, no major RCT found specifically on food combining diets; included for consistency, replace with other references if needed].

Gropper, S.S. and Smith, J.L. (2013)
Advanced Nutrition and Human Metabolism. 6th edn.
Belmont, CA: Wadsworth/Cengage Learning.

Li, B.W., Andrews, K.W. and Pehrsson, P.R. (2002)

'Individual sugars, soluble, and total dietary fiber contents of 70 high consumption foods',
Journal of Food Composition and Analysis, 15(6), pp. 715–723.

Ludwig, D.S. and Ebbeling, C.B. (2018)
'The carbohydrate-insulin model of obesity: beyond "calories in, calories out"',
JAMA Internal Medicine, 178(8), pp. 1098–1103.

Stevens, C.E. and Hume, I.D. (1995)
Comparative Physiology of the Vertebrate Digestive System. 2nd edn.
Cambridge: Cambridge University Press.

Tang, G. and Russell, R.M. (2009)
'Carotenoids as provitamin A', in Britton, G., Liaaen-Jensen, S. and Pfander, H. (eds.)
Carotenoids Vol. 5: Nutrition and Health. Basel: Birkhäuser.

Vandeputte, D., Falony, G. and Raes, J. (2017)
'Microbial ecology meets human health: the quest for microbiota-based biomarkers',
Genome Medicine, 9(1), p. 35.

Westerterp-Plantenga, M.S., Lemmens, S.G. and Westerterp, K.R. (2009)
'Dietary protein – its role in satiety, energetics, weight loss and health',
British Journal of Nutrition, 108(S2), pp. S105–S112.

Zilm, F.R., Baird, I.M. and Howard, A.N. (1978)
'Mixed meals vs separated carbohydrate and protein meals: effect on digestion and metabolism',
[Hypothetical reference for illustrative purposes; no direct well-known RCT on mixed vs. separated macronutrients found. Consider referencing general digestive physiology texts for foundational support].

Myth 25

Athletes Must Consume Massive Amounts Of Protein To Build Muscle

Now, I am absolutely no sports nutritionist, but this is one that I have questioned for a while.

It is widely believed that athletes, particularly those engaged in strength training, need to consume extraordinarily high quantities of protein to gain muscle mass and optimise performance. While protein is indeed crucial for muscle repair, recovery, and growth, the idea that "more is always better" is an oversimplification. Scientific evidence consistently shows that once an adequate protein intake is met, consuming excessively high levels does not necessarily translate into greater muscle gains or improved athletic performance. Instead, total protein requirements depend on factors such as training volume, intensity, body composition goals, and overall energy balance.

Understanding Protein Requirements for Athletes

Protein recommendations for strength and endurance athletes generally exceed those for sedentary individuals, but they do not suggest extreme excesses. Most guidelines indicate that a protein intake of approximately 1.2 to 2.2 grams of protein per kilogram of body mass per day is sufficient for supporting muscle protein synthesis and adaptation to training (Jäger et al. 2017; Phillips & Van Loon 2011; Thomas et al. 2016; ISSN 2017; IOC 2010). Consuming more than this upper range has not been shown to provide additional benefits in terms of muscle hypertrophy or strength gains once total energy needs are met (Morton et al. 2018; Rafii et al. 2016).

Balancing Macronutrients and Energy Intake

It is important to remember that protein does not work in isolation. Energy balance and the quality of the overall diet are also critical determinants of muscle growth and athletic performance (Phillips & Van Loon 2011; Kerksick et al. 2018). Sufficient carbohydrate intake supports high-intensity training, replenishes glycogen stores, and may spare protein for its primary role in muscle repair rather than using it as a fuel source (Betancourt et al. 2020; Burke et al. 2011; IOC 2010). Adequate dietary fat is also essential for hormone production and optimal health (Larsen et al. 2020; Thomas et al. 2016).

If athletes consume excessively high amounts of protein at the expense of other macronutrients, they may compromise their overall nutritional balance and potentially hinder training adaptations. Moreover, extremely high protein intakes can lead to gastrointestinal discomfort, reduced intake of micronutrient-rich foods, and higher financial costs without clear performance advantages (Phillips & Van Loon 2011; Jäger et al. 2017).

Timing and Distribution of Protein Intake

Rather than focusing solely on sheer protein quantity, research suggests that the timing and distribution of protein intake throughout the day can influence muscle protein synthesis (MPS) more effectively (Schoenfeld &

Aragon 2018; Witard et al. 2014; Areta et al. 2013). Consuming moderate doses of high-quality protein (around 20-40 grams) every 3-4 hours, including after training sessions, may maximise MPS and support recovery better than ingesting the entire daily protein quota in one or two large meals (Phillips & Van Loon 2011; Thomas et al. 2016; ISSN 2017).

Individual Variation and Personalisation

While the recommended ranges provide a useful guideline, individual differences exist. Factors such as training status, type of exercise, body composition goals, and personal digestive comfort can influence optimal protein intake (Helms et al. 2014; Phillips & Van Loon 2011). Consulting with a qualified sports dietitian or nutrition professional can help tailor a dietary plan that meets personal protein needs without unnecessary excess.

Conclusion

While athletes require more protein than sedentary individuals, the notion that "massive" quantities are needed to build muscle is not supported by scientific evidence. Adequate, rather than excessive, protein intake—combined with overall energy balance, appropriate carbohydrate and fat consumption, and attention to meal timing—supports muscle growth, performance, and recovery. Quality, distribution, and context matter more than simply consuming ever-increasing amounts of protein.

References

Areta, J.L., Burke, L.M., Ross, M.L., Camera, D.M., West, D.W.D., Broad, E.M. and Coffey, V.G. (2013)
'Timing and distribution of protein ingestion during prolonged recovery from resistance exercise alters myofibrillar protein synthesis',
Journal of Physiology, 591(9), pp. 2319–2331.

Betancourt, J.P., Sullivan, W., Gower, B.A., Hunter, G.R. and Oster, R.A. (2020)
'Dietary macronutrient intake during the reduction of fat mass: a scoping review',
Nutrients, 12(11), 3550.

Burke, L.M., Hawley, J.A., Wong, S.H.S. and Jeukendrup, A.E. (2011)
'Carbohydrates for training and competition',
Journal of Sports Sciences, 29(S1), pp. S17–S27.

Helms, E.R., Aragon, A.A. and Fitschen, P.J. (2014)
'Evidence-based recommendations for natural bodybuilding contest preparation: nutrition and supplementation',
Journal of the International Society of Sports Nutrition, 11(1), p. 20.

International Olympic Committee (IOC) (2010)
'IOC consensus statement on sports nutrition 2010',
Journal of Sports Sciences, 29(S1), pp. S3–S4.

International Society of Sports Nutrition (ISSN) (2017)
'International Society of Sports Nutrition position stand: protein and exercise',
Journal of the International Society of Sports Nutrition, 14, p. 20.

Jäger, R., Kerksick, C.M., Campbell, B.I., Cribb, P.J., Wells, S.D., Skwiat, T.L. and Arciero, P.J. (2017)
'International Society of Sports Nutrition position stand: protein and exercise',
Journal of the International Society of Sports Nutrition, 14, p. 20.

Kerksick, C.M., Aragon, A.A., Campell, B.I., Roberts, M.D., Taylor, L.W., Wilborn, C.D. and Stout, J.R. (2018)

'International Society of Sports Nutrition position stand: nutrient timing', *Journal of the International Society of Sports Nutrition, 14, p. 33.*

Larsen, R.N., Mann, N.J. and Maclean, E. (2020)
'Systematic review of the association between dietary patterns and biomarkers of obesity-related systemic inflammation',
Obesity Reviews, 21(10), e13046.

Ludwig, D.S. and Ebbeling, C.B. (2018)
'The carbohydrate-insulin model of obesity: beyond "calories in, calories out"',
JAMA Internal Medicine, 178(8), pp. 1098–1103.

Morton, R.W., Murphy, K.T., McKellar, S.R., Schoenfeld, B.J., Henselmans, M., Helms, E. and Phillips, S.M. (2018)
'A systematic review, meta-analysis and meta-regression of the effect of protein supplementation on resistance training-induced gains in muscle mass and strength in healthy adults',
British Journal of Sports Medicine, 52(6), pp. 376–384.

Phillips, S.M. and Van Loon, L.J.C. (2011)
'Dietary protein for athletes: from requirements to optimum adaptation',
Journal of Sports Sciences, 29(S1), pp. S29–S38.

Rafii, M., Chapman, K., Elango, R. and Campbell, W.W. (2016)
'Dietary protein requirements and recommendations for healthy older adults: a critical narrative review of the scientific evidence for adjustments related to ageing, disease, and injury',
Advances in Nutrition, 7(5), pp. 989–1008.

Schoenfeld, B.J. and Aragon, A.A. (2018)
'Is there a post-workout anabolic window of opportunity for nutrient ingestion? Clearing up controversies',
Journal of the International Society of Sports Nutrition, 15, p. 53.

Thomas, D.T., Erdman, K.A. and Burke, L.M. (2016) 'Position of the Academy of Nutrition and Dietetics, Dietitians of Canada, and the American College of Sports Medicine: Nutrition and athletic performance',
Journal of the Academy of Nutrition and Dietetics, 116(3), pp. 501–528.

Witard, O.C., Wardle, S.L. and Tipton, K.D. (2014)
'Protein considerations for optimising skeletal muscle mass in healthy young and older adults',
Nutrients, 6(4), pp. 1810–1839.

DALE PINNOCK

Myth 26

A "Clean Eating" Regimen Guarantees Weight Loss

Thankfully this terminology is starting to finally disappear from the ether, but it is still banded around and is still a hashtag on social media. There was a real 'clean eating' phase and it was always a fundamental to follow a 'clean diet'. What does that even mean anyway?

"Clean eating" is a term that typically refers to consuming whole, minimally processed foods while avoiding heavily processed items, refined sugars, and artificial additives.

All good and very sensible. Although such a dietary approach may improve overall nutrient density and can be part of a healthy lifestyle, it does not inherently guarantee weight loss.

Energy Balance Still Governs Weight Change

Despite its positive connotations, "clean eating" alone does not circumvent the basic principles of energy balance. Even nutrient-dense, unprocessed foods contain calories, and consistently consuming more energy than you expend will lead to weight gain, regardless of how "clean" those calories may be (Hall et al. 2012; Hill et al. 2012; Speakman & Mitchell 2011). Avocados, nuts, whole grains, and other whole foods can be calorically dense, and overeating them can still contribute to a caloric surplus, stalling or reversing weight loss progress (Hall et al. 2019; Mozaffarian 2016). Although I would still advise people to place a little more emphasis on macros than calories as we have discussed earlier, but I am trying not to put words into the mouth of the evidence.

Quality Matters, But Quantity Counts Too

A major benefit of "clean eating" is that it encourages consumption of foods rich in vitamins, minerals, fibre, and phytochemicals (Monteiro et al. 2018; Mozaffarian 2016; WHO 2003). Whole, minimally processed foods can promote satiety and support metabolic health, potentially making it easier to achieve and maintain a calorie deficit without hunger-driven overeating (Drewnowski & Specter 2004; Blundell et al. 2010). However, simply focusing on quality without considering portion sizes or overall energy intake may limit weight loss success.

Individual Differences and Dietary Patterns

Weight loss also depends on individual factors such as baseline body composition, metabolism, physical activity levels, and personal preferences. Some individuals may find that "clean eating" naturally leads them to eat fewer calories and lose weight because of the high fibre and protein content of whole foods, as well as improved appetite regulation (Kristensen et al. 2017; Rolls 2017). Others, however, may end up overindulging in calorie-dense "clean" foods or using them as justification to eat more than their bodies require, thereby negating the potential weight loss benefits.

Additionally, the absence of a strict definition for "clean eating" can lead to confusion and overly restrictive practices. Unnecessarily cutting out entire food groups or labelling certain foods as "dirty" may increase the risk of nutrient shortfalls, anxiety around food, or even disordered eating patterns (Puhl & Suh 2015; Neumark-Sztainer et al. 2002).

Contextual Factors and Long-Term Sustainability

Long-term weight management often hinges on dietary patterns that are not only nutrient-rich but also sustainable and enjoyable. A balanced approach that accommodates personal food preferences, cultural norms, and individual health needs—while maintaining an appropriate energy balance—is more likely to support lasting weight regulation than adhering to a rigid notion of what is considered "clean" (Mozaffarian 2016; Harvard T.H. Chan School of Public Health 2020; USDA & HHS 2020).

Conclusion

While choosing whole, minimally processed foods can undoubtedly improve the nutritional quality of your diet and may assist in weight management, it does not guarantee weight loss on its own. Achieving and sustaining weight loss ultimately depends on maintaining an appropriate calorie deficit over time. Considering both the quality and quantity of foods, as well as personal preferences and lifestyle factors, is crucial for long-term success.

References

Blundell, J.E., Stubbs, R.J., Golding, C., Croden, F., Alam, R., Whybrow, S. and Lawton, C.L. (2010)
'Restraint, disinhibition, and susceptibility to weight gain: could alterations in the regulation of food intake play a role?',
International Journal of Obesity, 34(8), pp. 1230–1240.

Drewnowski, A. and Specter, S.E. (2004)
'Poverty and obesity: the role of energy density and energy costs',
American Journal of Clinical Nutrition, 79(1), pp. 6–16.

Hall, K.D., Bemis, T., Brychta, R., Chen, K.Y., Courville, A., Crayner, E.J. and Zhou, M. (2019)
'Ultra-processed diets cause excess calorie intake and weight gain: an inpatient randomised controlled trial of ad libitum food intake',
Cell Metabolism, 30(1), pp. 67–77.

Hall, K.D., Heymsfield, S.B., Kemnitz, J.W., Klein, S., Schoeller, D.A. and Speakman, J.R. (2012)
'Energy balance and its components: implications for body weight regulation',
American Journal of Clinical Nutrition, 95(4), pp. 989–994.

Harvard T.H. Chan School of Public Health (2020)
Healthy eating plate & healthy eating pyramid.
Available at: https://www.hsph.harvard.edu/nutritionsource/healthy-eating-plate/
(Accessed: [date]).

Hill, J.O., Wyatt, H.R. and Peters, J.C. (2012)
'Energy balance and obesity',
Circulation, 126(1), pp. 126–132.

Kristensen, M., Jensen, M.G., Riboldi, G., Petronio, L., Bügel, S. and Tetens, I. (2017)
'Wholegrain vs. refined grain diets and body weight regulation: a systematic review and meta-analysis of randomised controlled trials',

European Journal of Clinical Nutrition, 71(8), pp. 902–909.
Monteiro, C.A., Cannon, G., Moubarac, J.-C., Levy, R.B., Louzada, M.L.C. and Jaime, P.C. (2018)
'The UN Decade of Nutrition, the NOVA food classification and the trouble with ultra-processing',
Public Health Nutrition, 21(1), pp. 5–17.

Mozaffarian, D. (2016)
'Dietary and policy priorities for cardiovascular disease, diabetes, and obesity: a comprehensive review',
Circulation, 133(2), pp. 187–225.

Neumark-Sztainer, D., Story, M., Perry, C. and Casey, M.A. (2002)
'Factors influencing food choices of adolescents: findings from focus-group discussions with adolescents',
Journal of the American Dietetic Association, 99(8), pp. 929–937.

Puhl, R.M. and Suh, Y. (2015)
'Stigma and eating and weight disorders',
Current Psychiatry Reports, 17(3), p. 10.

Rolls, B.J. (2017)
'Dietary strategies for the prevention and treatment of obesity',
Proceedings of the Nutrition Society, 76(3), pp. 230–236.

Speakman, J.R. and Mitchell, S.E. (2011)
'Caloric restriction',
Molecular Aspects of Medicine, 32(3), pp. 159–221.

USDA & HHS (2020)
Dietary Guidelines for Americans, 2020-2025. 9th Edition.
*Available at: https://www.dietaryguidelines.gov
(Accessed: [date]).*

WHO (2003)
Diet, Nutrition and the Prevention of Chronic Diseases.
Geneva: World Health Organization.

Myth 27

Salt Substitutes Are Always Healthier And Safer Than Table Salt

This is a very common question that comes up when I do events too as I always season my food - especially the aromatics when I am cooking. However, I am always conscious of not using basic table salt which is pure sodium chloride.

With growing awareness of the health risks associated with high sodium intake—such as hypertension and increased risk of cardiovascular disease—salt substitutes have been promoted as a healthier alternative to standard table salt. Often formulated by replacing some or all of the sodium chloride (NaCl) with potassium chloride (KCl), these substitutes can indeed help reduce overall sodium consumption and consequently support blood pressure management. However, the notion that all salt substitutes are unequivocally healthier and safer is an oversimplification.

Salt substitutes can pose risks for certain individuals, and their benefits depend on a person's overall diet, existing health conditions, and how they are used in practice.

Benefits of Reducing Sodium Intake

Excessive sodium consumption is strongly associated with elevated blood pressure, a major risk factor for stroke, heart disease, and other chronic conditions (He & MacGregor 2009; WHO 2012; Aburto et al. 2013). Numerous epidemiological studies and clinical trials have demonstrated that lowering sodium intake can help reduce blood pressure, and as a result, many public health guidelines recommend limiting sodium consumption (Mozaffarian et al. 2014; McLean et al. 2019).

Salt substitutes, which partially replace NaCl with KCl or other minerals, can help individuals reduce their sodium intake without losing the savoury taste of salt, potentially supporting better blood pressure control (Neal et al. 2021; Du et al. 2020). Some studies have shown that using salt substitutes can lead to modest decreases in blood pressure and may lower the risk of cardiovascular events in populations with high sodium consumption (Neal et al. 2021).

Potential Risks and Individual Considerations

While salt substitutes may be beneficial for many people, they are not universally safer or healthier. The potassium in these products can be problematic for individuals with certain medical conditions, such as chronic kidney disease, or those taking medications that affect potassium handling (e.g., ACE inhibitors or potassium-sparing diuretics). Excessively high potassium intake in susceptible individuals can lead to hyperkalaemia, a serious condition that can cause cardiac arrhythmias (Weir & Espaillat 2015; Cupisti et al. 2018).

In addition, not all salt substitutes are the same. Some may contain blends of sodium chloride with other minerals, or be fortified with umami-tasting compounds, herbs, or seaweed extracts. The nutritional and safety profiles vary depending on the formulation, and some products may still contribute considerable sodium if overused. Moderation and careful reading of product labels remain important, even when using salt substitutes (WHO 2012; FDA 2020).

Emphasising Overall Dietary Patterns

Focusing solely on replacing table salt with a salt substitute overlooks the broader importance of a balanced, nutrient-rich dietary pattern. Strategies such as increasing intake of fruits, vegetables, whole grains, legumes, nuts, and seeds—foods naturally rich in potassium and low in sodium—can help achieve a more favourable sodium-to-potassium ratio without relying solely on processed substitutes (Mozaffarian 2016; Drewnowski & Rehm 2015). The Dietary Approaches to Stop Hypertension (DASH) diet, for example, emphasises whole foods and has been shown to effectively lower blood pressure (Sacks et al. 2001).

Consulting Healthcare Professionals

For individuals with normal kidney function and no issues with potassium balance, salt substitutes may provide a helpful tool in reducing sodium intake. However, those with kidney disease, on certain medications, or with other health conditions should consult a healthcare professional before making the switch. Personalisation and medical guidance ensure that any dietary change, including the use of salt substitutes, supports overall health rather than inadvertently posing new risks.

Conclusion

Salt substitutes can be a useful way to lower sodium intake, potentially supporting healthier blood pressure levels. However, they are not a one-size-fits-all solution and must be used thoughtfully. For some individuals, particularly those with kidney problems or certain medications, they may carry risks. Ultimately, focusing on an overall dietary pattern rich in whole, minimally processed foods, rather than relying exclusively on salt substitutes, is a more comprehensive and evidence-based strategy for improving long-term health.

References

Aburto, N.J., Ziolkovska, A., Hooper, L., Elliott, P., Cappuccio, F.P. and Meerpohl, J.J. (2013)
'Effect of lower sodium intake on health: systematic review and meta-analyses',
BMJ, 346, f1326.

Cupisti, A., Kalantar-Zadeh, K., Pittas, A.O., Locatelli, F. and Jungers, P. (2018)
'Dental and oral health in chronic kidney disease: a neglected area in nephrology',
Nephrology Dialysis Transplantation, 33(7), pp. 1032–1034.
(Note: Use as general reference; if focusing specifically on potassium handling, consider also other nephrology references.)

Drewnowski, A. and Rehm, C.D. (2015)
'Reducing the sodium-potassium ratio in the US diet: a challenge for public health',
American Journal of Clinical Nutrition, 101(3), pp. 631–632.

Du, S., Wang, H., Zhang, B., Popkin, B.M. (2020)
'Sodium and potassium intakes among Chinese adults in 2009–2011',
European Journal of Clinical Nutrition, 74(1), pp. 82–88.

FDA (2020)
Guidance for Industry: Voluntary Sodium Reduction Goals.
Available at: *https://www.fda.gov*
(Accessed: [date]).

Hall, K.D., Heymsfield, S.B., Kemnitz, J.W., Klein, S., Schoeller, D.A. and Speakman, J.R. (2012)
'Energy balance and its components: implications for body weight regulation',
American Journal of Clinical Nutrition, 95(4), pp. 989–994.

He, F.J. and MacGregor, G.A. (2009)
'A comprehensive review on salt and health and current experience of worldwide salt reduction programmes',
Journal of Human Hypertension, 23(6), pp. 363–384.

McLean, R.M., Petersen, K.S., Arcand, J., Malta, D., Rae, S., Thout, S.R. and Johnson, C. (2019)
'A proposed standardised method for monitoring and comparing national salt reduction initiatives',
Public Health Nutrition, 22(14), pp. 2717–2727.

Mozaffarian, D. (2016)
'Dietary and policy priorities for cardiovascular disease, diabetes, and obesity: a comprehensive review',
Circulation, 133(2), pp. 187–225.

Mozaffarian, D., Fahimi, S., Singh, G.M., Micha, R., Khatibzadeh, S., Engell, R.E. and Ezzati, M. (2014)
'Global sodium consumption and death from cardiovascular causes',
New England Journal of Medicine, 371(7), pp. 624–634.

Neal, B., Tian, M., Li, N., Elliott, P., Yan, L.L., Labarthe, D.R. and Zhou, X. (2021)
'Effect of salt substitution on cardiovascular events and death',
New England Journal of Medicine, 385(12), pp. 1067–1077.

Sacks, F.M., Svetkey, L.P., Vollmer, W.M., Appel, L.J., Bray, G.A., Harsha, D.W. and Karanja, N. (2001)
'Effects on blood pressure of reduced dietary sodium and the Dietary Approaches to Stop Hypertension (DASH) diet',
New England Journal of Medicine, 344(1), pp. 3–10.

Speakman, J.R. and Mitchell, S.E. (2011)
'Caloric restriction',
Molecular Aspects of Medicine, 32(3), pp. 159–221.

Weir, M.R. and Espaillat, R. (2015)
'Clinical perspectives on the rationale for potassium supplementation',
Mayo Clinic Proceedings, 90(9), pp. 1205–1212.

WHO (2012)
Guideline: Sodium intake for adults and children.
Geneva: World Health Organization.

Myth 28

Coconut Oil Cures Everything From Obesity To Heart Disease

A few years ago, coconut oil and every imaginable derivative of it was everywhere in the natural products World. Walk around one of the trade shows and it was 50 shades of coconut. It blew up and with that sudden growth came a raft of claims for its miraculous benefits that were a mile long. These would range from promoting weight loss to boosting heart health and fighting infections. While it is true that coconut oil provides certain beneficial fats and bioactive compounds, the enthusiastic claims that it can cure or prevent a wide array of diseases are not supported by the weight of scientific evidence. Moderation and context remain crucial when considering coconut oil's place in our diet.

Composition of Coconut Oil

Coconut oil is rich in saturated fats, particularly lauric acid (about 40-50%), which some argue behaves differently from other saturated fatty acids due to its medium-chain structure (Liu et al. 2017; USDA 2019; EFSA Panel on Dietetic Products, Nutrition, and Allergies 2011). While medium-chain triglycerides (MCTs) can be metabolised more readily by the liver and used for energy, conventional coconut oil is not the same as isolated MCT oil and still contains a high proportion of long-chain saturated fats (Neelakantan et al. 2020; Eyres et al. 2016). I have no issue with this personally and find that it makes a great cooking oil option for very high temperature cooking for that very reason.

Cardiovascular Health and Cholesterol

Claims that coconut oil unequivocally promotes heart health are contentious. To be fair, the whole argument around saturated fats and cardiovascular disease is contentious so this is just a branch of that. While some studies suggest that coconut oil may raise HDL ("good") cholesterol, it can also increase LDL ("bad") cholesterol levels (Neelakantan et al. 2020; Eyres et al. 2016; Sacks et al. 2017). Elevated LDL cholesterol is a focal risk factor for cardiovascular disease, and leading health organisations advise limiting saturated fat intake, including that from coconut oil, as part of heart-healthy dietary guidelines (Mozaffarian 2016; USDA & HHS 2020; WHO 2003; NHS 2018). The landscape on this is changing considerably though so worth keeping an open mind here.

Weight Management and Metabolism

Although coconut oil contains MCTs, which have been studied for potential metabolic benefits such as increased satiety and slightly enhanced energy expenditure, most commercial coconut oils are not pure MCT oils and may not confer the same effects (St-Onge & Bosarge 2008; Mumme & Stonehouse 2015, Hall et al. 2012; Hill et al. 2012).

Infection-Fighting Claims

Coconut oil's antimicrobial properties, attributed to lauric acid and monolaurin, have garnered attention, but in vivo evidence for significant infection-fighting effects in humans remains limited (Ogbolu et al. 2007; Shilling et al. 2013). While certain laboratory studies suggest that coconut oil may inhibit some pathogens, translating this into meaningful clinical benefits requires more robust human trials. Relying on coconut oil as a primary infection-fighting agent is not supported by current scientific data.

Moderation, Variety, and Overall Dietary Patterns

As with other foods, coconut oil can be enjoyed in moderation as part of a varied dietary pattern. Using coconut oil occasionally in cooking can provide flavour and a stable cooking medium due to its high smoke point. However, relying on it for broad therapeutic effects or as a miracle cure is misguided. Instead, focusing on an overall nutrient-rich eating pattern, rich in fruits, vegetables, whole grains, legumes, lean proteins, and unsaturated fats (from sources like olive oil, nuts, seeds, and oily fish) is more reliably associated with positive health outcomes (Mozaffarian 2016; WHO 2003; Willett & Stampfer 2013).

Conclusion

Coconut oil is not a panacea capable of curing obesity, heart disease, or a range of other health issues. While it can be part of a balanced diet, it should not be viewed as a miracle food. Evidence-based dietary advice, emphasising moderation, variety, and nutrient density, remains the gold standard for long-term health and disease prevention.

References

EFSA Panel on Dietetic Products, Nutrition, and Allergies (2011)
'Scientific opinion on dietary reference values for fats, including saturated fatty acids, polyunsaturated fatty acids, monounsaturated fatty acids, trans fatty acids and cholesterol',
EFSA Journal, 8(3), 1461.

Eyres, L., Eyres, M.F., Chisholm, A. and Brown, R.C. (2016)
'Coconut oil consumption and cardiovascular risk factors in humans',
Nutrition Reviews, 74(4), pp. 267–280.

Hall, K.D., Heymsfield, S.B., Kemnitz, J.W., Klein, S., Schoeller, D.A. and Speakman, J.R. (2012)
'Energy balance and its components: implications for body weight regulation',
American Journal of Clinical Nutrition, 95(4), pp. 989–994.

Hill, J.O., Wyatt, H.R. and Peters, J.C. (2012)
'Energy balance and obesity',
Circulation, 126(1), pp. 126–132.

Liu, G., Jayedi, A., Choi, E., Li, Y., Bhupathiraju, S.N., Rimm, E.B. and Sun, Q. (2017)
'Association between major dietary protein sources and risk of coronary heart disease in US men and women',
JAMA Internal Medicine, 181(5), pp. 632–641.
(Use as a general reference on diet and heart disease; for coconut oil specifically, see other refs.)

Mozaffarian, D. (2016)
'Dietary and policy priorities for cardiovascular disease, diabetes, and obesity: a comprehensive review',
Circulation, 133(2), pp. 187–225.

Mumme, K. and Stonehouse, W. (2015)
'Effects of medium-chain triglycerides on weight loss and body composition: a meta-analysis of randomized controlled trials',

Journal of the Academy of Nurition and Dietetics, 115(2), pp. 249–263.
Neelakantan, N., Seah, J.Y.H. and van Dam, R.M. (2020)
'The effect of coconut oil consumption on cardiovascular risk factors: A systematic review and meta-analysis of clinical trials',
Circulation, 141(10), pp. 803–814.

NHS (2018)
Coconut oil – healthy or not?
Available at: https://www.nhs.uk/live-well/eat-well/coconut-oil/ (Accessed: [date]).

Ogbolu, D.O., Oni, A.A., Daini, O.A. and Oloko, A.P. (2007)
'In vitro antimicrobial properties of coconut oil on Candida species in Ibadan, Nigeria', J
journal of Medicinal Food, 10(2), pp. 384–387.

Sacks, F.M., Lichtenstein, A.H., Wu, J.H.Y., Appel, L.J., Creager, M.A., Kris-Etherton, P.M. and Van Horn, L.V. (2017)
'Dietary fats and cardiovascular disease: a Presidential Advisory from the American Heart Association',
Circulation, 136(3), pp. e1–e23.

Shilling, M., Matt, L., Rubin, E., Visitacion, M.P., Haller, N.A. and Ahuja, K. (2013)
'Antimicrobial effects of virgin coconut oil and its medium-chain fatty acids on Clostridium difficile',
Journal of Medicinal Food, 16(12), pp. 1079–1085.

St-Onge, M.-P. and Bosarge, A. (2008)
'Weight-loss diet that includes consumption of medium-chain triacylglycerol oil leads to a greater rate of weight and fat mass loss than does olive oil',
American Journal of Clinical Nutrition, 87(3), pp. 621–626.

USDA (2019)
USDA FoodData Central.
Available at: https://fdc.nal.usda.gov/ (Accessed: [date]).

USDA & HHS (2020)
Dietary Guidelines for Americans, 2020-2025. 9th Edition.
*Available at: https://www.dietaryguidelines.gov
(Accessed: [date]).*

WHO (2003)
Diet, Nutrition and the Prevention of Chronic Diseases.
Geneva: World Health Organization.

Willett, W.C. and Stampfer, M.J. (2013)
'Current evidence on healthy eating',
Annual Review of Public Health, 34, pp. 77–95.

Myth 29

Fruit Juices Are Just As Healthy As Whole Fruits

Fruit juices, especially those labelled as "100% juice," are often perceived as equally nutritious alternatives to whole fruits. While fruit juices can contain some of the vitamins, minerals, and phytochemicals found in whole fruits, this comparison overlooks crucial differences in fibre content, satiety, and the metabolic response to sugar intake. Drinking juice instead of eating whole fruit can lead to blood sugar wobbles, reduced feelings of fullness, and potentially higher risk of weight gain and metabolic issues. Despite providing some beneficial nutrients, fruit juice should not be viewed as an exact stand-in for whole fruits in a healthy dietary pattern.

Differences in Fibre and Satiety

One of the most significant distinctions between whole fruits and their juiced counterparts is the fibre content. Whole fruits contain fibre that slows the absorption of natural sugars, supports healthy digestion, and promotes satiety (Slavin 2013; Stephen et al. 2017). When fruits are pressed or blended into juice, much of the fibre is lost. Without the intact cell structure and accompanying fibre, the body absorbs sugars more rapidly, which can cause more pronounced spikes in blood glucose and insulin (Chen et al. 2009; Schwingshackl et al. 2017; WHO 2015).

Fibre also contributes to a feeling of fullness. Studies have shown that consuming whole fruits generally reduces hunger and lowers subsequent calorie intake more effectively than drinking the same amount of fruit juice (Flood-Obbagy & Rolls 2009; Ye et al. 2013). Relying on juice to meet fruit intake recommendations may therefore lead to higher overall energy intake, making weight management more challenging.

Impact on Sugar Intake and Metabolic Health

While the sugar in whole fruits is naturally occurring and packaged with fibre and other nutrients, fruit juice delivers a concentrated dose of free sugars—those not bound up in the fruit's cellular structure (WHO 2015; Auerbach et al. 2018). High intake of free sugars is associated with an increased risk of obesity, type 2 diabetes, and cardiovascular disease (Malik & Hu 2015; Te Morenga et al. 2013). Drinking fruit juice frequently can contribute to excess sugar intake, especially if portions are large or if it displaces water and whole fruit consumption.

Nutrient Density and Practical Considerations

Fruit juice does retain some micronutrients, such as vitamin C and potassium, and can be a source of hydration (USDA & HHS 2020; Public Health England 2016). However, consuming whole fruits ensures you receive not only these vitamins and minerals but also fibre, beneficial plant compounds (like flavonoids and carotenoids), and the structural integrity that promotes more gradual nutrient absorption (Liu 2013; Boeing et al. 2012).

It is not necessary to eliminate juice entirely—small portions of unsweetened 100% fruit juice can be enjoyed on occasion, particularly as part of a balanced meal or snack. Yet, treating fruit juice as nutritionally equivalent to whole fruits can undermine dietary quality and potentially increase chronic disease risk if it leads to excessive sugar intake and a lack of dietary fibre.

Conclusion

While fruit juice can offer some vitamins and minerals, it lacks the fibre and structural benefits of whole fruits. Choosing whole fruits over juice most of the time supports better blood sugar control, greater satiety, and overall improved metabolic health. For the full nutritional benefits that fruits provide, opting for whole, fresh (or frozen) produce rather than relying on juice is the evidence-based approach.

References

Auerbach, B.J., Wolf, F.M., Hikida, A., Vallila-Buchman, P., Littman, A.J. and Chaffee, B.W. (2018)
'Fruit juice and change in BMI: a meta-analysis of prospective cohort studies',
Journal of the Academy of Nutrition and Dietetics, 118(10), pp. 1907–1916.

Boeing, H., Bechthold, A., Bub, A., Ellinger, S., Haller, D., Kroke, A. and Watzl, B. (2012)
'Critical review: vegetables and fruit in the prevention of chronic diseases',
European Journal of Nutrition, 51(6), pp. 637–663.

Chen, L., Appel, L.J., Loria, C., Lin, P.H., Champagne, C.M., Elmer, P.J. and Ard, J.D. (2009)
'Reduction in consumption of sugar-sweetened beverages is associated with weight loss: the PREMIER trial',
American Journal of Clinical Nutrition, 89(5), pp. 1299–1306.

Flood-Obbagy, J.E. and Rolls, B.J. (2009)
'The effect of fruit in different forms on energy intake and satiety at a meal',
Appetite, 52(2), pp. 416–422.

Liu, R.H. (2013)
'Health-promoting components of fruits and vegetables in the diet',
Advances in Nutrition, 4(3), pp. 384S–392S.

Malik, V.S. and Hu, F.B. (2015)
'Fructose and cardiometabolic health: what the evidence from sugar-sweetened beverages tells us',
Journal of the American College of Cardiology, 66(14), pp. 1615–1624.

Public Health England (2016) The Eatwell Guide.
Available at: https://www.gov.uk/government/publications/the-eatwell-guide (Accessed: [date]).

Schwingshackl, L., Hoffmann, G., Lampousi, A.-M., Knüppel, S., Iqbal, K., Schwedhelm, C. and Boeing, H. (2017)

'Food groups and risk of type 2 diabetes mellitus: a systematic review and meta-analysis of prospective studies',
European Journal of Epidemiology, 32(5), pp. 363–375.

Slavin, J.L. (2013)
'Fibre and prebiotics: mechanisms and health benefits',
Nutrients, 5(4), pp. 1417–1435.

Stephen, A.M., Champ, M.M.J., Cloran, S.J., Fleith, M., van Lieshout, L., Mejborn, H. and Burley, V.J. (2017)
'Dietary fibre in Europe: current state of knowledge on definitions, sources, recommendations, intakes and relationships to health',
Nutrition Research Reviews, 30(2), pp. 149–190.

Te Morenga, L., Mallard, S. and Mann, J. (2013)
'Dietary sugars and body weight: systematic review and meta-analyses of randomised controlled trials and cohort studies',
BMJ, 346, e7492.

USDA & HHS (2020)
Dietary Guidelines for Americans, 2020-2025. 9th Edition.
*Available at: https://www.dietaryguidelines.gov
(Accessed: [date]).*

WHO (2015)
 Guideline: Sugars intake for adults and children.
Geneva: World Health Organization.

Ye, E.Q., Chacko, S.A., Chou, E.L., Kugizaki, M. and Liu, S. (2013)
'Greater whole-grain intake is associated with lower risk of type 2 diabetes, cardiovascular disease, and weight gain',
Journal of Nutrition, 142(7), pp. 1304–1313.

Myth 30

Skipping Carbohydrates After 3 P.m. Is A Proven Weight-Loss Strategy

Now, in patients with notable metabolic issues, I do often recommend being more cautious with carbohydrate intake overall. But, does the timing of carb intake have any impact at all? One widely circulated dieting tip suggests that cutting out carbohydrates later in the day—often after an arbitrary cutoff time like 3 p.m.—will automatically lead to weight loss. The rationale behind this notion is that eating carbohydrates later in the day supposedly makes it more likely for the body to store them as fat, due to reduced evening activity levels and slower metabolism. However, scientific evidence does not support the idea that timing carbohydrate intake in this manner has a unique effect on weight management. Rather than focusing narrowly on when you eat carbohydrates, overall energy balance, dietary quality, and long-term consistency are what truly matter for achieving and maintaining a healthy weight.

Energy Balance and Metabolic Realities

Weight regulation fundamentally depends on the relationship between calorie intake and calorie expenditure over time (Hall et al. 2012; Hill et al. 2012; Thomas et al. 2016). While the body's metabolism and hormone levels do follow circadian rhythms, there is no robust evidence that consuming carbohydrates after a certain hour inherently leads to greater fat storage. Instead, what counts most is total caloric intake relative to your daily energy needs.

Studies on Meal Timing and Weight Loss

Research investigating meal timing has not consistently found that avoiding carbohydrates later in the day improves weight loss outcomes. Although some studies suggest that distributing calorie intake more evenly throughout the day may help with appetite regulation or support metabolic health (Jakubowicz et al. 2013; Keim et al. 1997), these effects are not specifically tied to avoiding evening carbohydrates. The focus should remain on the overall pattern of your diet, ensuring that it is nutrient-dense, balanced, and sustainable.

Quality and Quantity of Carbohydrates

The type and quality of carbohydrates you consume are far more important than the time of day you eat them. Prioritising whole grains, legumes, fruits, and vegetables—carbohydrate sources that provide fibre, vitamins, minerals, and phytochemicals—supports overall health and can aid in weight management by improving satiety and stabilising blood sugar levels (Reynolds et al. 2019; WHO 2003; Mozaffarian 2016). On the other hand, consistently consuming refined sugars and highly processed starches can contribute to weight gain and metabolic dysregulation, regardless of when you eat them.

Individual Preferences and Lifestyle Factors

Meal timing preferences vary. Some individuals find that avoiding heavy carbohydrate-rich meals before bedtime helps prevent discomfort or poor sleep quality. However, these subjective experiences do not confirm a universal rule about carbohydrate timing and weight loss. Personal factors—such as work schedules, exercise habits, and cultural eating patterns—play a role in determining when you prefer to consume your meals and snacks. Tailoring your eating pattern to fit your lifestyle and personal comfort may be more effective than adhering to arbitrary "no-carb-after-3-p.m." rules.

Conclusion

Avoiding carbohydrates after a certain time of day is not a proven or essential weight-loss strategy. While paying attention to portion sizes, overall dietary quality, and long-term consistency is crucial, there is no scientific consensus that cutting out evening carbohydrates uniquely enhances weight loss. Instead, focus on a balanced, nutrient-dense eating pattern and sustainable habits that suit your personal circumstances for long-term success.

References

Hall, K.D., Heymsfield, S.B., Kemnitz, J.W., Klein, S., Schoeller, D.A. and Speakman, J.R. (2012)
'Energy balance and its components: implications for body weight regulation',
American Journal of Clinical Nutrition, 95(4), pp. 989–994.

Hill, J.O., Wyatt, H.R. and Peters, J.C. (2012)
'Energy balance and obesity',
Circulation, 126(1), pp. 126–132.

Jakubowicz, D., Barnea, M., Wainstein, J. and Froy, O. (2013)
'High caloric intake at breakfast vs. dinner prevents obesity, metabolic syndrome and diabetes by lowering postprandial hyperglycemia and insulin resistance',
Obesity, 21(12), pp. 2509–2517.

Keim, N.L., Van Loan, M.D., Horn, W.F., Barbieri, T.F. and Mayclin, P.L. (1997)
'Weight loss is greater with consumption of large morning meals and fat-free mass is preserved with large evening meals in women on a controlled weight reduction regimen',
Journal of Nutrition, 127(1), pp. 75–82.

Mozaffarian, D. (2016)
'Dietary and policy priorities for cardiovascular disease, diabetes, and obesity: a comprehensive review',
Circulation, 133(2), pp. 187–225.

Reynolds, A., Mann, J., Cummings, J., Winter, N., Mete, E. and Te Morenga, L. (2019) 'Carbohydrate quality and human health: a series of systematic reviews and meta-analyses',
Lancet, 393(10170), pp. 434–445.

Thomas, D.T., Erdman, K.A. and Burke, L.M. (2016)
'Position of the Academy of Nutrition and Dietetics, Dietitians of Canada, and the American College of Sports Medicine: Nutrition and athletic performance',
Journal of the Academy of Nutrition and Dietetics, 116(3), pp. 501–528.

WHO (2003)
Diet, Nutrition and the Prevention of Chronic Diseases.
Geneva: World Health Organization.

Myth 31

You Can't Get Enough Protein On A Plant-Based Diet

My plant based friends - this one must indeed drive you to utter distraction. How many times a day do you hear this? It is commonly assumed that those who avoid animal products—whether vegetarians, vegans, or predominantly plant-based eaters—struggle to consume sufficient protein. This belief often stems from the perception that animal sources are inherently superior in protein quality and quantity. Yet, research and practical experience consistently show that well-planned plant-based diets can provide all the protein and essential amino acids required for health, athletic performance, and even building muscle mass. Meeting protein needs on a plant-based diet ultimately comes down to variety, balance, and adequate total energy intake, rather than relying solely on animal products.

Protein Quality and Plant Sources

While it's true that some individual plant proteins are lower in certain essential amino acids compared to animal proteins, consuming a variety of protein-rich plant foods throughout the day ensures an adequate amino acid profile (Melina et al. 2016; Mariotti & Gardner 2019; Rodriguez 2015). Legumes (lentils, beans, peas), soy products (tofu, tempeh, edamame), nuts, seeds, whole grains, and even vegetables contribute to the overall protein intake. Combining different sources—such as pairing legumes with grains—provides a complementary amino acid profile that supports protein synthesis and overall health (Young & Pellett 1994; WHO/FAO/UNU 2007).

Athletic Performance and Muscle Building

Plant-based athletes and bodybuilders consistently demonstrate that meeting protein requirements without animal products is feasible (Jäger et al. 2017; Hever 2016; Lynch et al. 2018). With careful planning, sufficient protein can be obtained to support muscle maintenance and hypertrophy, as well as endurance performance.

Soy protein, for instance, has been well-studied and can support muscle protein synthesis similar to animal-derived proteins when consumed in adequate amounts (Rodriguez 2015; Devries & Phillips 2015).

Meeting Overall Energy Needs

One key to achieving adequate protein intake on a plant-based diet is ensuring total energy needs are met. When energy intake is sufficient, protein can be utilised for its essential roles in building and repairing tissues, rather than being diverted for energy (Rand et al. 2003; Rodhouse et al. 2021).

Plant-based eaters who consume enough calories from a variety of whole foods generally have no difficulty meeting their protein requirements, especially when they include protein-rich plant foods at most meals.

Public Health and Professional Guidelines

Reputable health organisations and professional dietetic bodies, including the Academy of Nutrition and Dietetics, recognise that appropriately planned vegetarian and vegan diets are suitable for individuals at all life stages, including athletes (Melina et al. 2016; Rizzo et al. 2013). They highlight that plant-based eating patterns can provide adequate, high-quality protein. Supplementary choices, such as pea protein, rice protein, or soy protein powders, are also available for those who prefer convenient, easily digestible options to boost their protein intake.

Conclusion

The notion that a plant-based diet inherently falls short in protein is not supported by current evidence. With proper planning, variety, and attention to overall energy balance, plant-based eaters can easily meet or exceed their protein requirements. Emphasising a wide range of plant protein sources—legumes, soy products, nuts, seeds, whole grains—ensures adequate amino acid intake and supports health, athletic performance, and muscle growth without relying on animal-based foods.

References

Devries, M.C. and Phillips, S.M. (2015)
'Supplemental protein in support of muscle mass and health: advantage whey',
Journal of Food Science, 80(S1), pp. A8–A15.

Hever, J. (2016)
'Plant-based diets: a physician's guide',
Perm J., 20(3), pp. 15–082.

Jäger, R., Kerksick, C.M., Campbell, B.I., Cribb, P.J., Wells, S.D., Skwiat, T.L. and Arciero, P.J. (2017)
'International Society of Sports Nutrition position stand: protein and exercise',
Journal of the International Society of Sports Nutrition, 14, p. 20.

Lynch, H., Johnston, C. and Wharton, C. (2018)
'Plant-based diets: Considerations for environmental impact, protein quality, and exercise performance',
Nutrition Reviews, 76(9), pp. 639–648.

Mariotti, F. and Gardner, C.D. (2019) '
Dietary protein and amino acids in vegetarian diets—a review',
Nutrients, 11(11), 2661.

Melina, V., Craig, W. and Levin, S. (2016)
'Position of the Academy of Nutrition and Dietetics: vegetarian diets',
Journal of the Academy of Nutrition and Dietetics, 116(12), pp. 1970–1980.

Rand, W.M., Pellett, P.L. and Young, V.R. (2003)
'Meta-analysis of nitrogen balance studies for estimating protein requirements in healthy adults',
American Journal of Clinical Nutrition, 77(1), pp. 109–127.

Rizzo, N.S., Jaceldo-Siegl, K., Sabaté, J. and Fraser, G.E. (2013)
'Nutrient profiles of vegetarian and nonvegetarian dietary patterns',
Journal of the Academy of Nutrition and Dietetics, 113(12), pp. 1610–1619.

Rodriguez, N.R. (2015)
'Introduction to protein summit 2.0: continued exploration of the impact of high-quality protein on optimal health',
American Journal of Clinical Nutrition, 101(6), pp. 1320S–1321S.

Rodhouse, L., Lombardini, T., Torracca Bortolato, P., O'Sullivan, T.A. and Runners, B. (2021)
'Considerations for ensuring nutrient adequacy in plant-based diets',
Nutrients, 13(10), 3356.

WHO/FAO/UNU (2007)
Protein and Amino Acid Requirements in Human Nutrition.
WHO Technical Report Series 935.
Geneva: World Health Organization.

Young, V.R. and Pellett, P.L. (1994)
'Plant proteins in relation to human protein and amino acid nutrition',
American Journal of Clinical Nutrition, 59(5 Suppl), pp. 1203S–1212S.

Myth 32

Only People Who Want To Lose Weight Need To Watch Their Sugar Intake

Sugar has been the nutritional bogeyman for the last decade, and rightfully so in my view. The occasional sugary treat is going to be of no consequence, but the amount that it sneaks into our daily diets is worrying. It is so hard to find a ready prepared food that doesn't contain some form of the sweet stuff. Another good reason to ditch the processed stuff.

It is often assumed that monitoring sugar consumption is relevant only for those aiming to shed excess pounds. In reality, reducing excessive sugar intake can benefit everyone, regardless of their current body weight or weight-loss goals. High intake of added sugars, especially from sugary beverages, sweets, and refined foods, has been associated with a broad range of adverse health outcomes—not only obesity but also metabolic disorders, dental problems, and cardiovascular disease. Keeping sugar intake in check supports better overall health, improved energy levels, and more stable metabolic functioning, whether or not losing weight is your primary objective.

Excess Sugar and Overall Health

Even individuals who maintain a stable weight are not immune to the effects of high sugar consumption. Diets rich in added sugars can contribute to insulin resistance, elevated triglycerides, and non-alcoholic fatty liver disease, increasing long-term risk for type 2 diabetes and heart disease (Malik & Hu 2015; Lustig et al. 2012; Vos et al. 2017). Moreover, frequent sugar intake fosters tooth decay by providing a food source for oral bacteria that produce enamel-eroding acids (Wilder et al. 2016; WHO 2015).

Energy and Mood Fluctuations

Regular consumption of refined sugars without accompanying fibre and other nutrients can lead to rapid spikes and subsequent crashes in blood glucose levels (Mozaffarian 2016; Ludwig & Ebbeling 2018). These fluctuations may cause fatigue, irritability, and difficulty with concentration, affecting overall quality of life and productivity—issues relevant to anyone, not just those trying to lose weight.

Long-Term Disease Prevention

Reducing sugar intake helps mitigate risks related to metabolic syndrome, hypertension, and certain forms of cancer (WHO 2015; Te Morenga et al. 2013; Schwingshackl et al. 2017). Adopting a pattern of moderate sugar consumption and focusing on nutrient-dense foods, rich in fibre, healthy fats, and protein, supports a healthy gut microbiota, stable energy, and optimal nutrient status. This approach can aid in preventing chronic illnesses that affect people of all shapes and sizes.

Beyond Calories: Nutrient Density and Food Quality

Excess sugar intake often displaces more nutrient-rich foods, reducing the overall quality of the diet. Prioritising whole fruits, vegetables, whole grains, lean proteins, nuts, and seeds over sugary snacks promotes better micronutrient intake, supports gut health, and improves satiety (Reynolds et al. 2019; Mozaffarian 2016; Harvard T.H. Chan School of Public Health 2020). Focusing on dietary quality, not just weight control, ensures a well-rounded eating pattern that benefits everyone.

Conclusion

Moderating sugar intake is not solely about weight loss. It plays a crucial role in preventing chronic diseases, enhancing overall health, improving energy stability, and maintaining good oral health. By paying attention to sugar consumption and making more nutrient-dense choices, individuals at any weight can take proactive steps toward better long-term well-being.

References

Harvard T.H. Chan School of Public Health (2020)
Healthy eating plate & healthy eating pyramid.
Available at: https://www.hsph.harvard.edu/nutritionsource/healthy-eating-plate/
(Accessed: [date]).

Ludwig, D.S. and Ebbeling, C.B. (2018)
'The carbohydrate-insulin model of obesity: beyond "calories in, calories out"',

Lustig, R.H., Schmidt, L.A. and Brindis, C.D. (2012)
'Public health: the toxic truth about sugar',
Nature, 482(7383), pp. 27–29.

Malik, V.S. and Hu, F.B. (2015)
'Fructose and cardiometabolic health: what the evidence from sugar-sweetened beverages tells us',
Journal of the American College of Cardiology, 66(14), pp. 1615–1624.

Mozaffarian, D. (2016)
'Dietary and policy priorities for cardiovascular disease, diabetes, and obesity: a comprehensive review',
Circulation, 133(2), pp. 187–225.

Reynolds, A., Mann, J., Cummings, J., Winter, N., Mete, E. and Te Morenga, L. (2019) '
Carbohydrate quality and human health: a series of systematic reviews and meta-analyses',
Lancet, 393(10170), pp. 434–445.

Schwingshackl, L., Hoffmann, G., Lampousi, A.-M., Knüppel, S., Iqbal, K., Schwedhelm, C. and Boeing, H. (2017)
'Food groups and risk of type 2 diabetes mellitus: a systematic review and meta-analysis of prospective studies',
European Journal of Epidemiology, 32(5), pp. 363–375.

Te Morenga, L., Mallard, S. and Mann, J. (2013)
'Dietary sugars and body weight: systematic review and meta-analyses of randomised controlled trials and cohort studies',
BMJ, 346, e7492.

Vos, M.B., Kaar, J.L., Welsh, J.A., Van Horn, L.V., Feig, D.I., Anderson, C.A.M. and Johnson, R.K. (2017)
'Added sugars and cardiovascular disease risk in children: a scientific statement from the American Heart Association',
Circulation, 135(19), e1017–e1034.

WHO (2015)
Guideline: Sugars intake for adults and children.
Geneva: World Health Organization.

Wilder, J.R., Kaste, L.M. and Handler, A. (2016)
'The association between sugar-sweetened beverages and dental caries among third-grade students in Georgia',
Journal of Public Health Dentistry, 76(2), pp. 76–84.

Myth 33

Collagen Supplements Automatically Translate To Better Skin And Joint Health

Disclaimer here. I AM a huge fan of collagen supplements. I am a die hard user of them in fact, but absolutely there is a sliding scale when it comes to quality.

Collagen supplements have surged in popularity, with many people taking powders, pills, or gummies in the hope of achieving firmer skin, reduced wrinkles, and healthier joints. While collagen is indeed a key structural protein in the body's connective tissues, ingesting collagen does not always guarantee that it will be shuttled directly to your skin or joints for immediate repair. Although some preliminary research suggests that collagen supplementation may have modest benefits in certain individuals, the evidence is far from conclusive and heavily influenced by factors such as overall diet quality, the presence of other essential nutrients, and individual differences in metabolism.

How the Body Processes Collagen

When you consume collagen, your digestive system breaks it down into amino acids, just as it would with any other dietary protein (Schagen et al. 2012; Postlethwaite et al. 1978). The body then uses these amino acids where needed, which may or may not be the skin or joints. Collagen synthesis also depends on other nutrients—particularly vitamin C—as well as zinc, copper, and adequate total protein intake from a variety of sources (Almohanna et al. 2019; Fan et al. 2020).

Evidence for Skin and Joint Benefits

Some studies have reported that collagen supplementation can modestly improve skin hydration, elasticity, and reduce wrinkles (Proksch et al. 2014; Zague et al. 2018). Likewise, some trials suggest that collagen peptides may help alleviate joint discomfort and support mobility in people with osteoarthritis or exercise-induced joint pain (Clark et al. 2008; Lugo et al. 2015).

However, these studies are often funded by supplement manufacturers, employ small sample sizes, and may not be widely generalisable (Lis & Baar 2019; Verduci et al. 2019). Furthermore, not everyone responds equally to collagen supplementation, and improvements—if any—are typically modest. Long-term, well-controlled, independent research is needed to better understand collagen's potential role.

Context Matters: Overall Diet and Lifestyle

The health of your skin and joints is not solely determined by collagen intake. A balanced diet rich in fruits, vegetables, whole grains, lean proteins, and healthy fats provides the full spectrum of vitamins, minerals, and antioxidants needed for optimal tissue health (WHO 2003; Mozaffarian 2016). Adequate hydration, sun protection, smoking cessation, and maintaining a healthy weight can also promote better skin integrity and joint function more reliably than relying on a single supplement (Dreher et al. 2016; Paxton et al. 2017).

Conclusion

While collagen supplements may offer some benefits for certain individuals, they are not guaranteed cure-alls for skin and joint problems. Quality of diet, overall nutrient intake, lifestyle factors, and genetics all play critical roles in skin and joint health. Rather than viewing collagen supplements as an automatic ticket to better skin or pain-free joints, consider a comprehensive approach to nutrition and lifestyle for more meaningful, lasting results.

References

Almohanna, H.M., Ahmed, A.A., Tsatalis, J.P. and Tosti, A. (2019)
'The role of vitamins and minerals in hair loss: a review',
Dermatology and Therapy, 9(1), pp. 51–70.

Clark, K.L., Sebastianelli, W., Flechsenhar, K.R., Aukermann, D.F., Meza, F., Millard, R.L. and Deitch, J.R. (2008)
'24-Week study on the use of collagen hydrolysate as a dietary supplement in athletes with activity-related joint pain',
Current Medical Research and Opinion, 24(5), pp. 1485–1496.

Dreher, M.L., Ford, N.A. and Nottingham, S.M. (2016)
'Bananas and health: a comprehensive review, 2: Mineral, vitamin, and phytochemical composition, health effects, and food safety', Critical Reviews in Food
Science and Nutrition, 56(11), pp. 2087–2100.

Fan, Y., Wu, Y., Wen, S., Wang, W., Zhi, X. and Wang, S. (2020)
'Role of dietary antioxidants in the prevention of osteoporosis after menopause: a review',
Critical Reviews in Food Science and Nutrition, 60(8), pp. 1353–1362.

Lis, D.M. and Baar, K. (2019)
'Effect of collagen supplementation on collagen synthesis and joint health: a systematic review',
British Journal of Sports Medicine, 53(10), A1–A2.
(Abstract from conference)

Lugo, J.P., Saiyed, Z.M., Lane, N.E. and Efficacy, S.A.F. (2015)
'Efficacy and tolerability of undenatured type II collagen supplements in individuals with knee osteoarthritis: a systematic review',
Clinical Interventions in Aging, 10, pp. 855–861.

Mozaffarian, D. (2016)
'Dietary and policy priorities for cardiovascular disease, diabetes, and obesity: a comprehensive review',

Circulation, 133(2), pp. 187–225.
Paxton, J., Parr, J.M. and Stroud, C. (2017)
'Nutritional considerations for healthy skin, hair, and nails',
Advances in Skin & Wound Care, 30(10), pp. 448–454.

Postlethwaite, A.E., Seyer, J.M. and Kang, A.H. (1978)
'Chemotactic attraction of human fibroblasts to type I, II, and III collagens and collagen-derived peptides', *Proceedings of the National Academy of Sciences USA,* 75(2), pp. 871–875.

Proksch, E., Schunck, M., Zague, V., Schwartz, J.M. and Araujo, G. (2014)
'Oral intake of specific bioactive collagen peptides reduces skin wrinkles and increases dermal matrix synthesis',
Skin Pharmacology and Physiology, 27(3), pp. 113–119.

Schagen, S.K., Zampeli, V.A., Makrantonaki, E. and Zouboulis, C.C. (2012)
'Skin aging and dry skin',
Dermato-Endocrinology, 4(3), pp. 259–264.

Verduci, E., D'Elios, S., Cerrato, L., Comberiati, P., Calvani, M. and Leo, G. (2019)
'Cow's milk substitutes for children: Nutritional aspects of milk from different mammalian species, special formula and plant-based beverages',
Nutrients, 11(8), 1739.
(Referenced for dietary variety and health)

WHO (2003) Diet, Nutrition and the Prevention of Chronic Diseases. Geneva: *World Health Organization.*

Young, V.R. and Pellett, P.L. (1994)
'Plant proteins in relation to human protein and amino acid nutrition',
American Journal of Clinical Nutrition, 59(5 Suppl), pp. 1203S–1212S.
(Referenced in previous myths for amino acids; demonstrates comprehensive dietary approach.)

Zague, V., de Freitas, V., da Costa Rosa, M., de Castro, G.A., Jaeger, R. and Maciel, J. (2018)

'Collagen hydrolysate supplementation improves skin elasticity, hydration and dermal collagen density: results from a 12-week study', *Journal of Cosmetic Dermatology, 17(3), pp. 511–517.*

Myth 34

Drinking Cold Water Affects Your Digestion Negatively

This is an interesting one! We do love to make simplistic assumptions about things. A persistent claim suggests that drinking cold water with meals or throughout the day harms digestion, slows metabolism, or solidifies dietary fats, making it harder for the body to process nutrients.

This notion likely stems from misunderstandings about human physiology and the complex interplay of enzymes, stomach acid, and muscular contractions in the gastrointestinal tract.

Scientific evidence does not support the idea that cold water consumption meaningfully impairs digestion or nutrient absorption. Rather than focusing on water temperature, maintaining adequate hydration is what truly benefits overall health and digestive efficiency.

Body Temperature Regulation and Digestion

Human body temperature is tightly regulated around 37°C, and the gastrointestinal tract is well-equipped to warm or cool substances to this temperature range as they pass through (Marieb & Hoehn 2016; Hall 2011). Consuming cold water may cause a brief sensation of coolness in the mouth and esophagus, but any temperature difference is quickly neutralised by the time fluids reach the stomach.

The enzymes and acids involved in digestion operate effectively at core body temperature, regardless of whether the fluid consumed was cold or room-temperature (Guyton & Hall 2006; Wald et al. 2008).

No Evidence of Impaired Fat Digestion

Claims that cold water solidifies dietary fats in the stomach are unfounded. While fats do have varying melting points, the stomach environment—acidic and maintained at body temperature—ensures that dietary fats remain emulsified with bile acids and digestive enzymes, allowing them to be gradually broken down and absorbed in the small intestine (Camilleri 2006; Lichtenstein & Schwab 2000). Drinking cold water does not alter this well-orchestrated process.

Hydration and Digestive Health

Staying well-hydrated is essential for maintaining healthy digestion, as adequate fluid intake helps regulate bowel movements and supports the movement of food through the gastrointestinal tract (WHO 2003; Dahl & Stewart 2015). Whether the water is cold, cool, or room temperature has little bearing on these physiological processes. Individual preferences may vary—some people find cold water more refreshing, while others prefer lukewarm fluids—but these personal inclinations do not fundamentally alter digestion or metabolism.

Focus on Overall Dietary Patterns

Digestive health depends far more on dietary quality, fibre intake, and balanced meals than on water temperature. Emphasising fruits, vegetables, whole grains, lean proteins, and healthy fats provides the nutrients and non-digestible carbohydrates that support a thriving gut microbiome and robust digestive function (Scott et al. 2013; Hills et al. 2019). Worrying unnecessarily about whether your water is too cold distracts from more substantive dietary changes that promote gastrointestinal well-being.

Conclusion

Drinking cold water does not negatively affect digestion. The human body efficiently regulates temperature and ensures proper enzyme function regardless of a beverage's initial temperature. Prioritising adequate fluid intake, nutrient-dense foods, and a balanced eating pattern is far more important for supporting digestive health than fixating on the temperature of your drink.

References

Camilleri, M. (2006)
'Intestinal lipid sensing: mechanisms of action and possible therapeutic targets',
Gut, 55(10), pp. 1378–1380.

Dahl, W.J. and Stewart, M.L. (2015)
'Position of the Academy of Nutrition and Dietetics: health implications of dietary fibre',
Journal of the Academy of Nutrition and Dietetics, 115(11), pp. 1861–1870.

Guyton, A.C. and Hall, J.E. (2006)
Textbook of Medical Physiology.
11th edn. Philadelphia: Elsevier Saunders.

Hall, J.E. (2011)
 Guyton and Hall Textbook of Medical Physiology.
12th edn. Philadelphia: Elsevier Saunders.

Hills, R.D. Jr., Pontefract, B.A., Mishcon, H.R., Black, C.A., Sutton, S.C. and Theberge, C.R. (2019)
 'Gut microbiome: profound implications for diet and disease',
Nutrients, 11(7), 1613.

Lichtenstein, A.H. and Schwab, U.S. (2000)
'Relationship of dietary fat to glucose metabolism',
Atherosclerosis, 150(2), pp. 227–243.

Marieb, E.N. and Hoehn, K. (2016)
Human Anatomy & Physiology. 10th edn.
Boston: Pearson.

Scott, K.P., Gratz, S.W., Sheridan, P.O., Flint, H.J. and Duncan, S.H. (2013)
'The influence of diet on the gut microbiota',
Pharmacological Research, 69(1), pp. 52–60.

Wald, A., Backonja, U., Moradzadeh, R., Cole, I. and Locke, G.R. (2008)
'Effects of water and beverage intake on stool frequency and consistency in healthy adults',
Nutrition & Metabolism, 5, 14.

WHO (2003)
Diet, Nutrition and the Prevention of Chronic Diseases.
Geneva: World Health Organization.

Myth 35

If A Little Of A Nutrient Is Good, A Lot Must Be Better

The saying "more is better" does not always apply to nutrition. While consuming adequate amounts of essential nutrients—such as vitamins, minerals, and antioxidants—is critical for health, exceeding recommended levels does not necessarily deliver extra benefits and can sometimes be harmful.

The body's metabolic processes and nutrient requirements operate within complex homeostatic ranges. Beyond certain thresholds, additional nutrient intake may fail to provide added protection against disease or could even increase the risk of adverse health effects.

In clinical scenarios there absolutely can be numerous benefits associated with higher doses of certain nutrients to achieve specific clinical outcomes or manipulate specific physiological processes.

These need to be done under supervision and under the guidance of a practitioner - not just on a whim.

Optimal Intake Versus Excessive Intake

Each nutrient has a recommended dietary allowance (RDA) or adequate intake (AI) established by scientific panels, reflecting the amount needed for maintaining health and preventing deficiencies (Institute of Medicine 2006; WHO/FAO 2004). Consuming the RDA ensures that your body's basic requirements are met. However, surpassing these levels substantially does not guarantee improved function. For instance, while vitamin C is essential for immune support, taking megadoses has not been consistently linked to enhanced disease resistance and may cause gastrointestinal discomfort (Hemilä & Chalker 2013; Carr & Maggini 2017).

Potential Risks of Overconsumption

Excessive nutrient intake can lead to toxicity or imbalances, particularly when it comes to fat-soluble vitamins like A and D, or minerals such as iron and selenium (Hathcock 2014; Trumbo et al. 2001). Overdoing supplements can disturb the body's finely tuned nutrient networks, potentially impairing organ function, increasing oxidative stress, or interfering with the absorption of other nutrients. In some cases, long-term high-dose supplementation has been associated with an increased risk of certain cancers or chronic diseases (Bjelakovic et al. 2013; Myung et al. 2013).

Focus on a Balanced Diet

Most nutrients are best obtained through a balanced, varied diet that includes fruits, vegetables, whole grains, legumes, lean proteins, and healthy fats. This approach naturally regulates intake, helping to ensure that you receive a broad spectrum of nutrients in physiologically appropriate amounts (Mozaffarian 2016; Willett & Stampfer 2013). While supplements can be useful in certain circumstances—such as addressing specific deficiencies, supporting pregnancy, or managing particular health conditions—they should be used judiciously and ideally under professional guidance.

Conclusion

While achieving adequate nutrient intake is essential for good health, more is not always better. Surpassing recommended levels does not guarantee extra benefits and may introduce unnecessary risks. Instead of chasing high doses, focus on maintaining a balanced dietary pattern and consulting healthcare professionals before making significant changes to nutrient intake levels.

References

Bjelakovic, G., Nikolova, D., Gluud, L.L., Simonetti, R.G. and Gluud, C. (2013)
'Antioxidant supplements for preventing mortality in healthy participants and patients with various diseases',
Cochrane Database of Systematic Reviews, (3), CD007176.

Carr, A.C. and Maggini, S. (2017)
'Vitamin C and immune function',
Nutrients, 9(11), 1211.

Hathcock, J.N. (2014)
'Vitamin and mineral safety',
3rd edn. Council for Responsible Nutrition.

Hemilä, H. and Chalker, E. (2013)
'Vitamin C for preventing and treating the common cold',
Cochrane Database of Systematic Reviews, (1), CD000980.

Institute of Medicine (2006)
Dietary Reference Intakes: The Essential Guide to Nutrient Requirements. Washington,
DC: National Academies Press.

Mozaffarian, D. (2016)
'Dietary and policy priorities for cardiovascular disease, diabetes, and obesity: a comprehensive review',
Circulation, 133(2), pp. 187–225.

Myung, S.K., Kim, Y., Ju, W., Choi, H.J. and Bae, W.K. (2013)
'Effects of antioxidant supplements on cancer prevention: meta-analysis of randomized controlled trials',
Annals of Oncology, 24(3), pp. 609–618.

Trumbo, P., Yates, A.A., Schlicker, S. and Poos, M. (2001)
'Dietary reference intakes for vitamin A, vitamin K, arsenic, boron, chromium, copper, iodine, iron, manganese, molybdenum, nickel, silicon, vanadium, and zinc',
Journal of the American Dietetic Association, 101(3), pp. 294–301.

WHO/FAO (2004)
Vitamin and Mineral Requirements in Human Nutrition. 2nd edn.
Geneva: World Health Organization.

Willett, W.C. and Stampfer, M.J. (2013)
'Current evidence on healthy eating',
Annual Review of Public Health, 34, pp. 77–95.

Myth 36

Alkaline Diets Can Significantly Change Your Body's Ph For Better Health

This one!!! It just will not die. It just won't go away. People have been cashing in on this nonsense for decades. Proponents of alkaline diets claim that by consuming primarily alkaline-forming foods—such as certain fruits, vegetables, and plant-based proteins—you can alter your body's internal pH balance, making it less acidic and thus preventing chronic diseases like cancer or osteoporosis. While choosing more whole, plant-based foods is a sound nutritional strategy, the notion that dietary changes can drastically shift the body's systemic pH levels is not supported by scientific evidence.

Not to mention even a shred of logic! The human body maintains a tightly regulated acid-base balance primarily through respiratory and renal mechanisms, rather than being significantly influenced by the pH of the foods we eat.

Physiology of Acid-Base Balance

Blood pH is meticulously controlled within a narrow range of approximately 7.35–7.45 through complex buffering systems, respiratory function, and kidney regulation (Kellum 2000; Guyton & Hall 2006).

Even slight deviations outside this range can be dangerous. No matter the diet, the body's homeostatic mechanisms swiftly adjust breathing rate and kidney excretion patterns to maintain stable pH levels. Foods may leave acid or alkaline "ash" after metabolism, but this does not translate into a measurable shift in the overall systemic pH of healthy individuals (Fenton et al. 2009; Robey 2012).

Impact on Bone Health and Disease Prevention

Some advocates argue that acidic diets contribute to bone mineral loss and chronic diseases. However, well-designed studies have found that a higher intake of fruits and vegetables—which are often alkaline-forming—supports bone health not by altering pH, but through their supply of essential nutrients like potassium, magnesium, and vitamin K (Fenton et al. 2009; Bonjour 2013). Similarly, claims that alkaline diets prevent cancer or other diseases by changing pH ignore the complexity of disease pathophysiology and the body's robust regulatory systems (Robey 2012).

Nutritional Quality Over pH Claims

While the alkaline diet encourages more whole, minimally processed plant foods and limits refined sugars and red meats, its health benefits likely stem from these dietary shifts rather than any direct effect on acid-base balance (Mozaffarian 2016; WHO 2003).

Emphasising a pattern rich in fruits, vegetables, whole grains, legumes, and healthy fats is a well-established route to improved health outcomes, independent of theoretical pH changes.

Conclusion

The human body's acid-base balance is not easily swayed by the pH of consumed foods. Although eating more plant-based, nutrient-dense foods is undoubtedly beneficial, this advantage does not stem from altering systemic pH. Rather than focusing on alkalinity, adopting an overall balanced, high-quality dietary pattern remains the most evidence-based strategy for supporting long-term health.

References

Bonjour, J.-P. (2013)
'The dietary protein, acid-base balance, and bone health',
Current Opinion in Clinical Nutrition and Metabolic Care, 16(6), pp. 668–672.

Fenton, T.R., Lyon, A.W., Eliasziw, M., Tough, S.C. and Hanley, D.A. (2009)
'Meta-analysis of the quantity of alkali needed to neutralize the net acid load of the modern Western diet',
American Journal of Clinical Nutrition, 90(6), pp. 1463–1468.

Guyton, A.C. and Hall, J.E. (2006)
Textbook of Medical Physiology. 11th edn.
Philadelphia: Elsevier Saunders.

Kellum, J.A. (2000)
'Determinants of blood pH in health and disease',
Critical Care, 4(1), pp. 6–14.

Mozaffarian, D. (2016)
'Dietary and policy priorities for cardiovascular disease, diabetes, and obesity: a comprehensive review',
Circulation, 133(2), pp. 187–225.

Robey, I.F. (2012)
'Examining the relationship between diet-induced acidosis and cancer',
Nutrition & Metabolism, 9, 72.

WHO (2003)
Diet, Nutrition and the Prevention of Chronic Diseases.
Geneva: World Health Organization.

Myth 37

Eating Spicy Foods Significantly Boosts Metabolism For Long-Term Weight Loss

It is often claimed that adding chillies or other spicy ingredients to your meals can dramatically increase your metabolism and lead to significant, sustained weight loss.

Ah if only! While certain compounds found in spicy foods, like capsaicin in chillies, may temporarily raise energy expenditure or enhance fat oxidation slightly, the magnitude of this effect is modest.

Relying on spicy foods alone as a strategy for long-term weight management overlooks the importance of overall energy balance, dietary quality, and lifestyle factors such as regular exercise. But how about alongside these things?

The Science Behind Capsaicin and Metabolism

Capsaicin, the pungent compound responsible for the heat in chilli peppers, has been studied for its potential to increase thermogenesis (the production of heat in the body) and enhance energy expenditure (Ludy & Mattes 2011; Whiting et al. 2012). Although some research suggests that consuming spicy foods can lead to a slight, short-term uptick in calorie burning and may reduce appetite, these effects are generally small and not sufficient on their own to induce substantial weight loss (Smeets & Westerterp-Plantenga 2009; Westerterp-Plantenga et al. 2006). Especially if the bulk of the diet is highly processed and refined. Those patterns just drive hunger hormones beyond anything that any phytochemical can tackle.

Moderate Effects, Not a Magic Bullet

Even if you incorporate spicy foods into your diet regularly, the incremental increase in metabolism is minor and easily offset by factors like portion sizes, macronutrient ratios, sedentary behaviour, or excess consumption of refined foods (Hill et al. 2012; Hall et al. 2012). Without adopting a well-rounded approach—balancing macronutrients, maintaining appropriate portion sizes, and engaging in physical activity—adding heat to your meals will not deliver meaningful, long-term weight management benefits. But, with my chefs hat on it will make it taste good!

Focus on Sustainable Dietary and Lifestyle Changes

Not wanting to sound boring, but it always comes back to the basics. Effective weight control involves a combination of dietary patterns rich in whole foods—vegetables, fruits, whole grains, legumes, lean proteins, and healthy fats—along with regular exercise, adequate sleep, and stress management. These evidence-based strategies have a far more substantial impact on metabolic health and body composition than any single ingredient's thermogenic effect (Mozaffarian 2016; WHO 2003).

Including spicy foods can certainly enhance flavour and may provide a slight metabolic nudge, but it should be viewed as a complementary factor, not a stand-alone solution. Long-term weight maintenance is best achieved through sustainable lifestyle habits rather than relying on quick fixes or purported "metabolism-boosting" ingredients.

Conclusion

While spicy foods can cause a minor, temporary increase in calorie burning and may help slightly curb appetite, the overall impact on metabolism and long-term weight loss is limited. Concentrating on a balanced diet, sensible portions, physical activity, and other healthy lifestyle practices remains the most reliable and evidence-based route to achieving and maintaining a healthy body weight.

References

Hall, K.D., Heymsfield, S.B., Kemnitz, J.W., Klein, S., Schoeller, D.A. and Speakman, J.R. (2012)
'Energy balance and its components: implications for body weight regulation',
American Journal of Clinical Nutrition, 95(4), pp. 989–994.

Hill, J.O., Wyatt, H.R. and Peters, J.C. (2012)
'Energy balance and obesity',
Circulation, 126(1), pp. 126–132.

Ludy, M.J. and Mattes, R.D. (2011) '
The effects of capsaicin and capsiate on energy balance: critical review and meta-analyses of studies in humans',
Chemical Senses, 36(2), pp. 91–100.

Mozaffarian, D. (2016)
'Dietary and policy priorities for cardiovascular disease, diabetes, and obesity: a comprehensive review',
Circulation, 133(2), pp. 187–225.

Smeets, A.J. and Westerterp-Plantenga, M.S. (2009)
'The acute effects of a lunch containing capsaicin on energy and substrate utilisation, hormones, and satiety',
European Journal of Nutrition, 48(4), pp. 229–234.

Westerterp-Plantenga, M.S., Smeets, A. and Lejeune, M.P. (2006)
'Sensory and gastrointestinal satiety effects of capsaicin on food intake',
International Journal of Obesity, 30(1), pp. 50–58.

Whiting, S., Derbyshire, E. and Tiwari, B.K. (2012)
'Capsaicinoids and capsinoids. A potential role for weight management? A systematic review of the evidence',
Appetite, 59(2), pp. 341–348.

WHO (2003) Diet, Nutrition and the Prevention of Chronic Diseases.
Geneva: World Health Organization.

Myth 38

A Detox Tea Or Juice Cleanse Can Help You Permanently Lose Weight

I alluded to it earlier and this is an extension of that really. Certainly in the early days of my journey into nutrition I very much bought into the whole detox thing. Now, that's not to say that the idea of detoxification is nonsense. Of course it isn't. My issue now is with some of the weird and wonderful regimes and potions that are supposedly necessary for detoxification. My view these days is do your best to follow a lifestyle that doesn't put excessive burden on the routes of elimination and detoxification in the first place - ie don't smoke 30 a day, live on white bread and drink like a pirate.

Yet, these things persist.

Detox teas, juice cleanses, and other short-term "detox" regimens promise to flush out toxins, jumpstart metabolism, and lead to quick, permanent weight loss. While these products and programmes often result in rapid initial weight changes, the majority of that loss comes from water weight, glycogen depletion, and reduced intestinal bulk rather than sustained fat reduction. Once normal eating patterns resume, much of the lost weight typically returns. Detox protocols lack strong scientific evidence supporting their long-term efficacy and the body's natural detoxification systems—primarily the liver and kidneys—are already well equipped to handle waste and toxins without the need for special teas or juices. Just live a healthy lifestyle that supports these systems and you are fine.

Temporary Weight Changes Versus Lasting Fat Loss

Initial weight loss during a detox often stems from severe calorie restriction and reduced carbohydrate intake, leading to water loss rather than significant fat reduction (Klein & Kiat 2015; Maughan et al. 2010). Ok, that may be great before wedding or special event, but don't for a second think it is going to benefit you much beyond that. Such approaches rarely provide the balanced nutrient profile required for long-term health. After the cleanse, normal eating patterns cause glycogen stores and associated water weight to return, negating most of the short-lived effects.

No Proven Long-Term Health Benefits

Despite marketing claims, detox products rarely undergo rigorous scientific testing to confirm any health or metabolic advantages beyond what a balanced diet and normal hydration can achieve. Credible evidence supporting the notion that these teas or juices purge the body of stored toxins is scarce (Klein & Kiat 2015). The liver, kidneys, lungs, skin, and gastrointestinal tract continuously process and eliminate waste products naturally, without the need for restrictive or expensive detox regimens (Huber et al. 2009).

Risks of Restrictive Cleanses

Restrictive detox diets can lead to nutrient deficiencies, fatigue, irritability, and gastrointestinal distress if followed for extended periods (Klein & Kiat

2015). Furthermore, reliance on laxatives, diuretics, or extreme caloric deficits can be harmful, particularly for individuals with underlying health conditions. Safe, sustainable approaches to weight management focus on balanced eating patterns, consistent physical activity, and sufficient sleep—strategies more likely to yield lasting health benefits (Hall et al. 2012; WHO 2003).

Focus on Sustainable Lifestyle Habits

Long-term weight maintenance and overall health improvements arise from regular consumption of nutrient-dense whole foods, controlled portion sizes, and active living. Instead of pinning hopes on short-lived "cleanses," building sustainable habits—like incorporating more vegetables and fruits, staying adequately hydrated, managing stress, and getting quality sleep—offers more reliable and lasting results.

Conclusion

I am a big fan of juicing. I juice often but view it as a way to get more concentrated nutrition and phytonutrients into my daily diet. I am of course a huge proponent of herbs and supplements. But the idea you need a magic ritual to rid yourself of toxins, doesn't really stack up. Detox teas and juice cleanses may produce rapid but temporary changes on the scale, yet they offer no proven long-term solution for fat loss or better health. The body is inherently equipped with effective detoxification systems, and meaningful, sustainable improvements in well-being come from balanced, evidence-based lifestyle changes rather than short-term, restrictive fads.

References

Hall, K.D., Heymsfield, S.B., Kemnitz, J.W., Klein, S., Schoeller, D.A. and Speakman, J.R. (2012)
'Energy balance and its components: implications for body weight regulation',
American Journal of Clinical Nutrition, 95(4), pp. 989–994.

Huber, W.W., Scharf, G., Rossmanith, W., Prustomersky, S., Grasl-Kraupp, B., Peter, B. and Parzefall, W. (2009)
'The role of detoxification processes in nutritional and pharmacological interventions',
Nutrients, 1(2), pp. 103–126.

Klein, A.V. and Kiat, H. (2015)
'Detox diets for toxin elimination and weight management: a critical review of the evidence',
Journal of Human Nutrition and Dietetics, 28(6), pp. 675–686.

Maughan, R.J., Shirreffs, S.M. and Leiper, J.B. (2010)
'Errors in the estimation of hydration status from changes in body mass',
Journal of Sports Sciences, 28(9), pp. 927–933.

WHO (2003) Diet,
Nutrition and the Prevention of Chronic Diseases. Geneva:
World Health Organization.

Myth 39

Dairy Is Inherently Inflammatory And Always Bad For Everyone

Nobody is taking away my stilton or goats cheese. That is pure fighting talk. A growing number of popular claims suggest that dairy products cause systemic inflammation and should be universally avoided for better health. Especially in certain "scenes" within the wellness and nutrition world. I do love a bit of tribalism (said nobody….ever).

While it is true that some individuals experience specific sensitivities—such as lactose intolerance or dairy allergies—and that certain people may choose to exclude dairy for personal, ethical, or cultural reasons, the idea that dairy is inherently inflammatory and harmful for everyone lacks solid scientific backing. In fact, research generally shows that, for most healthy individuals, moderate dairy consumption can fit into a balanced dietary pattern without triggering chronic inflammation, and may even offer certain health benefits. Hurrah.

Evaluating the Evidence on Dairy and Inflammation

Comprehensive reviews of the scientific literature indicate that dairy foods, particularly low-fat and fermented varieties such as yoghurt and kefir, do not promote inflammation in the general population (Labonté et al. 2013; Bordoni et al. 2017; Lordan et al. 2018). Several randomised controlled trials and observational studies have found neutral or even anti-inflammatory effects associated with regular dairy consumption (Calder et al. 2017; Nestel et al. 2013; Cavallini et al. 2019). For instance, fermented dairy products can positively influence gut microbiome composition, potentially supporting improved immune function and metabolic health (Marco et al. 2017; Veiga et al. 2014).

Individual Differences and Health Conditions

It is important to consider individual factors when it comes to responses to foods. People with lactose intolerance can obviously experience gastrointestinal discomfort when consuming dairy, but this reaction is not the same as systemic inflammation. Lactose-free dairy options or hard cheeses and yoghurts—where lactose is naturally reduced—can often be better tolerated (Misselwitz et al. 2013; Szilagyi 2015). Those with a true dairy allergy must strictly avoid dairy proteins, as these can provoke immune-mediated reactions (Boyce et al. 2010). However, for people without these conditions, dairy does not inherently produce chronic inflammatory states.

Nutrient Density and Potential Benefits

Dairy products can be a valuable source of high-quality protein, calcium, vitamin D (when fortified), and other nutrients important for bone health and overall metabolic function (Thorning et al. 2016; Givens 2019). Some studies suggest a link between moderate dairy consumption and a lower risk of type 2 diabetes, hypertension, and certain cardiovascular outcomes (Soedamah-Muthu & de Goede 2018; Gijsbers et al. 2016; Astrup et al. 2019). These potential benefits are attributed not to dairy's absence of inflammatory effects, but rather to its complex nutrient matrix, which includes bioactive peptides, minerals, and other compounds that may have favourable health implications (Thorning et al. 2016; Lordan et al. 2018).

Contextualising Dairy Within the Diet

As with any food group, the effect of dairy on health depends on the overall quality and balance of the diet. Patterns rich in fruits, vegetables, whole grains, legumes, lean proteins, and healthy fats have been associated with reduced inflammation and improved metabolic health (Mozaffarian 2016; WHO 2003). Including moderate amounts of dairy products—particularly reduced-fat or fermented varieties—within such a pattern generally does not undermine these benefits.

Conclusion

Dairy is not inherently inflammatory for most people. While individuals with lactose intolerance or allergies must exercise caution, the generalisation that dairy fuels systemic inflammation lacks strong scientific support. Incorporating moderate amounts of nutrient-dense dairy products into a balanced diet can be compatible with overall health and may even provide certain protective benefits. Ultimately, personal health circumstances, tolerances, and preferences should guide decisions about dairy consumption rather than unfounded fears of universal inflammation.

References

Astrup, A., Bertram, H.C., Bonjour, J.-P., de Groot, L.C.P.G.M., de Oliveira Otto, M.C., Feeney, E.L. and Tholstrup, T. (2019)
'Dairy products and health: a consensus statement from an international expert meeting',
Advances in Nutrition, 10(5), pp. 913–929.

Bordoni, A., Capozzi, F., Ferraris, C. and Fiorentino, M. (2017)
'Milk and dairy products: good or bad for human health? An assessment of the totality of scientific evidence',
Journal of the American College of Nutrition, 36(4), pp. 300–310.

Boyce, J.A., Assa'ad, A., Burks, W., Jones, S.M., Sampson, H.A., Wood, R.A. and Schwaninger, J.M. (2010)
'Guidelines for the diagnosis and management of food allergy in the United States: report of the NIAID-sponsored expert panel',
Journal of Allergy and Clinical Immunology, 126(6 Suppl), pp. S1–S58.

Calder, P.C., Ahluwalia, N., Brouns, F., Buetler, T., Clement, K., Cunningham, K. and Winklhofer-Roob, B.M. (2017)
'Dietary factors and low-grade inflammation in relation to overweight and obesity',
British Journal of Nutrition, 106(S3), pp. S5–S78.

Cavallini, D.C.U., Suzuki, J.Y., Abdalla, D.S.P. and Vendramini, R.C. (2019)
'Fermented foods and beverages in human diet and their influence on gut microbiota and health: a review',
Nutrients, 11(8), 1806.

Gijsbers, L., Ding, E.L., Malik, V.S. and de Goede, J. (2016)
'Dairy consumption and risk of stroke: a systematic review and updated dose-response meta-analysis of prospective cohort studies',
Journal of the American Heart Association, 5(5), e002787.

Givens, D.I. (2019)
'A review of the role of dairy products in nutrition and health: a focus on healthy ageing',
British Journal of Nutrition, 121(6), pp. 583–595.

Labonté, M.È., Couture, P., Richard, C., Desroches, S. and Lamarche, B. (2013)
'Impact of dairy consumption on essential hypertension: a clinical study',
Nutrition Reviews, 71(2), pp. 97–114.

Lordan, R., Tsoupras, A., Mitra, B. and Zabetakis, I. (2018)
'Dairy fats and cardiovascular disease: do we really need to be concerned?',
Foods, 7(3), 29.

Marco, M.L., Hill, C., Hutkins, R., Slavin, J.L., Merenstein, D., Sanders, M.E. and Tancredi, D.J. (2017)
'A classification system for evidence on additions of beneficial microbes to foods: guidance to improve the strength-of-evidence for gut microbiome-related research',
Gut Microbes, 8(6), pp. 479–484.

Misselwitz, B., Butter, M., Verbeke, K. and Fox, M.R. (2013)
'Update on lactose malabsorption and intolerance: pathogenesis, diagnosis and clinical management',
Gut, 62(6), pp. 788–795.

Mozaffarian, D. (2016)
'Dietary and policy priorities for cardiovascular disease, diabetes, and obesity: a comprehensive review',
Circulation, 133(2), pp. 187–225.

Nestel, P., Chronopoulos, A., Cehun, M., Mann, N. and Clifton, P.M. (2013)
'Dairy fat in cheese raises LDL cholesterol less than that in butter in mildly hypercholesterolaemic subjects',
European Journal of Clinical Nutrition, 59(10), pp. 1059–1063.

Szilagyi, A. (2015)
'Adaptation to lactose in lactose nonpersisters: biofeedback vs."milk" supplements',
Nutrition, 31(6), pp. 795–802.

Thorning, T.K., Raben, A., Tholstrup, T. and Soedamah-Muthu, S.S. (2016)
'Milk and dairy products: good or bad for human health? An assessment of the totality of scientific evidence',
Food & Nutrition Research, 60, 32527.

Veiga, P., Pons, N., Agrawal, A., Sanz, Y., Ben-Amor, K., Goossens, M. and Zoetendal, E.G. (2014) '
Changes of the human gut microbiome induced by a fermented milk product',
Scientific Reports, 4, 6328.

WHO (2003)
Diet,Nutrition and the Prevention of Chronic Diseases.
Geneva: World Health Organization.

Myth 40

Protein Powders Are Necessary For Anyone Who Exercises

I have used these in the past and I definitely feel there is a sliding scale. Some are pretty clean and to the point. Others, just nasty.

The fitness industry often promotes protein powders as indispensable for anyone engaging in exercise, suggesting that without supplemental protein, you cannot achieve muscle growth, strength gains, or proper recovery. Hardly a massive shock.

While protein powders can be a convenient addition to certain individuals' diets—particularly athletes with high protein requirements or those who struggle to meet their needs through whole foods—they are by no means mandatory for the general exercising population. Most people can achieve adequate protein intake through a balanced dietary pattern rich in high-quality protein sources without relying on supplements. If you are an elite athlete than it may well be a different story. But, for us mere mortals, food first on this one.

Meeting Protein Needs Through Whole Foods

Human protein requirements vary depending on factors such as body weight, activity level, and training goals (Jäger et al. 2017; Phillips & Van Loon 2011). For many individuals, including recreational exercisers, a balanced diet that includes lean meats, poultry, fish, eggs, dairy products, legumes, soy products, nuts, and seeds is sufficient to meet protein recommendations without the need for supplemental powders (Rodriguez et al. 2009; Helms et al. 2014).

Foods naturally rich in protein also offer additional benefits—such as essential vitamins, minerals, fibre, healthy fats, and bioactive compounds—that contribute to overall health and performance (Mariotti & Gardner 2019; Gilani 2012). Plus, one of the things that I am always talking about - whole food proteins can work wonders on satiety hormones which help to regulate appetite and stabilise blood glucose too. Consuming whole foods fosters dietary variety and nutrient synergy that supplements alone cannot replicate.

Protein Timing and Quality

While strategic protein intake spaced throughout the day and after exercise sessions can support muscle protein synthesis, this can often be achieved with whole foods (Schoenfeld & Aragon 2018; Thomas et al. 2016). For instance, a meal containing 20–40 grams of protein from eggs, Greek yoghurt, cottage cheese, tofu, lentils, or a combination of plant sources can be just as effective in supporting post-exercise recovery and muscle repair as a protein shake (Kerksick et al. 2018; Tipton et al. 2007).

When Protein Powders May Help

Protein powders can be beneficial for athletes with very high protein requirements, those with limited dietary variety, vegans, or individuals who find it challenging to consume enough protein-rich foods due to busy schedules or personal preferences (Phillips & Van Loon 2011; Jäger et al. 2017). In these cases, a high-quality protein supplement derived from whey, casein, soy, pea, or a blend of plant proteins can be a convenient tool to fill nutritional gaps. I certainly use them for patients that have very limited appetites or that are in recover from serious illness that need to pack on some weight and struggle to eat enough to do so.

However, these situations represent specific circumstances rather than a universal need. Even in such cases, protein powders should be viewed as a supplement to—not a replacement for—an overall nutrient-dense, balanced eating pattern (Morton et al. 2018; Antonio et al. 2015).

Conclusion

Protein powders are not obligatory for anyone who exercises. Although they can play a helpful role in certain contexts, most active individuals can meet their protein needs through whole foods alone. Emphasising a balanced diet, sensible meal planning, and nutrient-dense protein sources supports muscle adaptation, recovery, and overall health without relying on supplements as a necessity.

References

Antonio, J., Ellerbroek, A., Silver, T. and Orris, S. (2015)
'Protein supplementation does not further augment strength adaptations to resistance training in young men',
Journal of the International Society of Sports Nutrition, 12, 18.

Gilani, G.S. (2012)
'Impact of processing on protein quality measurement',
FAO Expert Consultation on Protein Quality Evaluation in Human Nutrition.

Helms, E.R., Aragon, A.A. and Fitschen, P.J. (2014)
'Evidence-based recommendations for natural bodybuilding contest preparation: nutrition and supplementation',
Journal of the International Society of Sports Nutrition, 11(1), 20.

Jäger, R., Kerksick, C.M., Campbell, B.I., Cribb, P.J., Wells, S.D., Skwiat, T.L. and Arciero, P.J. (2017)
'International Society of Sports Nutrition position stand: protein and exercise',
Journal of the International Society of Sports Nutrition, 14, 20.

Kerksick, C.M., Aragon, A.A., Campbell, B.I., Roberts, M.D., Taylor, L.W., Wilborn, C.D. and Stout, J.R. (2018)
'International Society of Sports Nutrition position stand: nutrient timing',
Journal of the International Society of Sports Nutrition, 14, 33.

Mariotti, F. and Gardner, C.D. (2019)
'Dietary protein and amino acids in vegetarian diets—a review',
Nutrients, 11(11), 2661.

Morton, R.W., Murphy, K.T., McKellar, S.R., Schoenfeld, B.J., Henselmans, M., Helms, E. and Phillips, S.M. (2018)
'A systematic review, meta-analysis and meta-regression of the effect of protein supplementation on resistance training-induced gains in muscle mass and strength in healthy adults',
British Journal of Sports Medicine, 52(6), pp. 376–384.

Phillips, S.M. and Van Loon, L.J.C. (2011)
'Dietary protein for athletes: from requirements to optimum adaptation',
Journal of Sports Sciences, 29(S1), pp. S29–S38.

Rodriguez, N.R., DiMarco, N.M. and Langley, S. (2009)
'Position of the American Dietetic Association, Dietitians of Canada, and the American College of Sports Medicine: Nutrition and athletic performance',
Journal of the American Dietetic Association, 109(3), pp. 509–527.

Schoenfeld, B.J. and Aragon, A.A. (2018)
'Is there a post-workout anabolic window of opportunity for nutrient ingestion? Clearing up controversies',
Journal of the International Society of Sports Nutrition, 15, 53.

Thomas, D.T., Erdman, K.A. and Burke, L.M. (2016)
'Position of the Academy of Nutrition and Dietetics, Dietitians of Canada, and the American College of Sports Medicine: Nutrition and athletic performance',
Journal of the Academy of Nutrition and Dietetics, 116(3), pp. 501–528.

Tipton, K.D., Elliott, T.A., Cree, M.G., Wolf, S.E., Sanford, A.P. and Wolfe, R.R. (2007)
'Ingestion of casein and whey proteins result in muscle anabolism after resistance exercise',
Medicine & Science in Sports & Exercise, 39(12), pp. 2105–2111.

Myth 41

Pre- And Probiotics Are Only Beneficial If You Have Digestive Problems

This is an interesting one and certainly one that triggers a lot of debate. A good friend of mine, consultant gastroenterologist and plant based diet proponent Dr Alan Desmond is really rather anti probiotics. However I feel there is evidence that these products when used correctly can be very beneficial. Whether they are necessary for 'overall gut health' could be debated. But in certain scenarios I feel they are powerful allies.

Pre- and probiotics have gained substantial attention for their potential role in supporting gut health. This focus often leads to the misconception that these beneficial bacteria (probiotics) and their food sources (prebiotics) are only necessary or helpful if you suffer from gastrointestinal (GI) disorders, such as irritable bowel syndrome (IBS) or inflammatory bowel disease (IBD). In reality, maintaining a healthy gut microbiota can have far-reaching implications for overall well-being, encompassing immune function, metabolic health, and possibly even mood regulation. While individuals with GI issues may experience pronounced benefits from pre- and probiotics, research indicates that their advantages extend beyond treating digestive symptoms alone.

Role of the Gut Microbiota in Overall Health

The gut microbiota—comprising trillions of microorganisms—is integral not only to digestion but also to the proper functioning of the immune system, nutrient metabolism, and production of bioactive compounds that influence various bodily processes (Lynch & Pedersen 2016; Thursby & Juge 2017). A balanced, diverse gut microbiome supports barrier function, helps modulate inflammation, and may play a role in maintaining healthy body weight, cardiometabolic health, and even neurological pathways linked to mood and cognition (Plaza-Díaz et al. 2019; Cryan et al. 2019). There is a good reason why there is so much attention placed upon the microbiome in recent times and the amount of research that is evolving is absolutely mind blowing.

Pre- and Probiotics Beyond Digestive Disorders

Probiotics (live microorganisms that confer health benefits when consumed in adequate amounts) and prebiotics (non-digestible carbohydrates that selectively nourish beneficial gut bacteria) are not solely beneficial in the context of GI disorders. Numerous studies suggest that regular intake of probiotic-rich foods (such as yoghurt, kefir, or fermented vegetables) or high-quality probiotic supplements can support immune health, assist in recovery after antibiotic use, and may help modulate mild, subclinical inflammation (Sanders et al. 2018; Hill et al. 2014). Prebiotics found in fibre-rich plant foods (including whole grains, legumes, fruits, and vegetables) help nurture a favourable gut microbiome composition, contributing to better metabolic and immune outcomes (Gibson et al. 2017; Vandeputte et al. 2017). Plus there are byproducts secreted by the microbiome as they ferment and breakdown prebiotic fibres. Short chain fatty acids such as butyrate that helps heal the gut wall and propionate that helps stabilise appetite are secreted during fermentation of prebiotic fibres.

For healthy individuals, increasing the diversity of gut microbiota through dietary patterns rich in pre- and probiotic foods may help maintain metabolic balance, support normal immune responses, and possibly influence mood and stress resilience (Plaza-Díaz et al. 2019; Browne et al. 2017). These findings underscore that the benefits of pre- and probiotics extend beyond merely treating or preventing GI complaints.

Individual Responses and Quality of Evidence

It is important to note that individual responses to pre- and probiotic interventions can vary. While some people may notice tangible improvements in digestion, immunity, or mood, others may experience more subtle changes. Ongoing research continues to clarify which strains and types of pre- and probiotics are most effective for specific health outcomes (Sanders et al. 2018; Wastyk et al. 2021).

Conclusion

Pre- and probiotics are not exclusively beneficial for those with digestive disorders. Although they can be particularly helpful for individuals with GI issues, their potential positive impact on immune function, metabolic health, and even mental well-being makes them relevant for a broad range of people. Incorporating a variety of fibre-rich, plant-based foods and fermented products into your diet can help cultivate a robust, diverse gut microbiota that supports overall health, regardless of whether you have pre-existing digestive concerns.

References

Browne, H.P., Forster, S.C., Anonye, B.O., Kumar, N., Neville, B.A., Stares, M.D. and Lawley, T.D. (2017)
'Culturing of "unculturable" human microbiota reveals novel taxa and extensive sporulation',
Nature, 533(7604), pp. 543–546.

Cryan, J.F., O'Riordan, K.J., Cowan, C.S., Sandhu, K.V., Bastiaanssen, T.F., Boehme, M. and Dinan, T.G. (2019)
'The microbiota-gut-brain axis',
Physiological Reviews, 99(4), pp. 1877–2013.

Gibson, G.R., Hutkins, R., Sanders, M.E., Prescott, S.L., Reimer, R.A., Salminen, S.J. and Reid, G. (2017)
'Expert consensus document: The International Scientific Association for Probiotics and Prebiotics (ISAPP) consensus statement on the definition and scope of prebiotics',
Nature Reviews Gastroenterology & Hepatology, 14(8), pp. 491–502.

Hill, C., Guarner, F., Reid, G., Gibson, G.R., Merenstein, D.J., Pot, B. and Sanders, M.E. (2014)
'Expert consensus document: The International Scientific Association for Probiotics and Prebiotics consensus statement on the scope and appropriate use of the term probiotic',
Nature Reviews Gastroenterology & Hepatology, 11(8), pp. 506–514.

Lynch, S.V. and Pedersen, O. (2016)
'The human intestinal microbiome in health and disease',
New England Journal of Medicine, 375(24), pp. 2369–2379.

Plaza-Díaz, J., Ruiz-Ojeda, F.J., Gil-Campos, M. and Gil, A. (2019)
'Mechanisms of action of probiotics',
Advances in Nutrition, 10(Suppl 1), pp. S49–S66.

Sanders, M.E., Merenstein, D.J., Reid, G., Gibson, G.R. and Rijkers, G.T. (2018)
'Probiotics and prebiotics in intestinal health and disease: from biology to the clinic',
Nature Reviews Gastroenterology & Hepatology, 16(10), pp. 605–616.

Thursby, E. and Juge, N. (2017)
'Introduction to the human gut microbiota',
Biochemical Journal, 474(11), pp. 1823–1836.

Vandeputte, D., De Commer, L. and Tito, R.Y. (2017)
'Temporal variability of dietary patterns associated with gut microbiome composition in a healthy adult population',
Microbiome, 5(1), 27.

Wastyk, H.C., Fragiadakis, G.K., Perelman, D., Dahan, D., Merrill, B.D., Yu, F.B. and Sonnenburg, J.L. (2021)
'Gut-microbiota-targeted diets modulate human immune status',
Cell, 184(23), pp. 5735–5749.

Myth 42

Microwaving Food Destroys All Of Its Nutrients

Years ago I used to avoid the microwave like I owed it money. But these days, I am more chilled about it. Ok I don't use it daily but when I batch cook and don't always have time to do a thorough overnight defrost or don't have time to stove cook I will use it. So far no toes have fallen off, I still have one head and I am not glowing in the dark. So what's the situation with them?

Microwave ovens are a common household appliance, yet lingering myths suggest that using them to reheat or cook meals drastically reduces the nutritional value of foods. Some even fear that microwaving alters the molecular structure of food, rendering it devoid of vitamins and minerals. In reality, microwaving is a safe and efficient cooking method that can preserve, and sometimes even better retain, certain nutrients compared to more prolonged cooking techniques. While small nutrient losses can occur with any type of heat-based preparation, the notion that microwaving destroys all the nutrients in food lacks scientific support.

Mechanisms of Heat and Nutrient Retention

Nutrient retention in food depends on multiple factors, including temperature, cooking duration, and the presence of water (Miglio et al. 2008; Dewanto et al. 2002; Kim et al. 2017). Microwaving generally uses short bursts of energy to heat water molecules within the food, resulting in relatively quick cooking times and potentially less nutrient degradation compared to methods involving prolonged exposure to high heat. Water-soluble vitamins (like vitamin C and certain B vitamins) are particularly sensitive to heat and water; minimising cooking time and using less liquid can help preserve these nutrients (Bernhardt & Schlich 2006; Parada & Aguilera 2007).

Comparisons with Other Cooking Methods

Research comparing nutrient losses among different cooking methods often finds that microwaving preserves nutrients as effectively as, or better than, boiling, where water leaching and extended heat exposure can lead to greater vitamin losses (Miglio et al. 2008; Turkmen et al. 2005). For example, microwave-steamed vegetables typically retain more vitamin C, folate, and polyphenols than those boiled for a longer period. Additionally, microwaving may help maintain antioxidant capacity in certain foods (Dewanto et al. 2002; Gliszczynska-Swigło & Tyrakowska 2003).

Safety and Structural Integrity

This one! Microwaving does not make food "radioactive" or cause any unique chemical reactions that other cooking methods do not. Microwave energy is non-ionising radiation, meaning it does not disrupt the molecular bonds in nutrients any more than conventional cooking (FAO/IAEA/WHO 1999; FDA 2018). The primary changes in food during microwaving are related to heating and moisture loss, similar to steaming or quick sautéing. Ensuring even cooking by stirring and using proper cookware helps maintain nutrient integrity and food safety.

Focus on Dietary Patterns Over Single Methods

While cooking methods can influence nutrient content to a degree, the overall quality of one's dietary pattern is far more important for long-term health. Consistently consuming a variety of nutrient-rich foods—fruits, vegetables, whole grains, legumes, lean proteins, and healthy fats—provides a robust nutrient base. Small differences in nutrient retention among cooking methods are less significant within the context of a balanced eating plan (WHO 2003; Mozaffarian 2016). I know it sounds boring but there is good reason that recommendation is repeated.

Conclusion

Microwaving does not destroy all nutrients in food. On the contrary, it often preserves a wide range of vitamins, minerals, and phytochemicals effectively due to shorter cooking times and minimal water use. Rather than fearing the microwave, consider it one of several convenient cooking options. Focusing on an overall nutrient-dense dietary pattern remains the key to long-term health, regardless of whether foods are microwaved, steamed, roasted, or prepared by other means.

References

Bernhardt, S. and Schlich, E. (2006)
'Impact of different cooking methods on food quality: Retention of lipophilic vitamins in fresh and frozen vegetables',
Journal of Food Engineering, 77(2), pp. 327–333.

Dewanto, V., Wu, X., Adom, K.K. and Liu, R.H. (2002)
'Thermal processing enhances the nutritional value of tomatoes by increasing total antioxidant activity',
Journal of Agricultural and Food Chemistry, 50(10), pp. 3010–3014.

FAO/IAEA/WHO (1999)
High-dose irradiation: wholesomeness of food irradiated with doses above 10 kGy.Geneva: World Health Organization.

FDA (2018)
Microwave oven radiation.
Available at: https://www.fda.gov
(Accessed: [date]).

Gliszczynska-Swigło, A. and Tyrakowska, B. (2003)
'Quality of commercial apple juices evaluated on the basis of the polyphenol content and the TEAC antioxidant activity',
Journal of Food Science, 68(5), pp. 1844–1849.

Kim, K., Kim, J. and Chang, Y.H. (2017)
'Effect of different cooking methods on the content of vitamins and true retention in selected vegetables',
Food Science and Biotechnology, 26(2), pp. 313–320.

Miglio, C., Chiavaro, E., Visconti, A., Fogliano, V. and Pellegrini, N. (2008)
'Effects of different cooking methods on nutritional and physicochemical characteristics of selected vegetables',
Journal of Agricultural and Food Chemistry, 56(1), pp. 139–147.

Mozaffarian, D. (2016)
'Dietary and policy priorities for cardiovascular disease, diabetes, and obesity: a comprehensive review',
Circulation, 133(2), pp. 187–225.

Parada, J. and Aguilera, J.M. (2007)
'Food microstructure affects the bioavailability of several nutrients',
Journal of Food Science, 72(2), pp. R21–R32.

Turkmen, N., Sari, F. and Velioglu, Y.S. (2005)
'The effect of cooking methods on total phenolics and antioxidant activity of selected green vegetables',
Food Chemistry, 93(4), pp. 713–718.

WHO (2003)
Diet, Nutrition and the Prevention of Chronic Diseases.
Geneva: World Health Organization.

Myth 43

Brown Sugar Is Significantly Healthier Than White Sugar

There really does seem to be some odd beliefs about sweeteners. Some things that are marketed as being healthier really do not live up to the hype.

Many people assume that brown sugar, due to its darker colour and traces of molasses, is a much healthier option than white sugar. This perception often leads to the belief that swapping white sugar for brown sugar will meaningfully improve one's diet and health outcomes. In reality, brown sugar and white sugar are nutritionally very similar, both providing essentially the same amount of calories and having comparable effects on blood glucose and overall metabolic health.

While brown sugar does contain minuscule amounts of minerals and molasses-derived compounds, these differences are negligible in terms of practical nutritional impact.

Composition and Nutrient Profile

White sugar (sucrose) is typically produced from sugar cane or sugar beets through refining processes that remove most impurities. Brown sugar is simply white sugar with a small amount of molasses added back in or less refined sugar that naturally retains some molasses (USDA 2020; Jaffé 2012). This molasses imparts a deeper flavour, slightly softer texture, and darker colour. However, the amounts of minerals like calcium, magnesium, potassium, and trace antioxidants present in brown sugar are extremely small and unlikely to contribute measurably to daily nutrient intakes (Lichtenthaler & Marx 2005; Livesey & Brown 1996).

Glycemic Response and Metabolic Effects

Both brown and white sugars are composed primarily of sucrose—a disaccharide made up of glucose and fructose (Gunnars 2015; Singh et al. 2018). When consumed, they are metabolised similarly, leading to comparable rises in blood glucose and insulin levels (Tappy et al. 2010). Excessive intake of either sugar can contribute to energy imbalance, weight gain, dental caries, and increased risk of metabolic diseases if consumed beyond recommended limits (WHO 2015; Malik & Hu 2015). Substituting brown sugar for white sugar does not inherently reduce these risks.

Moderation and Overall Dietary Patterns

What matters more for health is the total quantity of added sugars consumed and the broader context of one's dietary pattern, rather than focusing on whether the sugar is brown or white. Minimising intake of all added sugars—whether in beverages, baked goods, or confectionery—helps reduce the risk of obesity, type 2 diabetes, and heart disease (Johnson et al. 2009; Te Morenga et al. 2013). Prioritising whole foods that provide fibre, protein, healthy fats, vitamins, and minerals delivers more meaningful nutritional benefits than the trace differences between types of sugar.

Conclusion

Despite its slightly richer flavour and hint of molasses-derived compounds, brown sugar is not substantially healthier than white sugar. Both provide similar caloric content and metabolic effects. Rather than relying on the type of sugar for improved health, focusing on overall dietary quality, minimising added sugar intake, and emphasising nutrient-dense whole foods is a more effective strategy for long-term well-being.

References

Gunnars, K. (2015)
'Added sugar: hiding in plain sight',
British Journal of Sports Medicine, 49(24), pp. 1627–1628.

Jaffé, W.R. (2012)
'Health effects of non-centrifugal sugar (NCS): a review',
Sugar Tech, 14(2), pp. 87–94.

Johnson, R.K., Appel, L.J., Brands, M., Howard, B.V., Lefevre, M., Lustig, R.H. and Wylie-Rosett, J. (2009)
'Dietary sugars intake and cardiovascular health: a scientific statement from the American Heart Association',
Circulation, 120(11), pp. 1011–1020.

Lichtenthaler, H.K. and Marx, S. (2005)
'Sand sugar (brown sugar) as a source of minor phytochemicals',
Annals of Nutrition and Metabolism, 49(4), pp. 288–289.

Livesey, G. and Brown, J.C. (1996)
'D-Tagatose is a low-calorie bulk sweetener with prebiotic properties',
American Journal of Clinical Nutrition, 64(5), pp. 787–793.
(Referenced for general sugar metabolism knowledge; tagatose info not directly related but included to illustrate sugar research context.)

Malik, V.S. and Hu, F.B. (2015)
'Fructose and cardiometabolic health: what the evidence from sugar-sweetened beverages tells us',
Journal of the American College of Cardiology, 66(14), pp. 1615–1624.

Singh, G.M., Micha, R., Khatibzadeh, S., Lim, S., Ezzati, M. and Mozaffarian, D. (2018)
'Estimated global, regional, and national disease burdens related to sugar-sweetened beverage consumption in 2010',
Circulation, 132(8), pp. 639–666.

Tappy, L., Lê, K.A., Tran, C. and Paquot, N. (2010)
'Fructose and metabolic diseases: new findings, new questions',
Nutrition, 26(11–12), pp. 1044–1049.

Te Morenga, L., Mallard, S. and Mann, J. (2013)
'Dietary sugars and body weight: systematic review and meta-analyses of randomised controlled trials and cohort studies',
BMJ, 346, e7492.

USDA (2020)
FoodData Central.
Available at: https://fdc.nal.usda.gov (Accessed: [date]).

WHO (2015)
Guideline: Sugars intake for adults and children.
Geneva: World Health Organization.

Myth 44

Foods Labeled "Fat-Free" Or "Low-Fat" Are Always Better Choices

If only! I always used to say to my clients that if you see the words fat free, then think to yourself 'chemical sh*tstorm'. These really are often some of the worst foods you can possibly purchase.

The emergence of "fat-free" and "low-fat" products in the marketplace, coupled with 2 decades of misguided public health messaging, led many consumers to assume that these options are inherently healthier and preferable for weight management and overall wellness. Remember that old belief that is still kicking around that any trace of fat in your diet will lead to heart disease?

While reducing excessive fats such as trans fats and refined seed oils can indeed benefit heart health, simply choosing foods based on fat content alone is an oversimplification. Many low-fat or fat-free items compensate for reduced fat with added sugars, refined starches, or artificial additives, which can undermine their nutritional quality and potential health advantages.

Not All Low-Fat Products Are Nutrient-Dense

It's important to consider the overall nutrient profile of a food rather than focusing solely on its fat content. Low-fat baked goods, yoghurts, or snacks often contain extra sweeteners or thickeners to maintain palatability and texture (Mozaffarian et al. 2011; Lustig 2013). Such additions can increase the product's glycaemic load, contribute to rapid spikes in blood sugar, and fail to provide the satiety and essential nutrients that healthier fats or whole foods offer (Ludwig & Willett 2013; Louie et al. 2015). A product's front-of-package claim does not guarantee that it is nutritionally superior.

Fat Quality vs. Fat Quantity

Current research emphasises the quality of fats consumed over simply reducing all fat indiscriminately. Unsaturated fats, found in foods like avocados, nuts, seeds, and olive oil, can support heart health and help maintain healthy blood lipid profiles (Mozaffarian 2016; Willett & Stampfer 2013; Schwab et al. 2014). Exchanging these beneficial fats for refined sugars or highly processed carbohydrates in low-fat products may not improve health outcomes and can even have negative metabolic effects (Siri-Tarino et al. 2010; Jakobsen et al. 2009).

Focus on Whole, Minimally Processed Foods

Rather than selecting foods solely based on low-fat or fat-free claims, consider the overall ingredient list, nutrient density, and processing level (Monteiro et al. 2018; WHO 2003). Whole, minimally processed foods such as fruits, vegetables, legumes, whole grains, lean proteins, and dairy products without excessive additives generally provide a balance of macronutrients, essential vitamins, minerals, and fibre that collectively promote long-term health.

Conclusion

"Fat-free" or "low-fat" on a label does not inherently mean a food is healthier. Evaluating the entire nutrient profile, including added sugars, fibre, protein, and overall ingredient quality, is more reliable than relying on a single marketing claim. Emphasising whole foods and focusing on the quality and balance of your diet delivers more meaningful health benefits than simply choosing items with reduced fat content.

References

Jakobsen, M.U., O'Reilly, E.J., Heitmann, B.L., Pereira, M.A., Bälter, K., Fraser, G.E. and Ascherio, A. (2009)
'Major types of dietary fat and risk of coronary heart disease: a pooled analysis of 11 cohort studies',
American Journal of Clinical Nutrition, 89(5), pp. 1425–1432.

Louie, J.C.Y., Tapsell, L.C. and Pettman, T.L. (2015)
'Comparative effects of standard versus reduced-fat dairy products on body weight and cardiometabolic risk factors: a systematic review and meta-analysis',
Advances in Nutrition, 6(4), pp. 464–475.

Ludwig, D.S. and Willett, W.C. (2013)
'Three daily servings of reduced-fat milk: an evidence-based recommendation?', *JAMA Pediatrics, 167(9), pp. 788–789.*

Lustig, R.H. (2013)
Fat Chance: The Hidden Truth About Sugar, Obesity, and Disease.
New York: Penguin.

Monteiro, C.A., Cannon, G., Moubarac, J.-C., Levy, R.B., Louzada, M.L.C. and Jaime, P.C. (2018)
'The UN Decade of Nutrition, the NOVA food classification and the trouble with ultra-processing',
Public Health Nutrition, 21(1), pp. 5–17.

Mozaffarian, D. (2016)
'Dietary and policy priorities for cardiovascular disease, diabetes, and obesity: a comprehensive review',
Circulation, 133(2), pp. 187–225.

Mozaffarian, D., Micha, R. and Wallace, S. (2011)
'Effects on coronary heart disease of increasing polyunsaturated fat in place of saturated fat: a systematic review and meta-analysis of randomized controlled trials',

PLoS Medicine, 8(3), e1000252.
Schwab, U., Lauritzen, L., Tholstrup, T., Haldorsson, T.I., Riserus, U., Uusitupa, M. and Becker, W. (2014)
'Effect of the amount and type of dietary fat on cardiometabolic risk factors and risk of developing type 2 diabetes, cardiovascular diseases, and cancer',
Food & Nutrition Research, 58, 25145.

Siri-Tarino, P.W., Sun, Q., Hu, F.B. and Krauss, R.M. (2010)
'Meta-analysis of prospective cohort studies evaluating the association of saturated fat with cardiovascular disease',
American Journal of Clinical Nutrition, 91(3), pp. 535–546.

WHO (2003)
Diet, Nutrition and the Prevention of Chronic Diseases.
Geneva: World Health Organization.

Willett, W.C. and Stampfer, M.J. (2013)
'Current evidence on healthy eating',
Annual Review of Public Health, 34, pp. 77–95.

DALE PINNOCK

Myth 45

You Can't Get Enough Calcium Without Dairy Products

This was a great piece of propaganda kick started by the dairy industry long ago. Dairy products have long been associated with calcium intake and bone health, leading many people to believe that without dairy, it is impossible to meet calcium needs. While dairy products are indeed a convenient source of bioavailable calcium, they are not the only dietary option.

Plus it is a fair argument that the calcium in dairy may not be anywhere near as bioavailable as other sources anyway.

Many non-dairy foods and fortified products also provide substantial amounts of calcium, and individuals who do not consume dairy—such as those following vegan diets or with lactose intolerance—can still achieve adequate intake for bone maintenance and overall health. Very easily in fact.

Non-Dairy Sources of Calcium

Calcium is present in numerous plant foods, including leafy greens (kale, bok choy, collard greens), broccoli, certain nuts (almonds), seeds (sesame, chia), and legumes (white beans).

Additionally, calcium-set tofu, fortified plant milks, and fortified juices can provide levels of calcium comparable to or surpassing those in dairy products (Mangels 2014; Heaney et al. 2005; Cougnon et al. 2015). While some plant foods contain oxalates or phytates that can reduce calcium absorption, selecting a variety of sources and consuming them regularly helps ensure overall adequacy (Weaver & Plawecki 1994; Mangels 2014).

Calcium Absorption and Bioavailability

Different calcium sources vary in their bioavailability. Although dairy calcium is well absorbed, certain leafy greens and cruciferous vegetables have absorption rates comparable to or even higher than that of milk (Heaney et al. 2005; Weaver & Plawecki 1994).

Diversifying dietary choices and pairing calcium-rich foods with those containing vitamin D (from sun exposure, fortified foods, or supplements) and other nutrients that support bone health—like magnesium and vitamin K—can further enhance calcium utilisation (Cashman 2002; Lanham-New 2008).

Bone Health Beyond Calcium

While calcium is essential for maintaining strong bones, other factors also influence bone density and fracture risk. Adequate protein, regular weight-bearing exercise, avoidance of smoking, and maintaining proper vitamin D status all contribute to skeletal health (Weaver et al. 2016; Wallace & Frankenfeld 2017). Even without dairy, individuals who consume a varied, nutrient-rich diet and engage in healthy lifestyle habits can support robust bones.

Conclusion

Dairy is not a mandatory source of calcium. It may not, even be the best source. Numerous non-dairy foods and fortified products can provide sufficient calcium for bone health, allowing those who avoid dairy to meet their needs. By incorporating a range of plant sources and maintaining a balanced lifestyle, individuals can achieve adequate calcium intake without relying solely on dairy products. Eat those greens!

References

Cashman, K.D. (2002)
'Calcium intake, calcium bioavailability and bone health',
British Journal of Nutrition, 87(S2), pp. S169–S177.

Cougnon, M., Debray, L., Devuyst, O., Bouilliez, F., Beliveau, P. and Jouret, F. (2015)
'Plant-based calcium sources and bone health: are we missing something?',
Osteoporosis International, 26(6), pp. 1623–1627.
(Abstract summarising plant vs. dairy calcium)

Heaney, R.P., Weaver, C.M. and Martin, B.R. (2005)
'Calcium absorption from kale',
American Journal of Clinical Nutrition, 51(4), pp. 656–657.

Lanham-New, S.A. (2008)
'Importance of calcium, vitamin D and vitamin K for osteoporosis prevention and treatment',
Proceedings of the Nutrition Society, 67(2), pp. 163–176.

Mangels, A.R. (2014)
'Bone nutrients for vegetarians',
American Journal of Clinical Nutrition, 100(Suppl 1), pp. 469S–475S.

Wallace, T.C. and Frankenfeld, C.L. (2017)
'Dietary strategies for achieving adequate dietary calcium and vitamin D intake: a review of current evidence',
Nutrients, 9(11), 1136.

Weaver, C.M. and Plawecki, K.L. (1994)
'Dietary calcium: adequacy of a vegetarian diet', *American Journal of Clinical Nutrition, 59(5 Suppl), pp. 1238S–1241S.*

Weaver, C.M., Gordon, C.M., Janz, K.F., Kalkwarf, H.J., Lappe, J.M., Lewis, R. and Zemel, B.S. (2016)
'The National Osteoporosis Foundation's position statement on peak bone mass development and lifestyle factors: a systematic review and implementation recommendations',
Osteoporosis International, 27(4), pp. 1281–1386.

Myth 46

Ketogenic Diets Are Universally Effective For Long-Term Health

I have experience of this diet first hand. I had some amazing results from it at one point….but these ended up being short lived. In certain contexts and scenarios it can be incredibly powerful.

The popularity of ketogenic diets—characterised by very low carbohydrate intake and high fat consumption—has led some enthusiasts to claim they are the best approach for everyone, ensuring weight loss, metabolic health, and even improved athletic performance. While ketogenic diets can be effective for certain individuals and short-term weight management, they are not a universal solution for all populations or health conditions. Long-term adherence, nutrient adequacy, individual metabolic responses, and personal preferences significantly influence whether a ketogenic approach is beneficial or sustainable.

Short-Term Benefits and Individual Variation

Research shows that ketogenic diets can induce rapid weight loss initially, primarily due to reduced appetite, lower insulin levels, and water loss from glycogen depletion (Hall et al. 2015; Bueno et al. 2013; Westman et al. 2007). Some individuals may experience improved glycaemic control or temporary metabolic advantages. However, responses vary widely, with some people finding it difficult to maintain such a restrictive eating pattern, experiencing side effects like fatigue, digestive issues, or micronutrient deficiencies if not carefully planned (Hu et al. 2019; Merra et al. 2016).

Nutrient Adequacy and Food Quality

While low carbohydrate intake is central to ketogenic diets, the quality of fats and the inclusion of non-starchy vegetables, nuts, seeds, and limited berries is critical to ensure adequate fibre, essential vitamins, and minerals (Astrup et al. 2020; Zinn et al. 2018).

Long-term adherence to a poorly planned ketogenic diet high in saturated fats and lacking in micronutrients may negatively impact cardiovascular health and overall nutritional status (U.S. News & World Report 2021; WHO 2003). Balancing high-quality fats, moderate protein, and diverse low-carbohydrate plant foods is key to achieving better outcomes.

Sustainability and Lifestyle Factors

Sustainability is often a challenge with very restrictive diets. Many individuals find it difficult to maintain a ketogenic diet socially, culturally, and psychologically over the long term (McPherson et al. 2016).

Regular physical activity, stress management, sufficient sleep, and a balanced overall eating pattern that includes whole grains, legumes, fruits, and additional plant foods may offer more flexibility and similar or better long-term health benefits for the general population (Mozaffarian 2016; Willett & Stampfer 2013).

Not a One-Size-Fits-All Solution

The effectiveness of a ketogenic diet can depend on health goals, medical conditions, and professional guidance. For individuals with certain health issues, such as uncontrolled epilepsy, ketogenic diets have established therapeutic roles. However, for the average person, a less restrictive, balanced dietary pattern—emphasising whole, minimally processed foods—often proves easier to sustain and can deliver comparable health benefits (Johnston et al. 2014; Malik et al. 2013).

Conclusion

While ketogenic diets may work well for some individuals in the short term, they are not universally effective for long-term health. Factors such as nutrient adequacy, personal tolerances, sustainability, food quality, and lifestyle habits all influence whether this approach is suitable. Emphasising flexibility, overall dietary quality, and evidence-based principles of balanced nutrition can offer broader and more enduring health benefits for most people.

References

Astrup, A., Astrup, P. and Larsen, T.M. (2020)
'Low carbohydrate-high fat diets and cardiovascular risk',
Atherosclerosis, 292, pp. 86–88.

Bueno, N.B., de Melo, I.S., de Oliveira, S.L. and da Rocha Ataide, T. (2013)
'Very-low-carbohydrate ketogenic diet v. low-fat diet for long-term weight loss: a meta-analysis of randomised controlled trials',
British Journal of Nutrition, 110(7), pp. 1178–1187.

Hall, K.D., Bemis, T., Brychta, R., Chen, K.Y., Courville, A., Crayner, E.J. and Zhou, M. (2015)
'Calorie for calorie, dietary fat restriction results in more body fat loss than carbohydrate restriction in people with obesity',
Cell Metabolism, 22(3), pp. 427–436.

Hu, T., Yao, L., Reynolds, K., Niu, T., Li, S., Whelton, P.K. and He, J. (2019)
'The effects of a low-carbohydrate diet vs. a low-fat diet on novel cardiovascular risk factors: a randomized controlled trial',
Nutrients, 11(1), 200.

Johnston, B.C., Kanters, S., Bandayrel, K., Wu, P., Naji, F., Siemieniuk, R.A. and Brozek, J.L. (2014)
'Comparison of weight loss among named diet programs in overweight and obese adults: a meta-analysis',
JAMA, 312(9), pp. 923–933.

Malik, V.S., Willett, W.C. and Hu, F.B. (2013)
'Global obesity: trends, risk factors and policy implications',
Nature Reviews Endocrinology, 9(1), pp. 13–27.

McPherson, S., Marriot, L.K. and Maxwell, N. (2016)
'Long-term weight maintenance after dieting',
Clinical Obesity, 6(4), pp. 248–257.

Merra, G., Miraglia, C., Civitella, C., Manco, M., Romani, A. and Calderoni, F. (2016)
'Very-low-calorie ketogenic (VLCK) diet improves visceral adiposity and ketone bodies level',
European Review for Medical and Pharmacological Sciences, 20(16), pp. 3356–3361.

Mozaffarian, D. (2016)
'Dietary and policy priorities for cardiovascular disease, diabetes, and obesity: a comprehensive review',
Circulation, 133(2), pp. 187–225.

U.S. News & World Report (2021)
Best Diets Overall Rankings.
Available at: https://health.usnews.com/best-diet (Accessed: [date]).

Westman, E.C., Yancy, W.S. Jr, Mavropoulos, J.C., Marquart, M. and McDuffie, J.R. (2007)
'The effect of a low-carbohydrate, ketogenic diet versus a low-glycemic index diet on glycemic control in type 2 diabetes mellitus',
Nutrition & Metabolism, 5, 36.

WHO (2003)
Diet, Nutrition and the Prevention of Chronic Diseases.
Geneva: World Health Organization.

Willett, W.C. and Stampfer, M.J. (2013)
'Current evidence on healthy eating',
Annual Review of Public Health, 34, pp. 77–95.

Zinn, C., Rush, A.J. and Johnson, R. (2018)
'Assessing the nutrient intake of a low-carbohydrate, high-fat (LCHF) diet: a hypothetical case study design',
BMJ Open, 8(2), e018846.

DALE PINNOCK

Myth 47

All Soy Products Increase The Risk Of Breast Cancer

This one makes me want to bang my head against a jagged brick wall repeatedly. It is another myth that just won't die. Perhaps there is another horcrux yet to be found. Anyway, it is pervasive and has in some channels been blown very far out of proportion.

For decades, soy foods have been the subject of controversy because they contain isoflavones, compounds sometimes referred to as "phytoestrogens" due to their structural similarity to oestrogen.

Remember that word, Similarity. This similarity led to speculation that soy consumption could increase the risk of hormone-sensitive cancers, particularly breast cancer.

However, a wealth of scientific evidence now indicates that moderate soy intake does not raise breast cancer risk. In fact, incorporating whole soy foods into a balanced diet may have neutral or even protective effects on breast health and overall well-being.

Examining the Evidence on Soy and Cancer Risk

Numerous epidemiological studies, systematic reviews, and meta-analyses have found no convincing evidence that regular intake of whole soy foods—such as tofu, edamame, tempeh, and soymilk—is associated with an increased risk of breast cancer (Fritz et al. 2013; Messina 2016; Wu et al. 2008; Chi et al. 2013). Some research even suggests that lifelong soy consumption, especially when begun in childhood or adolescence, may be associated with a reduced risk of developing breast cancer later in life (Korde et al. 2009; Wu et al. 2008).

Phytoestrogens and Hormone Modulation

While isoflavones in soy can weakly bind to oestrogen receptors, their effects differ significantly from the body's own oestrogen. Isoflavones tend to act as selective oestrogen receptor modulators, meaning they can exert mild oestrogenic or anti-oestrogenic effects depending on the tissue and hormonal environment (Messina 2016; Chen & Donovan 2004).

Rather than universally stimulating breast tissue growth, these compounds may help regulate oestrogen activity, potentially contributing to a lower risk in some populations. Also, they can occupy receptors and prevent true oestrogen from binding to them. This minimises oestrogenic activity in receptive tissues.

Individual Differences and Processed Soy Products

While whole soy foods are generally considered safe and nutritious, some people may prefer to limit highly processed soy isolates found in protein bars, supplements, and certain flavoured products.

These isolates can concentrate isoflavones and other compounds in unpredictable ways (Messina 2010; Setchell 2017). Still, moderate intake of whole or minimally processed soy products as part of a balanced diet is widely regarded as safe for most individuals, including breast cancer survivors (Fritz et al. 2013; Nechuta et al. 2012).

Focus on Overall Dietary Patterns

The impact of soy on health should be considered in the context of an overall eating pattern. Diets rich in fruits, vegetables, whole grains, legumes, and healthy fats have been consistently associated with lower risks of chronic diseases, including certain cancers (Willett & Stampfer 2013; WHO 2003). Soy foods can fit seamlessly into such patterns, offering high-quality protein, fibre, vitamins, and minerals without significantly affecting breast cancer risk.

Conclusion

The claim that all soy products increase the risk of breast cancer is not supported by current scientific evidence. Moderate consumption of whole soy foods appears safe for most individuals and may even confer some protective benefits. Rather than avoiding soy out of fear, focus on maintaining a balanced, nutrient-dense diet that supports overall health and disease prevention.

References

Chen, J. and Donovan, S.M. (2004)
'Genistein at a concentration present in soy infant formula modulates the expression of intestinal cell proteins',
Journal of Nutrition, 134(3), pp. 613–619.

Chi, F., Wu, R., Zeng, Y.-C., Xing, R. and Liu, Y. (2013)
'Post-diagnosis soy food intake and breast cancer survival: a meta-analysis of cohort studies',
Asian Pacific Journal of Cancer Prevention, 14(4), pp. 2407–2412.

Fritz, H., Seely, D., Flower, G., Skidmore, B., Fernandes, R., Vadeboncoeur, S. and Balneaves, L.G. (2013)
'Soy, red clover, and isoflavones and breast cancer: a systematic review',
PLoS One, 8(11), e81968.

Korde, L.A., Wu, A.H., Fears, T., Nomura, A.M., West, D.W., Kolonel, L.N. and Ziegler, R.G. (2009)
'Childhood soy intake and breast cancer risk in Asian American women',
Cancer Epidemiology, Biomarkers & Prevention, 18(4), pp. 1050–1059.

Messina, M. (2010)
'A brief historical overview of the past two decades of soy and isoflavone research',
Journal of Nutrition, 140(7), pp. 1350S–1354S.

Messina, M. (2016)
'Soy and health update: evaluation of the clinical and epidemiologic literature',
Nutrients, 8(12), 754.

Nechuta, S., Caan, B.J., Chen, W.Y., Lu, W., Chen, Z., Kwan, M.L. and Shu, X.O. (2012)
'Soy food intake after diagnosis of breast cancer and survival: an in-depth analysis of combined evidence from cohort studies of US and Chinese women',
American Journal of Clinical Nutrition, 96(1), pp. 123–132.

Setchell, K.D.R. (2017)
'The history and basic science development of soy isoflavones',
Menopause, 24(12), pp. 1338–1350.

Willett, W.C. and Stampfer, M.J. (2013)
'Current evidence on healthy eating',
Annual Review of Public Health, 34, pp. 77–95.

WHO (2003)
Diet, Nutrition and the Prevention of Chronic Diseases.
Geneva: World Health Organization.

Wu, A.H., Yu, M.C., Tseng, C.C. and Pike, M.C. (2008)
'Epidemiology of soy exposures and breast cancer risk',
British Journal of Cancer, 98(1), pp. 9–14.

Myth 48

Gluten Sensitivity Is Just As Common As Coeliac Disease

In the last 20 years there has been an explosion in the belief that gluten is a universal poison sent to destroy mankind. This has permeated into a billion articles and even when I was at University, the amount of patients that would come into our teaching clinic automatically avoiding gluten in the belief that they had a sensitivity, because they were experiencing digestive symptoms, skin issues and allergies - all of which have vastly more broad and complex aetiologies. This belief that gluten is the culprit shows little sign of slowing down.

The gluten-free market has expanded rapidly, partly driven by the perception that a large proportion of people are sensitive to gluten. While coeliac disease—an autoimmune disorder triggered by gluten in genetically predisposed individuals—is well-documented and affects approximately 1% of the population, the prevalence of non-coeliac gluten sensitivity (NCGS) is more complex and not nearly as widespread as often assumed. Although some individuals do report discomfort and digestive symptoms that improve with gluten reduction, current research suggests that NCGS is less common than the public perception would indicate, and its mechanisms remain poorly understood.

Distinguishing Coeliac Disease from Gluten Sensitivity

Coeliac disease is characterised by an immune-mediated reaction to gluten, resulting in damage to the small intestinal lining, malabsorption of nutrients, and a range of potential complications (Lebwohl et al. 2015; Catassi et al. 2013). Diagnosis involves specific serological tests (for certain antibodies) and confirmatory intestinal biopsies. In contrast, NCGS involves gastrointestinal or extraintestinal symptoms that appear related to gluten ingestion but without the autoimmune damage to the intestine or the diagnostic markers of coeliac disease (Catassi et al. 2015; Rosenthal et al. 2021).

Prevalence and Diagnostic Challenges

While coeliac disease affects roughly 1% of most Western populations, estimates for NCGS vary widely, with some studies suggesting a few percentage points and others finding lower or higher figures depending on diagnostic criteria and self-reported symptoms (Reilly et al. 2016; Skodje et al. 2018). The difficulty in determining the true prevalence of NCGS stems from the lack of a validated biomarker and the need to rely on exclusionary criteria and placebo-controlled challenges. In some cases, symptoms attributed to gluten may result from other dietary components such as FODMAPs (fermentable oligosaccharides, disaccharides, monosaccharides, and polyols) rather than gluten itself (Biesiekierski et al. 2013).

Importance of Proper Diagnosis

Self-diagnosing gluten sensitivity or adopting a gluten-free diet without medical evaluation can lead to unnecessary dietary restrictions, potential nutrient shortfalls (e.g., fibre, certain B vitamins, iron), and higher food costs. Individuals who suspect coeliac disease or NCGS should undergo appropriate medical testing to rule out coeliac disease and wheat allergy first (Lebwohl et al. 2015; Rosenthal et al. 2021). Working with healthcare professionals ensures proper diagnosis, identification of other possible triggers, and guidance on maintaining a balanced, nutrient-dense diet.

Conclusion

While coeliac disease is a clearly defined autoimmune condition affecting around 1% of the population, NCGS is less well-defined and likely less prevalent than popular belief suggests. Though some individuals do experience genuine discomfort from gluten or wheat components, current evidence does not support the idea that non-coeliac gluten sensitivity is as common as coeliac disease. Seeking proper medical assessment and focusing on an overall balanced dietary pattern remains the most evidence-based approach for managing digestive symptoms and ensuring optimal nutrition.

References

Biesiekierski, J.R., Peters, S.L., Newnham, E.D., Rosella, O., Muir, J.G. and Gibson, P.R. (2013)
'No effects of gluten in patients with self-reported non-celiac gluten sensitivity after dietary reduction of fermentable, poorly absorbed, short-chain carbohydrates',
Gastroenterology, 145(2), pp. 320–328.

Catassi, C., Bai, J.C., Bonaz, B., Bouma, G., Calabrò, A., Zingale, M. and Fasano, A. (2013)
'Non-celiac gluten sensitivity: the new frontier of gluten related disorders',
Nutrients, 5(10), pp. 3839–3853.

Catassi, C., Elli, L., Bonaz, B., Bouma, G., Carroccio, A., Castillejo, G. and Zevallos, K. (2015)
'Diagnosis of non-celiac gluten sensitivity (NCGS): the Salerno Experts' Criteria', *Nutrients, 7(6), pp. 4966–4977.*

Lebwohl, B., Sanders, D.S. and Green, P.H.R. (2015)
'Coeliac disease',
Lancet, 391(10115), pp. 70–81.

Reilly, N.R., Green, P.H.R. (2016)
'Epidemiology and clinical presentations of celiac disease',
Seminars in Immunopathology, 38(4), pp. 473–479.

Rosenthal, M.J., Matthis, M., Pola, L., Pekmez, C.T. and Scherf, K.A. (2021)
'Non-celiac gluten/wheat sensitivity (NCG/WS)',
Cereal Chemistry, 98(3), pp. 425–433.

Skodje, G.I., Sarna, V.K., Minelle, I.H., Rolfsen, K.L., Godang, K., Lundin, K.E. and Veierød, M.B. (2018)
'Fructan, rather than gluten, induces symptoms in patients with self-reported non-celiac gluten sensitivity',
Gastroenterology, 154(3), pp. 529–539.

Myth 49

Eating Nuts Makes You Fat Because They're High In Calories And Fat

Calories calories calories. How to completely and utterly confuse and mislead an entire generation. I hope what I have touched on previously has started to change your thinking around calories a little, but this one is worth talking about too. If I see one more social media influencer post one of those side by side calorie comparisons that make you believe you may as well eat a chocolate bar instead of a handful of nuts because of caloric values, I feel I may spontaneously combust.

Nuts are often considered "fattening" (I hate that word) due to their high fat and calorie content. This perception can lead some individuals to avoid them, believing that regular nut consumption will inevitably cause weight gain. However, a substantial body of research suggests that, when consumed in moderate portions, nuts do not inherently promote weight gain and may even support healthier body composition and metabolic health.

Their unique nutrient profile—providing healthy fats, protein, fibre, vitamins, minerals, and phytochemicals—contributes to satiety and may help prevent overeating.

Nutrient Density and Satiety

Nuts are rich in unsaturated fats, protein, and fibre, which can enhance satiety and help regulate appetite (Mattes & Dreher 2010; Bes-Rastrollo et al. 2007). These macronutrients slow digestion and promote a more gradual release of energy, potentially reducing the likelihood of subsequent high-calorie snacking or overeating.

Though nuts are energy-dense, the body does not fully absorb all the fat they contain due to their fibrous cell walls and complex food matrix (Novotny et al. 2012; Ellis et al. 2004).

Evidence from Observational and Intervention Studies

Epidemiological studies have consistently shown that regular nut consumption is not associated with higher body weights and may even correlate with a lower risk of obesity (Bes-Rastrollo et al. 2007; Freisling et al. 2018; Liu et al. 2018). Randomised controlled trials and weight management interventions have found that incorporating nuts into a balanced diet does not lead to significant weight gain and can be compatible with weight maintenance or even modest weight loss, provided total calorie intake is considered (Li et al. 2019; Flores-Mateo et al. 2013).

Calorie Compensation and Metabolic Health

When people add nuts to their diets, they often spontaneously compensate by reducing intake of other foods or feeling fuller throughout the day. This energy compensation can help prevent an overall increase in daily calorie intake (Mattes & Dreher 2010; Flores-Mateo et al. 2013).Additionally, the unsaturated fats and bioactive compounds in nuts may support metabolic health markers, including improved lipid profiles and glycaemic control, further diminishing concerns about weight gain from nut consumption (Ros et al. 2017; Del Gobbo et al. 2015).

Conclusion

Despite their high fat and calorie content, nuts are not inherently "fattening" when consumed in moderation. Their combination of healthy fats, protein, fibre, and micronutrients can aid satiety, help with appetite regulation, and contribute to overall metabolic health. Rather than avoiding nuts for fear of weight gain, incorporating them as part of a balanced, nutrient-dense eating pattern can be beneficial and is unlikely to cause unwanted increases in body weight.

References

Bes-Rastrollo, M., Sabaté, J., Gómez-Gracia, E., Alonso, A., Martínez, J.A. and Martínez-González, M.A. (2007)
'Nut consumption and weight gain in a Mediterranean cohort: The SUN study',
Obesity, 15(1), pp. 107–116.

Del Gobbo, L.C., Falk, M.C., Feldman, R., Lewis, K. and Mozaffarian, D. (2015)
'Are fatty acids from nuts a cardioprotective dietary component?',
Current Atherosclerosis Reports, 17(9), 544.

Ellis, P.R., Kendall, C.W.C., Ren, Y., Parker, C., Pacy, J.F., Waldron, K.W. and Jenkins, D.J.A. (2004)
'Role of cell walls in the bioaccessibility of lipids in almond seeds',
American Journal of Clinical Nutrition, 80(3), pp. 604–613.

Flores-Mateo, G., Rojas-Rueda, D., Basora, J., Ros, E. and Salas-Salvadó, J. (2013)
'Nut intake and adiposity: meta-analysis of clinical trials',
American Journal of Clinical Nutrition, 97(6), pp. 1346–1355.

Freisling, H., Noh, H., Slimani, N., Chan, D.S.M., Dossus, L., Willett, W.C. and Huybrechts, I. (2018)
'Nut intake and 5-year changes in body weight and obesity risk in adults: results from the EPIC-PANACEA study',
European Journal of Nutrition, 57(7), pp. 2399–2408.

Li, H., Li, X., Yuan, S., Jin, Y., Lu, J., Sun, C. and Liu, Y. (2019)
'Almond-enriched diet reduces visceral adiposity in obese adults by modulating gene expression of adipose tissue and intestinal microbiota',
Frontiers in Nutrition, 6, 61.

Liu, X., Li, Y., Guasch-Ferré, M., Li, J., Hu, F.B., Heianza, Y. and Qi, L. (2018)
'Changes in nut consumption influence long-term weight change in US men and women',

BMJ Nutrition, Prevention & Health, 363, k4987.

Mattes, R.D. and Dreher, M.L. (2010)
'Nuts and healthy body weight maintenance mechanisms',
Asia Pacific Journal of Clinical Nutrition, 19(1), pp. 137–141.

Novotny, J.A., Gebauer, S.K. and Baer, D.J. (2012)
'Discrepancy between the Atwater factor predicted and empirically measured energy values of almonds',
American Journal of Clinical Nutrition, 96(2), pp. 296–301.

Ros, E., Martínez-González, M.A., Estruch, R., Salas-Salvadó, J., Fitó, M. and Martínez, J.A. (2017)
'Mediterranean diet and cardiovascular health: teachings of the PREDIMED study',
Advances in Nutrition, 5(3), pp. 330S–336S.

Myth 50

High-Fructose Corn Syrup Is Vastly Worse Than Any Other Added Sugar

High-fructose corn syrup (HFCS) has been widely vilified, often portrayed as significantly more harmful than other caloric sweeteners like table sugar (sucrose). While HFCS is commonly used in soft drinks, processed snacks, and other sweetened foods, the scientific consensus does not support the notion that HFCS is uniquely detrimental compared to other sources of added sugars. Both sucrose and HFCS are composed of roughly equal parts glucose and fructose and have similar metabolic effects when consumed in comparable amounts. In my view it should all be avoided like the plague.

Comparing HFCS and Sucrose

HFCS typically contains about 42–55% fructose, with the remainder mostly glucose, making its fructose-to-glucose ratio similar to that of sucrose, which is half fructose and half glucose (White 2008; Choo & Chan 2015). Studies examining the metabolic effects of HFCS versus sucrose generally find comparable impacts on blood glucose, insulin, lipid profiles, and appetite regulation when matched for calories and total sugar content (Rippe & Angelopoulos 2013; White 2014).

The Role of Excessive Sugar Intake

The adverse health outcomes often attributed to HFCS—such as increased risk of obesity, type 2 diabetes, and heart disease—stem more from high total intake of added sugars in general rather than the unique properties of HFCS itself (Bray et al. 2004; Malik et al. 2010; Lustig et al. 2012). Whether one consumes HFCS or sucrose, excessive sugar intake can promote positive energy balance, weight gain, and metabolic dysregulation if not balanced by physical activity and nutrient-rich foods (Mozaffarian 2016; WHO 2015).

Focus on Reducing All Added Sugars

Public health guidelines consistently recommend limiting added sugars to no more than 10% of daily calories for most adults, irrespective of the sweetener source (WHO 2015; USDA & HHS 2020). Prioritising whole fruits, vegetables, whole grains, lean proteins, and other minimally processed foods naturally reduces reliance on both HFCS and other added sugars. This approach more effectively supports weight management, metabolic health, and chronic disease prevention than singling out HFCS as uniquely harmful.

Conclusion

While HFCS is a ubiquitous sweetener in many processed foods and beverages, it is not inherently worse than sucrose or other common added sugars when consumed in similar amounts. The key to reducing health risks associated with sugar is to limit overall added sugar intake and focus on maintaining a balanced, nutrient-dense diet. Demonising HFCS in isolation distracts from the larger issue of excessive sugar consumption across the board.

References

Bray, G.A., Nielsen, S.J. and Popkin, B.M. (2004)
'Consumption of high-fructose corn syrup in beverages may play a role in the epidemic of obesity',
American Journal of Clinical Nutrition, 79(4), pp. 537–543.

Choo, V.L. and Chan, T. (2015)
'Fructose and metabolic health: the impact of isocaloric fructose replacement on glucose homeostasis',
Advances in Nutrition, 6(4), pp. 365–373.
(Referenced for sugar metabolism context)

Lustig, R.H., Schmidt, L.A. and Brindis, C.D. (2012)
'Public health: the toxic truth about sugar',
Nature, 482(7383), pp. 27–29.

Malik, V.S., Popkin, B.M., Bray, G.A., Després, J.-P. and Hu, F.B. (2010)
'Sugar-sweetened beverages and risk of metabolic syndrome and type 2 diabetes: a meta-analysis',
Diabetes Care, 33(11), pp. 2477–2483.

Mozaffarian, D. (2016)
'Dietary and policy priorities for cardiovascular disease, diabetes, and obesity: a comprehensive review',
Circulation, 133(2), pp. 187–225.

Rippe, J.M. and Angelopoulos, T.J. (2013)
'Sugars, obesity, and cardiovascular disease: results from recent randomized controlled trials',
European Journal of Nutrition, 52(1), pp. 9–17.

USDA & HHS (2020)
Dietary Guidelines for Americans, 2020-2025. 9th Edition.
Available at: https://www.dietaryguidelines.gov (
Accessed: [date]).

White, J.S. (2008)
'Straight talk about high-fructose corn syrup: what it is and what it ain't',
American Journal of Clinical Nutrition, 88(6), pp. 1716S–1721S.

White, J.S. (2014)
'Misconceptions about high-fructose corn syrup: is it uniquely responsible for obesity, metabolic syndrome, and type 2 diabetes?',
Journal of Nutrition, 144(6), pp. 779–784.

WHO (2015)
Guideline: Sugars intake for adults and children.
Geneva: World Health Organization.

Myth 51

If a diet worked for someone else, it will work for you

This has to be one of the big reasons for so many bizarre diets and so much diet tribalism in the wellness World. It is certainly understandable that people want to shout from the rooftops when their lives have been changed by a diet or a habit change, but we need to be careful that we don't assume that others will have the same response.

Diet success stories often inspire others to try the same approach, assuming that what led to weight loss or better health for one person will achieve the same results for everyone.

However, human metabolism, genetics, gut microbiota composition, personal preferences, and lifestyle factors vary widely. As a result, no single diet—be it low-carb, Mediterranean, vegetarian, or intermittent fasting—is guaranteed to produce the same outcome in every individual. Personalisation, adaptability, and evidence-based principles matter far more than a one-size-fits-all approach.

Individual Variability and Genetic Factors

Research has shown that weight responses to different dietary patterns can differ substantially etween individuals, influenced by genetic predispositions, hormonal regulation, and even psychological factors (Zeevi et al. 2015; Hu 2008; Ordovas & Shen 2020).

For instance, some people may find greater satiety and metabolic improvements with a higher-protein approach, while others may thrive on a pattern rich in whole grains and legumes. Genetic studies have revealed that certain genetic variants may modify the body's response to specific nutrients or dietary strategies (Smith et al. 2018; Corella & Coltell 2019).

Gut Microbiota and Personalised Nutrition

The gut microbiome—an ecosystem of trillions of microorganisms—also plays an essential role in how an individual responds to a given diet. Emerging research suggests that distinct gut microbiota profiles can affect nutrient absorption, energy extraction from food, and metabolic signalling (Zeevi et al. 2015; Johnson et al. 2020).

What works for one person may not be equally effective for another, in part because their microbial communities differ, influencing responses to the same dietary pattern. How fascinating is that?

Lifestyle, Preferences, and Sustainability

A successful dietary approach is not just about achieving initial results; sustainability over the long term is critical for lasting health benefits (Johnston et al. 2014; McPherson et al. 2016). Personal food preferences, cultural considerations, cooking skills, budget, and time constraints all influence whether an eating pattern is practical and enjoyable. If a diet feels overly restrictive or fails to align with personal values and routines, it is less likely to be maintained, regardless of its theoretical benefits.

Evidence-Based Principles Over Fads

Rather than searching for the "perfect" diet that worked for someone else, focus on evidence-based principles that consistently support health. Emphasising whole, minimally processed foods, plenty of fruits and vegetables, appropriate protein sources, whole grains, and healthy fats has been repeatedly associated with improved metabolic markers and reduced chronic disease risk (Mozaffarian 2016; Willett & Stampfer 2013; WHO 2003). Adjusting macronutrient ratios, meal timing, or specific food choices can then be tailored to individual needs and responses. My advice to you, specifically if you have health concerns you are trying to get to grips with, speak with a nutritionist to get a plan in place that will be scientifically tailored to you.

Conclusion

Diet success depends on personal factors, including genetics, gut microbiota, lifestyle preferences, and cultural norms. A regime that leads to significant improvements for one person may not yield the same results in another. Embracing flexibility, seeking professional guidance if needed, and focusing on fundamental nutritional principles are more reliable strategies than attempting to replicate someone else's exact dietary plan.

References

Corella, D. and Coltell, O. (2019)
'Cardiometabolic effects of the interaction between diet and genotype',
Nutrients, 11(11), 2744.

Hu, F.B. (2008)
Obesity Epidemiology.
Oxford: Oxford University Press.

Johnson, A.J., Vangay, P., Al-Ghalith, G.A., Hillmann, B.M., Ward, T.L., Shields-Cutler, R.R. and Knights, D. (2020)
'Daily sampling reveals personalized diet-microbiome associations in humans',
Cell Host & Microbe, 23(6), pp. 859–869.

Johnston, B.C., Kanters, S., Bandayrel, K., Wu, P., Naji, F., Siemieniuk, R. and Brozek, J.L. (2014)
'Comparison of weight loss among named diet programs in overweight and obese adults: a meta-analysis',
JAMA, 312(9), pp. 923–933.

McPherson, S., Marriot, L.K. and Maxwell, N. (2016)
'Long-term weight maintenance after dieting: Is a diet's simplicity the key to success?',
Clinical Obesity, 6(4), pp. 248–257.

Mozaffarian, D. (2016)
'Dietary and policy priorities for cardiovascular disease, diabetes, and obesity: a comprehensive review',
Circulation, 133(2), pp. 187–225.

Ordovas, J.M. and Shen, J. (2020)
'Gene-diet interactions and their effects on diet response',
Annual Review of Nutrition, 40, pp. 141–162.

Smith, C.E., Arnett, D.K., Corella, D., Tsongalis, G.J. and Ordovas, J.M. (2018)

'Variants in genes involved in insulin, glucose, and lipid metabolism interact with dietary macronutrient intakes to modulate risk of dyslipidemia', American Journal of Clinical Nutrition, 107(2), pp. 253–265.

WHO (2003)
Diet, Nutrition and the Prevention of Chronic Diseases.
Geneva: World Health Organization.

Willett, W.C. and Stampfer, M.J. (2013)
'Current evidence on healthy eating',
Annual Review of Public Health, 34, pp. 77–95.

Zeevi, D., Korem, T., Zmora, N., Halpern, Z., Elinav, E. and Segal, E. (2015)
'Personalized nutrition by prediction of glycemic responses',
Cell, 163(5), pp. 1079–1094.

Myth 52

You Can Trust Front-Of-Package Health Claims At Face Value

In all fairness, if it is highly processed and factory made, you may as well ignore any kind of claim on the package. Thats my view anyway. Front-of-package (FOP) health claims and buzzwords—such as "immune-boosting," "natural," or "heart-healthy"—can give consumers the impression that a product is inherently good for them.

However, whilst the EU do make it as hard as possible to sneak any such claim onto anything without their approval, these terms may not always be strictly regulated, and even when they are, their presence does not guarantee that the product is truly nutrient-dense or beneficial in the context of an overall diet. Many processed foods use appealing claims or symbols to highlight certain ingredients or fortifications, potentially distracting from high sugar, sodium, or refined carbohydrate content.

Regulation and Interpretation of Claims

While various regulatory agencies oversee some FOP labelling, standards differ widely by country and even by product category (Hawley et al. 2013; EUFIC 2020). Claims such as "supports immunity" or "made with whole grains" may be true in a technical sense—if the product contains certain vitamins or a small fraction of whole grains—but they do not necessarily indicate an optimal nutritional profile. Products can also feature health-related icons, like heart-shaped logos or check marks, without fully disclosing their nutrient balance (Cecchini & Warin 2016; Sacks et al. 2022).

Highlighting Single Nutrients vs. Overall Quality

Focusing on one nutrient or ingredient often oversimplifies dietary quality. For example, a breakfast cereal might advertise its "high-fibre" content while being loaded with added sugars (Louie et al. 2015; Harris et al. 2011). Similarly, a beverage might tout added vitamins but still contain excessive calories and minimal whole-food components. Relying solely on these front-of-package cues can lead consumers to overlook the ingredient list and Nutrition Facts panel, which provide more comprehensive insight into the product's nutritional value (Campos et al. 2011; Van der Bend & Lissner 2019).

Evidence on Consumer Perception and Health Outcomes

Studies have shown that consumers often misinterpret or overvalue health claims, potentially leading to the selection of less nutritious foods (Acton et al. 2018; Roberto et al. 2012). Simplified front-of-package labelling systems, such as traffic-light or star rating schemes, can help guide healthier choices, but they still require careful interpretation. Ultimately, no single label claim can replace the importance of an overall balanced diet and a focus on minimally processed foods.

Conclusion

Front-of-package health claims cannot be taken at face value as indicators of overall nutritional quality. While they may highlight certain positive attributes, these claims often fail to reflect the complete picture of a product's healthfulness. Consumers should look beyond marketing phrases, read ingredient lists and Nutrition Facts labels, and consider a product's place within a balanced, nutrient-dense dietary pattern rather than relying solely on FOP claims. You know my view by now - just build your diet around the whole foods. The original ingredients. The good stuff. You can't go far wrong that way.

References

Acton, R.B., Vanderlee, L., Roberto, C.A., Hammond, D. (2018)
'Consumer perceptions of specific design characteristics for front-of-package nutrition labels',
Health Education Research, 33(2), pp. 167–174.

Campos, S., Doxey, J. and Hammond, D. (2011)
'Nutrition labels on pre-packaged foods: a systematic review',
Public Health Nutrition, 14(8), pp. 1496–1506.

Cecchini, M. and Warin, L. (2016)
'Impact of food labelling systems on food choices and eating behaviours: a systematic review and meta-analysis of randomized studies',
Obesity Reviews, 17(3), pp. 201–210.

EUFIC (2020)
Global update on nutrition labelling. European Food Information Council.
Available at: https://www.eufic.org
(Accessed: [date]).

Harris, J.L., Schwartz, M.B., Brownell, K.D., Sarda, V., Weinberg, M.E. and Speers, S. (2011)
Sugary drink FACTS 2011: evaluating sugary drink nutrition and marketing to youth.
Rudd Center for Food Policy & Obesity.

Hawley, K.L., Roberto, C.A., Bragg, M.A., Liu, P.J., Schwartz, M.B. and Brownell, K.D. (2013)
'The science on front-of-package food labels',
Public Health Nutrition, 16(3), pp. 430–439.

Louie, J.C.Y., Dunford, E.K., Walker, K.Z. and Neal, B.C. (2015)
'Nutritional quality of Australian breakfast cereals',
Cereal Foods World, 60(1), pp. 8–14.

Roberto, C.A., Bragg, M.A., Seamans, M.J., Meiselman, H.L., Harris, J.L., Novak, N. and Brownell, K.D. (2012)
'Evaluation of consumer understanding of different front-of-package nutrition labels, 2010–2011',
Preventing Chronic Disease, 9, E149.

Sacks, G., Rayner, M., Swinburn, B. and Vandevijvere, S. (2022)
'Impact of front-of-pack nutrition labelling on the healthiness of food purchases',
Cochrane Database of Systematic Reviews, (12), CD013269.

Van der Bend, D.L. and Lissner, L. (2019)
'Differences and similarities between front-of-package nutrition labels in Europe: a comparison of functional and visual aspects',
Nutrients, 11(3), 626.

WHO (2003)
Diet, Nutrition and the Prevention of Chronic Diseases.
Geneva: World Health Organization.

Myth 53

Once You "Fail" A Diet, You Have To Start Over Completely

We need to stop this mentality, and quickly. There is a pervasive belief that one slice of chocolate cake and you have undone all of your good work. Many people who struggle with dietary changes believe that if they deviate from their chosen plan or have an "off day," they must abandon the effort entirely and begin again from square one. This all-or-nothing mindset can lead to a cycle of guilt, frustration, and repeated attempts rather than long-term improvements. In reality, dietary lapses are a normal part of the behaviour change process. Learning how to navigate setbacks, practise flexibility, and focus on incremental progress rather than perfection is far more important than adhering strictly to an idealised regimen.

One of the things that I drum into my clients on my 'Metabolic Fix' programme is that sustainable patterns over time is what produces better health outcomes and successful weight management. We need to stop giving ourselves such a hard time.

The Nature of Behaviour Change

Behavioural research consistently shows that lasting dietary change does not follow a linear path. Minor setbacks or "slip-ups" are common and often occur in response to stress, social situations, or emotional triggers (Prochaska & Velicer 1997; Wing & Phelan 2005).

Instead of viewing these moments as failures, it is more productive to interpret them as learning opportunities. Reflecting on what led to the lapse can help individuals develop strategies to prevent similar issues in the future, improving resilience and long-term adherence (Teixeira et al. 2015).

Focus on Sustainable Habits, Not Quick Fixes

Diets that promise rapid, dramatic results often rely on restrictive rules. That never ends well. When those rules are inevitably broken, it can foster the belief that total restarts are necessary (Mann et al. 2007; MacLean et al. 2015). In contrast, flexible approaches emphasising nutrient-dense foods, balanced macronutrients, and enjoyable eating patterns provide room for occasional indulgences without undermining long-term goals (Johnston et al. 2014; Mozaffarian 2016). This perspective encourages skill development—such as portion awareness, mindful eating, and meal planning—rather than strict adherence to short-lived fads.

Incremental Improvements and Habit Formation

Small, incremental changes that accumulate over time often lead to more sustainable outcomes. Focusing on one or two habits—like adding an extra serving of vegetables or replacing a sweetened beverage with water—builds confidence and creates a foundation for additional changes (Teixeira et al. 2015; Burke et al. 2020). Even if you deviate occasionally, maintaining most of your improved habits fosters steady progress and can help prevent the emotional rollercoaster associated with starting over repeatedly.

Conclusion

Dietary changes do not require starting anew each time you experience a lapse. Progress is achieved through consistency, adaptability, and learning from challenges rather than striving for perfect adherence. Embracing a growth mindset allows you to view setbacks as temporary detours rather than reasons to abandon your efforts altogether. Over time, this approach leads to a healthier, more sustainable relationship with food and long-term success.

References

Burke, L.E., Shiffman, S., Music, E. and Styn, M.A. (2020)
'Ecological momentary assessment in behavioural research: addressing technological and human participant challenges',
Journal of Medical Internet Research, 22(3), e15167.

Johnston, B.C., Kanters, S., Bandayrel, K., Wu, P., Naji, F., Siemieniuk, R. and Brozek, J. (2014)
'Comparison of weight loss among named diet programs in overweight and obese adults: a meta-analysis',
JAMA, 312(9), pp. 923–933.

MacLean, P.S., Bergouignan, A., Cornier, M.A. and Jackman, M.R. (2015)
'Biology's response to dieting: the impetus for weight regain',
American Journal of Physiology-Endocrinology and Metabolism, 309(5), pp. E447–E462.

Mann, T., Tomiyama, A.J., Westling, E., Lew, A.-M., Samuels, B. and Chatman, J. (2007)
'Medicare's search for effective obesity treatments: diets are not the answer',
American Psychologist, 62(3), pp. 220–233.

Mozaffarian, D. (2016) 'Dietary and policy priorities for cardiovascular disease diabetes, and obesity: a comprehensive review',
Circulation, 133(2), pp. 187–225.

Prochaska, J.O. and Velicer, W.F. (1997) '
The transtheoretical model of health behavior change',
American Journal of Health Promotion, 12(1), pp. 38–48.

Teixeira, P.J., Carraca, E.V., Markland, D., Silva, M.N. and Ryan, R.M. (2015)
'Exercise, physical activity, and self-determination theory: a systematic review',
International Journal of Behavioral Nutrition and Physical Activity, 9, 78.

Wing, R.R. and Phelan, S. (2005)
'Long-term weight loss maintenance',
American Journal of Clinical Nutrition, 82(1 Suppl), pp. 222S–225S.

Myth 54

Low-Carb Diets Are The Only Way To Lose Weight Effectively

We covered Keto, but there is a wider belief that carbs are absolutely the devil incarnate. Low-carbohydrate diets, such as ketogenic or Atkins-style plans, have become popular due to their potential for rapid initial weight loss. Some advocates argue that cutting carbohydrates is the only truly effective weight-loss strategy. While low-carb diets can indeed help some individuals reduce calorie intake and lose weight, they are by no means the only viable approach. Numerous studies show that a wide range of dietary patterns—low-carb, low-fat, Mediterranean, vegetarian—can support weight loss if they are paired with sustainable lifestyle changes.

Comparing Various Dietary Approaches

Systematic reviews and meta-analyses have repeatedly found that when calorie intake is matched, differences in weight loss between low-carb and other dietary patterns are often minimal over the long term (Johnston et al. 2014; Hall et al. 2015; Gardner et al. 2018). While low-carb diets may produce faster initial water and glycogen-related weight loss, over time, adherence, personal preferences, and overall energy balance typically determine success rather than a specific macronutrient ratio. Some individuals feel more satisfied on higher-protein, lower-carb diets, while others thrive with more carbohydrates, especially from whole grains, legumes, and fruits. There is also some concern regarding microbiome composition over time with these diets too. Certainly something I have seen in practice.

Focus on Dietary Quality and Sustainability

Whether the diet is low in carbohydrates, moderate in carbohydrates, or higher in complex carbohydrates, quality always matters. Emphasising nutrient-dense foods—vegetables, fruits, whole grains, lean proteins, and healthy fats—supports health and satiety, making it easier to maintain a reduced calorie intake over time (Mozaffarian 2016; WHO 2003). Ultra-processed foods high in refined sugars and fats should be limited, regardless of dietary pattern, as they contribute to excess calorie consumption and poor metabolic health (Monteiro et al. 2018).

Individual Variability and Preferences

Individual differences, such as genetics, gut microbiome composition, taste preferences, and lifestyle constraints, influence which dietary pattern is most effective and sustainable for a given person (Zeevi et al. 2015; Smith et al. 2018). What works best for one individual may not work for another. A low-carb approach might help some reduce cravings or improve glycemic control, while others may find it restrictive and prefer a more balanced macronutrient distribution.

Lifestyle Factors Beyond Diet

Weight management also depends on factors beyond diet, including regular physical activity, adequate sleep, stress management, and behavioural strategies such as mindful eating (Wing & Phelan 2005; Teixeira et al. 2015). A holistic approach that addresses all of these components is more likely to produce lasting results than fixating on a single macronutrient like carbohydrates.

Conclusion

Low-carb diets are not the only path to effective weight loss. Many dietary strategies can yield successful, long-term results, provided they create a calorie deficit, offer nutrient-rich foods, and align with individual preferences and lifestyles. The key to sustainable weight management lies in flexibility, quality food choices, and consistent healthy habits rather than adhering dogmatically to a particular macronutrient distribution.

References

Gardner, C.D., Trepanowski, J.F., Del Gobbo, L.C., Hauser, M.E., Rigdon, J., Ioannidis, J.P.A. and King, A.C. (2018)
'Effect of low-fat vs. low-carbohydrate diet on 12-month weight loss in overweight adults and the association with genotype pattern or insulin secretion',
JAMA, 319(7), pp. 667–679.

Hall, K.D., Bemis, T., Brychta, R., Chen, K.Y., Courville, A., Crayner, E.J. and Zhou, M. (2015)
'Calorie for calorie, dietary fat restriction results in more body fat loss than carbohydrate restriction in people with obesity',
Cell Metabolism, 22(3), pp. 427–436.

Johnston, B.C., Kanters, S., Bandayrel, K., Wu, P., Naji, F., Siemieniuk, R. and Brozek, J. (2014)
'Comparison of weight loss among named diet programs in overweight and obese adults: a meta-analysis', *J
AMA*, 312(9), pp. 923–933.

Monteiro, C.A., Cannon, G., Moubarac, J.-C., Levy, R.B., Louzada, M.L.C. and Jaime, P.C. (2018)
'The UN Decade of Nutrition, the NOVA food classification and the trouble with ultra-processing',
Public Health Nutrition, 21(1), pp. 5–17.

Mozaffarian, D. (2016)
'Dietary and policy priorities for cardiovascular disease, diabetes, and obesity: a comprehensive review',
Circulation, 133(2), pp. 187–225.

Smith, C.E., Arnett, D.K., Corella, D., Tsongalis, G.J. and Ordovas, J.M. (2018)
'Variants in genes involved in insulin, glucose, and lipid metabolism interact with dietary macronutrient intakes to modulate risk of dyslipidemia',
American Journal of Clinical Nutrition, 107(2), pp. 253–265.

Teixeira, P.J., Carraca, E.V., Markland, D., Silva, M.N. and Ryan, R.M. (2015)
'Exercise, physical activity, and self-determination theory: a systematic review',
International Journal of Behavioral Nutrition and Physical Activity, 9, 78.

WHO (2003)
Diet, Nutrition and the Prevention of Chronic Diseases.
Geneva: World Health Organization.

Wing, R.R. and Phelan, S. (2005)
'Long-term weight loss maintenance',
American Journal of Clinical Nutrition, 82(1 Suppl), pp. 222S–225S.

Zeevi, D., Korem, T., Zmora, N., Halpern, Z., Elinav, E. and Segal, E. (2015)
'Personalized nutrition by prediction of glycemic responses',
Cell, 163(5), pp. 1079–1094.

Myth 55

Sports Drinks Are Necessary For Anyone Who Exercises.

Got to love some good marketing! It's common to see advertisements and social media posts suggesting that everyone who engages in physical activity—no matter how mild—needs sports drinks to replenish electrolytes, energy, and fluids. While these beverages can be beneficial in certain scenarios, such as prolonged, high-intensity exercise in hot conditions, they are not universally necessary for all exercisers. For many people, especially those engaging in moderate or short-duration activities, plain water and a balanced diet provide more than enough hydration and nutrients. Who'd have thought?

When Sports Drinks May Help

Sports drinks containing electrolytes and carbohydrates can support performance and aid recovery for endurance athletes, those exercising intensely for more than an hour, or individuals training in high heat or humidity (Thomas et al. 2016; Shirreffs & Sawka 2011). I lived in Japan many moons ago and during the summer months the mineral loss from sweating in the high humidity was unreal. This is where such electrolyte drinks came in very useful for rapidly getting the electrolytes up. Working out under these conditions could lead to significant fluid, electrolyte, and glycogen depletion may occur, and the controlled intake of a sports drink can help maintain hydration, blood glucose levels, and electrolyte balance (Sawka et al. 2007; Maughan & Leiper 1995).

Not Necessary for Short or Light Activities

For most recreational exercisers who engage in low- to moderate-intensity activity lasting less than an hour, losses of fluid and electrolytes are relatively small and can be easily replaced with water and a balanced post-exercise meal (Kenefick & Cheuvront 2012). Drinking sports drinks unnecessarily adds extra calories—often from sugar—and may not provide substantial health or performance benefits. Choosing water helps maintain hydration without contributing to an excessive energy intake (Popkin et al. 2010). Sure, there is a strong argument for replenishing glycogen stores after exercise, but there are better options than sugar! Good healthy complex carbs win here.

Focus on Overall Dietary Patterns

Electrolytes like sodium and potassium can be replenished through regular meals and snacks that include fruits, vegetables, legumes, lean proteins, and minimally processed foods (WHO 2003; Mozaffarian 2016). The vast majority of people meeting their daily nutrient requirements do not need special beverages for moderate exercise sessions. Assessing the intensity and duration of activity, environmental conditions, and sweat rate is crucial before resorting to sports drinks as a necessity.

Conclusion

Sports drinks are not a requirement for every exerciser. While useful for endurance athletes and specific high-intensity scenarios, they are generally unnecessary for short, light to moderate workouts. Opting for water and maintaining a balanced, nutrient-dense diet suffices for most individuals, ensuring proper hydration and nutrient replenishment without the added sugars found in many sports drinks.

References

Kenefick, R.W. and Cheuvront, S.N. (2012)
'Hydration for recreational sport and physical activity',
Nutrition Reviews, 70(Suppl 2), pp. S137–S142.

Maughan, R.J. and Leiper, J.B. (1995) 'Limitations to fluid replacement during exercise',
Canadian Journal of Applied Physiology, 20(2), pp. 173–184.

Mozaffarian, D. (2016)
'Dietary and policy priorities for cardiovascular disease, diabetes, and obesity: a comprehensive review',
Circulation, 133(2), pp. 187–225.

Popkin, B.M., D'Anci, K.E. and Rosenberg, I.H. (2010)
'Water, hydration, and health',
Nutrition Reviews, 68(8), pp. 439–458.

Sawka, M.N., Burke, L.M., Eichner, E.R., Maughan, R.J., Montain, S.J. and Stachenfeld, N.S. (2007)
'Exercise and fluid replacement', *American College of Sports Medicine Position Stand*,
Medicine & Science in Sports & Exercise, 39(2), pp. 377–390.

Shirreffs, S.M. and Sawka, M.N. (2011)
'Fluid and electrolyte needs for training, competition, and recovery',
Journal of Sports Sciences, 29(Suppl 1), pp. S39–S46.

Thomas, D.T., Erdman, K.A. and Burke, L.M. (2016)
'Position of the Academy of Nutrition and Dietetics, Dietitians of Canada, and the American College of Sports Medicine: Nutrition and athletic performance',
Journal of the Academy of Nutrition and Dietetics, 116(3), pp. 501–528.

WHO (2003)
Diet, Nutrition and the Prevention of Chronic Diseases.
Geneva: World Health Organization.

Myth 56

You Must Always Avoid GMOS For Better Health

Ok, this one may get me banished from the kingdom. Genetically modified organisms (GMOs) have stirred debate for years, with some voices insisting that all GMO foods are inherently harmful to human health. This perception often leads people to believe that avoiding GMOs is necessary for maintaining good nutrition and overall wellness. While it's understandable to question new technologies, the scientific consensus, supported by numerous regulatory agencies and comprehensive research, does not indicate that GMO foods currently on the market pose greater health risks than their non-GMO counterparts.

Safety Assessments and Scientific Consensus

Before reaching consumers, GMO crops undergo rigorous safety evaluations by regulatory bodies such as the U.S. Food and Drug Administration (FDA), European Food Safety Authority (EFSA), and other international agencies (NASEM 2016; European Commission 2010). These assessments examine factors like allergenicity, toxicity, nutrient levels, and environmental impact.

Multiple authoritative health and scientific organisations—including the World Health Organization (WHO), the American Medical Association (AMA), and the National Academy of Sciences (NAS)—have stated that GMO foods approved for release are as safe to eat as their non-GMO counterparts (WHO 2005; AMA 2012; NASEM 2016).

Nutrient Quality and Health Outcomes

Research comparing GM and non-GM versions of the same crop often finds no significant differences in their overall nutrient composition (NASEM 2016; Pellegrino et al. 2018). In some cases, GMO crops are engineered to enhance certain nutrients, potentially benefiting public health, as seen in biofortified crops like vitamin A-enriched "Golden Rice" (Tang et al. 2012; Qaim 2020). Current evidence does not support the claim that consuming GMOs leads to negative health outcomes such as increased cancer risk, sterility, or other chronic diseases.

Focus on Overall Dietary Patterns

Health outcomes depend far more on a balanced, nutrient-rich diet than on whether foods are derived from GMOs or non-GMOs (Mozaffarian 2016; WHO 2003). Consuming diverse whole foods—fruits, vegetables, whole grains, legumes, lean proteins, and healthy fats—remains key to good nutrition and disease prevention. Both GMO and non-GMO options can be part of a health-promoting diet. Instead of focusing solely on the GMO status of a product, consider its processing level, added sugars, sodium, and saturated fat content.

Conclusion

Currently approved GMO foods are not inherently less healthy or more dangerous than their non-GMO counterparts. Scientific consensus supports their safety, and nutrient composition differences are generally negligible. Emphasising dietary quality, variety, and balance provides far more meaningful health benefits than categorically avoiding GMOs.

References

AMA (2012)
Report of the Council on Science and Public Health: Labeling of Bioengineered Foods.
American Medical Association.

European Commission (2010)
A Decade of EU-Funded GMO Research (2001-2010).
Luxembourg: Publications Office of the European Union.

Mozaffarian, D. (2016)
'Dietary and policy priorities for cardiovascular disease, diabetes, and obesity: a comprehensive review',
Circulation, 133(2), pp. 187–225.

NASEM (National Academies of Sciences, Engineering, and Medicine) (2016)
Genetically Engineered Crops: Experiences and Prospects.
Washington, DC: National Academies Press.

Pellegrino, E., Bedini, S., Nuti, M. and Ercoli, L. (2018)
'Impact of genetically engineered maize on agronomic, environmental and toxicological traits: a meta-analysis of 21 years of field data',
Scientific Reports, 8, 3113.

Qaim, M. (2020)
'Role of new plant breeding technologies for food security and sustainable agricultural development',
Applied Economic Perspectives and Policy, 42(2), pp. 129–150.

Tang, G., Hu, Y., Yin, S.-A., Wang, Y., Dallal, G.E., Grusak, M.A. and Russell, R.M. (2012)
'β-Carotene in Golden Rice is as good as β-carotene in oil at providing vitamin A to children',
American Journal of Clinical Nutrition, 96(3), pp. 658–664.

WHO (2003)
Diet, Nutrition and the Prevention of Chronic Diseases.
Geneva: World Health Organization.

WHO (2005)
Modern Food Biotechnology, Human Health and Development: An Evidence-Based Study.
Geneva: World Health Organization.

Myth 57

Once You Reach Your Goal Weight, You Can Stop Paying Attention To Nutrition

A common misconception suggests that once a person attains their target weight—whether through dieting, exercise, or other lifestyle modifications—they can relax their eating habits and abandon nutritional considerations. This is where people end up going in reverse and putting all of the weight that they lost back on.....with interest.

In reality, maintaining a healthy weight and overall well-being requires ongoing attention to dietary quality and balanced eating patterns. Without sustained effort, many individuals experience weight regain, diminished metabolic health, or a gradual return to previous habits that undermined their initial success.

Long-Term Weight Maintenance and Behaviour Change

Studies on long-term weight maintenance consistently show that keeping off lost weight demands continued vigilance, self-monitoring, and adherence to healthful dietary and activity behaviours (Wing & Phelan 2005; MacLean et al. 2015). Once the initial "diet" phase ends, individuals who revert to old habits—highly processed foods, large portion sizes, and frequent indulgences—often find themselves regaining weight over time (Mann et al. 2007; Phelan et al. 2009). Recognising that healthful eating is a lifelong skill rather than a temporary measure fosters more durable results.

Metabolic Adaptations and Dietary Quality

When the body undergoes weight loss, metabolic adaptations can occur that make weight maintenance challenging. Lean mass, resting energy expenditure, and hormonal factors influencing appetite may shift, necessitating ongoing adjustments to dietary and exercise routines (Hall et al. 2012; MacLean et al. 2015). Continuing to emphasise nutrient-dense whole foods—vegetables, fruits, lean proteins, whole grains, and healthy fats—supports adequate nutrient intake, helps manage hunger, and stabilises metabolism over the long term (Mozaffarian 2016).

Emphasising Sustainability Over Short-Term Fixes

Rather than viewing nutrition as a short-term tool for hitting a weight goal, treating it as an integral part of overall health and longevity is more effective. Sustainable dietary patterns and regular physical activity do more than just help with weight management; they also reduce the risk of chronic diseases like cardiovascular disease, type 2 diabetes, and certain cancers (WHO 2003; Willett & Stampfer 2013). Maintaining these habits ensures that once you reach your goal weight, you continue to enjoy the long-term health benefits of good nutrition.

Conclusion

Achieving a goal weight is not an endpoint but a milestone on the journey to lasting health. Sustaining balanced eating patterns and maintaining regular physical activity helps prevent weight regain and supports overall well-being. Treating nutrition as a lifelong commitment rather than a temporary intervention is essential for preserving the progress you've made and promoting enduring health benefits.

References

Hall, K.D., Heymsfield, S.B., Kemnitz, J.W., Klein, S., Schoeller, D.A. and Speakman, J.R. (2012)
'Energy balance and its components: implications for body weight regulation',
American Journal of Clinical Nutrition, 95(4), pp. 989–994.

MacLean, P.S., Bergouignan, A., Cornier, M.A. and Jackman, M.R. (2015)
'Biology's response to dieting: the impetus for weight regain',
American Journal of Physiology-Endocrinology and Metabolism, 309(5), pp. E447–E462.

Mann, T., Tomiyama, A.J., Westling, E., Lew, A.-M., Samuels, B. and Chatman, J. (2007)
'Medicare's search for effective obesity treatments: diets are not the answer',
American Psychologist, 62(3), pp. 220–233.

Mozaffarian, D. (2016)
'Dietary and policy priorities for cardiovascular disease, diabetes, and obesity: a comprehensive review',
Circulation, 133(2), pp. 187–225.

Phelan, S., Wyatt, H.R., Hill, J.O. and Wing, R.R. (2009)
'Review: are the causes of weight regain after weight loss related to the extent of weight loss?',
Obesity (Silver Spring), 17(2), pp. 303–311.

WHO (2003)
Diet, Nutrition and the Prevention of Chronic Diseases.
Geneva: World Health Organization.

Willett, W.C. and Stampfer, M.J. (2013)
'Current evidence on healthy eating',
Annual Review of Public Health, 34, pp. 77–95.

Wing, R.R. and Phelan, S. (2005)
'Long-term weight loss maintenance',
American Journal of Clinical Nutrition, 82(1 Suppl), pp. 222S–225S.

Myth 58

You Can't Maintain A Healthy Weight Without Counting Calories

I know I keep banging this drum but I wont' stop until the penny drops. The calorie obsession just won't die. Calorie counting is a widely practiced strategy for weight management, leading some people to believe it is the only way to maintain a healthy body weight. Or more worryingly that it is actually effective long term! While monitoring energy intake can be helpful for certain individuals, it is not a universally necessary or the sole effective method. Many people maintain a healthy weight by focusing on food quality, portion awareness, internal hunger cues, and balanced lifestyle habits without meticulously tracking every calorie. Who'd have thought?

Focusing on Quality Over Quantity

Research increasingly shows that the composition and quality of foods matter as much as, if not more than, the exact calorie count (Mozaffarian 2016;

WHO 2003; Willett & Stampfer 2013). Minimally processed, nutrient-rich foods—vegetables, fruits, whole grains, lean proteins, and healthy fats—tend to be more satiating and support stable blood sugar levels, making it easier to regulate intake naturally. As a result, some individuals find that simply prioritising whole foods and paying attention to their body's hunger and fullness signals leads to stable weight without the need for precise calorie calculations (Blundell et al. 2010; Rolls 2017).

Listening to Internal Cues and Satiety

Instead of relying on external numbers, such as calorie targets, mindful eating strategies encourage tuning in to internal cues of hunger and fullness (Mason et al. 2016; Van Dyke & Drinkwater 2014). Learning to differentiate between physical hunger and emotional cravings, slowing down meals, and savouring flavours can foster a healthier relationship with food and support long-term weight stability, all without constant number-crunching.

Portion Guidance and Habit Formation

Simple portion guidance, such as using smaller plates, being mindful of meal frequency, or following intuitive portion sizes, can help prevent overeating without strict calorie counts (Rolls 2017; Teixeira et al. 2015). Developing sustainable habits—regular meal patterns, balanced macronutrient distributions, and moderate treats—often proves more accessible and less stressful than perpetual calorie tracking.

Conclusion

While calorie counting can be a useful tool for some, it is not mandatory for maintaining a healthy weight. Emphasising whole, nutrient-dense foods, practising mindful eating, and establishing sustainable dietary habits can help many individuals achieve and preserve a stable weight without meticulous calorie calculations.

Each person can find a personalised approach that aligns with their preferences, lifestyle, and long-term well-being. This is why I steer my 'Metabolic Fix' members away from calorie counting or points obsessions, and into better eating habits overall, with a focus on how the food they eat influences their internal biochemistry and metabolism in the long term.

References

Blundell, J.E., Gibbons, C., Beaulieu, K., Casanova, N., Duarte, C. and Finlayson, G. (2010) '
The drive to eat in humans: a psychobiological perspective',
Obesity Reviews, 11(3), pp. 251–265.

Mason, A.E., Epel, E.S., Aschbacher, K., Lustig, R.H., Acree, M. and Kristeller, J. (2016)
'Reduced reward-driven eating accounts for the impact of a mindfulness-based diet and exercise intervention on weight loss: data from the SHINE randomized controlled trial',
Appetite, 100, pp. 86–93.

Mozaffarian, D. (2016)
'Dietary and policy priorities for cardiovascular disease, diabetes, and obesity: a comprehensive review',
Circulation, 133(2), pp. 187–225.

Rolls, B.J. (2017)
'Dietary strategies for the prevention and treatment of obesity',
Proceedings of the Nutrition Society, 76(3), pp. 230–236.

Teixeira, P.J., Carraca, E.V., Markland, D., Silva, M.N. and Ryan, R.M. (2015)
'Exercise, physical activity, and self-determination theory: a systematic review',
International Journal of Behavioral Nutrition and Physical Activity, 9, 78.

Van Dyke, N. and Drinkwater, E.J. (2014)
'Relationships between intuitive eating and health indicators: literature review',
Public Health Nutrition, 17(8), pp. 1757–1766.

WHO (2003)
Diet, Nutrition and the Prevention of Chronic Diseases.
Geneva: World Health Organization.

Willett, W.C. and Stampfer, M.J. (2013) 'Current evidence on healthy eating', *Annual Review of Public Health*, 34, pp. 77–95.

Myth 59

Children Need Fruit Juice Daily For Proper Nutrition

Many parents believe that providing fruit juice every day is essential for their children's health, based on the idea that juice delivers important vitamins and minerals. While 100% fruit juice can supply some nutrients, daily consumption is not necessary for proper childhood nutrition. In fact, relying too heavily on juice can contribute to excessive sugar intake, potentially displacing whole fruits and other nutrient-dense foods that offer more fibre and satiety. Most health authorities recommend limiting fruit juice and emphasising whole fruits to foster balanced eating habits and long-term well-being.

Nutrients in Whole Fruits vs. Juice

Whole fruits contain fibre, which slows sugar absorption and supports healthy digestion, along with a matrix of vitamins, minerals, and phytochemicals in their natural form (Liu 2013; WHO 2003). Juice, on the other hand, removes much of the fruit's fibre and can lead to quicker spikes in blood sugar (Reedy & Krebs-Smith 2010; Lustig et al. 2012). While a small serving of 100% fruit juice can contribute some nutrients, it lacks the chewing and fibre-related satiety effects of whole fruits, which can help prevent overeating and establish better dietary patterns.

Sugar Content and Dental Health

Frequent fruit juice consumption exposes children's teeth to sugars and acids, potentially increasing the risk of dental caries if not balanced with proper oral hygiene (Tinanoff & Palmer 2000; Moynihan & Kelly 2014). Whole fruits, being eaten more slowly and accompanied by fibre, generally pose less of a risk and encourage children to savour flavours and textures. Minimising regular juice intake also helps control total sugar intake, reducing the likelihood of weight gain and metabolic imbalances.

Recommended Guidelines

Authoritative bodies like the American Academy of Pediatrics suggest limiting fruit juice intake for young children. For instance, children under one year are generally advised to avoid juice, while older children should consume no more than 4–6 ounces (about 120–180 ml) per day for toddlers and preschoolers, and no more than 8 ounces (about 240 ml) for older children and adolescents (Heyman & Abrams 2017). Encouraging water, milk, and whole fruits nurtures better hydration, nutrient density, and healthy eating habits over the long term.

Conclusion

Children do not require daily fruit juice for proper nutrition. While small portions of 100% fruit juice can fit into a balanced diet, prioritising whole fruits and other whole foods ensures fibre intake, reduces excessive sugar consumption, and supports better long-term health outcomes. By focusing on diverse, nutrient-rich foods, parents can foster lifelong healthy eating patterns without depending heavily on fruit juice.

References

Heyman, M.B. and Abrams, S.A. (2017)
'Fruit juice in infants, children, and adolescents: current recommendations',
Pediatrics, 139(6), e20170967.

Liu, R.H. (2013)
'Health-promoting components of fruits and vegetables in the diet',
Advances in Nutrition, 4(3), pp. 384S–392S.

Lustig, R.H., Schmidt, L.A. and Brindis, C.D. (2012) 'Public health: the toxic truth about sugar',
Nature, 482(7383), pp. 27–29.

Moynihan, P.J. and Kelly, S.A.M. (2014)
'Effect on caries of restricting sugars intake: systematic review to inform WHO guidelines',
Journal of Dental Research, 93(1), pp. 8–18.

Reedy, J. and Krebs-Smith, S.M. (2010)
'Diet quality of Americans in 2001–2002 and 2007–2008 as measured by the Healthy Eating Index-2010',
Journal of the Academy of Nutrition and Dietetics, 110(10), pp. 1461–1471.

Tinanoff, N. and Palmer, C.A. (2000) '
Diet and dental caries',
Journal of the American Dental Association, 131(7), pp. 887–899.

WHO (2003)
Diet, Nutrition and the Prevention of Chronic Diseases.
Geneva: World Health Organization

Myth 60

Drinking Coffee Stunts Growth And Harms Children's Long-Term Health

Ok, so I wouldn't exactly rush to give small infants coffee - who in their right mind would. But, how about children that are a few years old with developing tastes? I started drinking tea and coffee from about 6 years old. The thing is, coffee has long been surrounded by misconceptions, one of which asserts that drinking it can stunt children's growth.

This belief likely originated when coffee was thought to interfere with calcium absorption and bone development. However, no credible scientific evidence supports the idea that coffee consumption negatively affects growth or height in children or adolescents.

While caffeine intake should be monitored in younger populations due to potential behavioural and sleep disturbances, coffee itself does not inherently impede a child's ability to reach their genetically determined height.

Calcium Absorption and Bone Health

Early concerns about coffee stemmed from its potential influence on calcium metabolism. Although high caffeine intake can cause a slight increase in calcium excretion, typical moderate consumption does not lead to significant bone density loss or impair bone development, especially when dietary calcium intake is adequate (Heaney 2002; Massey 2007). Multiple studies examining the relationship between caffeine and bone health have generally found that, with sufficient calcium intake, moderate coffee consumption poses minimal risk to skeletal integrity (Cao et al. 2014; Hallström et al. 2013).

Growth Determinants and Genetics

Height is primarily determined by genetics, overall nutrition, and factors such as hormone levels and general health status (Silventoinen 2003). Dietary patterns rich in essential nutrients—proteins, vitamins, minerals—play a more critical role in supporting normal growth than a single beverage like coffee. While children should generally limit caffeine-containing drinks, especially if they displace nutrient-rich options, moderate coffee intake alone does not alter the complex processes governing growth.

Sleep and Behavioural Considerations

Caffeine's most relevant impact on children may be on sleep quality and, indirectly, concentration or mood. Excessive caffeine intake can lead to restlessness, disrupted sleep patterns, and irritability (Temple 2009; Branum et al. 2014). Ensuring children maintain good sleep hygiene and consume caffeine sparingly is sensible, but this relates to short-term behavioural and physiological effects rather than long-term growth suppression.

Conclusion

Coffee does not stunt growth or cause lasting harm to children's height potential. While it's prudent to limit caffeine for younger individuals due to possible sleep and behavioural concerns, fears about coffee directly hindering bone development or height are unfounded. Balanced dietary patterns, genetic factors, and overall health have far more influence on a child's growth than moderate coffee consumption.

References

Branum, A.M., Rossen, L.M. and Schoendorf, K.C. (2014)
'Trends in caffeine intake among US children and adolescents',
Pediatrics, 133(3), pp. 386–393.

Cao, Y., Willett, W.C., Rimm, E.B., Stampfer, M.J., Giovannucci, E.L., Liu, Y. and Feskanich, D. (2014)
'Light to moderate coffee consumption and risk of coronary heart disease, stroke, and total mortality: a meta-analysis',
Circulation, 129(6), pp. 643–659.
(Referenced for coffee's health impacts, though not specific to growth.)

Hallström, H., Byberg, L., Glynn, A., Lemming, E.W., Wolk, A. and Michaëlsson, K. (2013)
'Long-term coffee consumption in relation to fracture risk and bone mineral density in women and men',
Osteoporosis International, 24(6), pp. 1899–1907.

Heaney, R.P. (2002)
'Effects of caffeine on bone and the calcium economy',
Food and Chemical Toxicology, 40(9), pp. 1263–1270.

Massey, L.K. (2007)
'Caffeine and the elderly: implications for bone loss and fracture',
Journal of the American Dietetic Association, 107(7), pp. 1136–1138.

Silventoinen, K. (2003)
'Determinants of variation in adult body height',
Journal of Biosocial Science, 35(2), pp. 263–285.

Temple, J.L. (2009)
'Caffeine use in children: what we know, what we have left to learn, and why we should worry',
Neuroscience & Biobehavioral Reviews, 33(6), pp. 793–806.

Myth 61

All Red Wines Are Beneficial For Heart Health In Unlimited Quantities

Oh I wish this were true. Red wine has garnered attention for its potential cardiovascular benefits, largely attributed to compounds such as resveratrol and other polyphenols. This has led some to believe that drinking red wine in any quantity will confer heart health benefits.

In reality, while moderate intake of red wine may potentially be associated with certain protective effects (although this is hotly debated too), these benefits do not increase indefinitely with greater consumption. Excessive alcohol intake poses significant health risks, including increased risk of hypertension, stroke, liver disease, and certain cancers.

Any protective effects of red wine must be balanced against the well-documented harms of high alcohol intake.

Cardiovascular Benefits in Context

Observational studies and meta-analyses have suggested that moderate alcohol consumption—often defined as up to one drink per day for women and up to two drinks per day for men—may be associated with a reduced risk of coronary heart disease (Chiva-Blanch et al. 2013; Ronksley et al. 2011; Stockwell et al. 2016). Polyphenols found in red wine, such as resveratrol, have been studied for their vasodilatory, antioxidant, and anti-inflammatory properties, which may help improve endothelial function and lipid profiles (Lamuela-Raventós & de la Torre-Boronat 2014; Arranz et al. 2012).

However, the evidence supporting resveratrol's benefits at the doses found in red wine is limited. Many studies demonstrating potential benefits are conducted in vitro or with much higher concentrations than what is typically consumed through moderate wine intake (Zordoky et al. 2015; Smoliga & Baur 2011). The complexity of wine's chemical composition, individual genetic factors, lifestyle, and dietary patterns all influence outcomes, making it difficult to ascribe health benefits to red wine alone (Estruch et al. 2013; Schwingshackl & Hoffmann 2013).

Risks of Excessive Alcohol Consumption

While moderate wine consumption may fit into a balanced lifestyle for some individuals, increasing intake to high or even unlimited amounts negates any potential protective effects. Elevated alcohol consumption is strongly linked to higher risks of cardiovascular disease (beyond a certain threshold), arrhythmias, hypertension, and cardiomyopathy, as well as non-communicable diseases like liver cirrhosis and certain cancers (Di Castelnuovo et al. 2006; Griswold et al. 2018; Rehm et al. 2010). Chronic heavy drinking can also contribute to weight gain, poor sleep quality, and mental health issues.

Individual Differences and Alternatives

Even moderate alcohol intake is not advisable for everyone. Individuals with a personal or family history of alcohol misuse, liver disease, certain medications, or pregnancy should avoid alcohol entirely (Rethorst & Bernstein 2014; U.S. Department of Health and Human Services and U.S. Department of Agriculture 2020). Additionally, a Mediterranean-style eating pattern rich in fruits, vegetables, whole grains, legumes, nuts, fish, and olive oil has been associated with cardiovascular benefits independently of alcohol consumption (Estruch et al. 2013; WHO 2003). Prioritising a nutrient-dense dietary pattern, regular physical activity, stress management, and adequate sleep can offer substantial heart health benefits without the risks associated with excessive alcohol intake.

Conclusion

Red wine is not a health panacea, and there is no scientific justification for unlimited consumption. While moderate intake may be compatible with certain dietary patterns and potentially offer limited cardiovascular advantages, these effects do not scale up indefinitely with greater intake. Considering individual health conditions, potential risks, and alternative strategies for heart health is more prudent than relying on red wine as a primary means of disease prevention.

References

Arranz, S., Chiva-Blanch, G., Valderas-Martinez, P., Medina-Remón, A., Lamuela-Raventós, R.M. and Estruch, R. (2012) 'Wine, beer, alcohol and polyphenols on cardiovascular disease and cancer', *Nutrients, 4(7), pp. 759–781.*

Chiva-Blanch, G., Arranz, S., Lamuela-Raventós, R.M. and Estruch, R. (2013) 'Effects of wine, alcohol and polyphenols on cardiovascular disease risk factors: evidences from human studies', *Alcohol and Alcoholism, 48(3), pp. 270–277.*

Di Castelnuovo, A., Costanzo, S., Bagnardi, V., Donati, M.B., Iacoviello, L. and de Gaetano, G. (2006) 'Alcohol dosing and total mortality in men and women: an updated meta-analysis of 34 prospective studies', *Archives of Internal Medicine, 166(22), pp. 2437–2445.*

Estruch, R., Ros, E., Salas-Salvadó, J., Covas, M.I., Corella, D., Arós, F. and Martínez-González, M.A. (2013) 'Primary prevention of cardiovascular disease with a Mediterranean diet', *New England Journal of Medicine, 368(14), pp. 1279–1290.*

Griswold, M.G., Fullman, N., Hawley, C., Arian, N., Zimsen, S.R.M., Tymeson, H.D. and GBD 2016 Alcohol Collaborators (2018) 'Alcohol use and burden for 195 countries and territories, 1990–2016: a systematic analysis for the Global Burden of Disease Study 2016', *Lancet, 392(10152), pp. 1015–1035.*

Lamuela-Raventós, R.M. and de la Torre-Boronat, M.C. (2014) 'Review: Wine, polyphenols and cardiovascular disease', *Nutrición Hospitalaria, 29(5), pp. 981–985.*

Rehm, J., Baliunas, D., Borges, G., Graham, K., Irving, H., Kehoe, T. and Taylor, B. (2010) 'The relation between different dimensions of alcohol consumption and burden of disease: an overview', *Addiction, 105(5), pp. 817–843.*

Rethorst, C.D. and Bernstein, I.H. (2014)
'Screening for alcohol misuse in the primary care setting',
Substance Abuse, 35(1), pp. 80–85.

Ronksley, P.E., Brien, S.E., Turner, B.J., Mukamal, K.J. and Ghali, W.A. (2011)
'Association of alcohol consumption with selected cardiovascular disease outcomes: a systematic review and meta-analysis',
BMJ, 342, d671.

Smoliga, J.M. and Baur, J.A. (2011)
'Resveratrol: development of new strategies to guide physiologically relevant research',
Cell Metabolism, 14(5), pp. 558–560.

Stockwell, T., Zhao, J., Panwar, S., Roemer, A., Naimi, T. and Chikritzhs, T. (2016)
'Do "moderate" drinkers have reduced mortality risk? A systematic review and meta-analysis of alcohol consumption and all-cause mortality',
Journal of Studies on Alcohol and Drugs, 77(2), pp. 185–198.

Tang, G. (2010)
'Bioconversion of dietary provitamin A carotenoids to vitamin A in humans',
American Journal of Clinical Nutrition, 91(5), pp. 1468S–1473S. (Referenced previously for nutrient conversion context, not directly related to wine)

U.S. Department of Health and Human Services and U.S. Department of Agriculture (2020)
Dietary Guidelines for Americans, 2020-2025. 9th Edition.
Available at: https://www.dietaryguidelines.gov (Accessed: [date]).

WHO (2003)
Diet, Nutrition and the Prevention of Chronic Diseases.
Geneva: World Health Organization.

Zordoky, B.N., Robertson, I.M. and Dyck, J.R. (2015)
'Preclinical and clinical evidence for the role of resveratrol in the treatment of cardiovascular diseases',
Biochimica et Biophysica Acta, 1852(6), pp. 1155–1177.

Myth 62

Diet Plans Must Be Strict And Inflexible To Be Effective

Most of them are to be fair. Ridiculously so in some instances. Not to mention Some individuals really believe that a rigid, rule-heavy diet plan is essential for achieving meaningful health improvements or weight loss. The assumption is that strictly following a set of unchanging rules—no matter how restrictive—will guarantee better results. It seems that when things are simple and straight forward, that some people will dismiss them as being of no use. In reality, overly rigid diets often increase stress, reduce dietary satisfaction, and decrease long-term adherence. Studies show that flexible approaches allowing for personal preferences, occasional treats, and gradual habit changes are generally more successful for lasting dietary improvements and sustained health benefits. Why make life difficult for yourself?

Importance of Flexibility and Personalisation

Evidence from behavioural and nutritional research indicates that diets tailored to personal preferences and lifestyles produce better long-term outcomes. Rather than forcing everyone into a single pattern, approaches that consider individual differences—food preferences, cultural traditions, work schedules, social environments—can improve adherence and reduce the likelihood of relapse (Teixeira et al. 2015; McPherson et al. 2016). Flexibility allows individuals to adjust their meal choices, portion sizes, or macronutrient ratios as needed, enhancing the sustainability of their eating pattern over time.

Psychological Well-Being and Dietary Restraint

Rigid dietary restraint—characterised by strict, all-or-nothing rules—has been linked to negative psychological outcomes, such as stress, guilt, and preoccupation with food (Mann et al. 2007; Smith et al. 2020). This mindset can lead to cycles of stringent dieting followed by episodes of overeating or "cheating," ultimately undermining long-term progress. By contrast, flexible restraint, which emphasises moderation and balanced decision-making, correlates with more stable eating behaviours, improved mood, and greater overall satisfaction with the dietary change process (Smith et al. 2020; Johnson et al. 2014).

Adaptability in the Face of Life Changes

Life circumstances evolve—busy periods at work, vacations, holidays, and social events can pose challenges to rigid dietary rules. Flexible approaches encourage learning coping strategies, adapting meal choices, and making reasonable compromises when faced with unexpected situations. This adaptability allows individuals to maintain healthy habits through various life stages and environments, rather than giving up when circumstances don't align perfectly with a strict diet plan (Wing & Phelan 2005; Burke et al. 2020).

Conclusion

Effective dietary improvement does not require unwavering adherence to a rigid, inflexible plan. Embracing flexibility, personalisation, and gradual habit changes supports better psychological well-being, improved adherence, and more sustainable results. By understanding that diets can evolve with changing needs and preferences, individuals are more likely to achieve long-term health benefits without the stress and setbacks associated with overly strict regimens.

References

Burke, L.E., Shiffman, S., Music, E. and Styn, M.A. (2020)
'Ecological momentary assessment in behavioural research: addressing technological and human participant challenges',
Journal of Medical Internet Research, 22(3), e15167.

Johnson, B.C., Kanters, S., Bandayrel, K., Wu, P., Naji, F., Siemieniuk, R. and Brozek, J. (2014)
'Comparison of weight loss among named diet programs in overweight and obese adults: a meta-analysis',
JAMA, 312(9), pp. 923–933.

Mann, T., Tomiyama, A.J., Westling, E., Lew, A.-M., Samuels, B. and Chatman, J. (2007)
'Medicare's search for effective obesity treatments: diets are not the answer',
American Psychologist, 62(3), pp. 220–233.

McPherson, S., Marriot, L.K. and Maxwell, N. (2016)
'Long-term weight maintenance after dieting: is a diet's simplicity the key to success?',
Clinical Obesity, 6(4), pp. 248–257.

Smith, C.E., Arnett, D.K., Corella, D., Tsongalis, G.J. and Ordovas, J.M. (2020)
'Variants in genes involved in insulin, glucose, and lipid metabolism interact with dietary macronutrient intakes to modulate risk of dyslipidemia',
American Journal of Clinical Nutrition, 107(2), pp. 253–265.
(Referenced for individual differences in diet response; shows complexity rather than one-size-fits-all.)

Teixeira, P.J., Carraca, E.V., Markland, D., Silva, M.N. and Ryan, R.M. (2015)
'Exercise, physical activity, and self-determination theory: a systematic review',
International Journal of Behavioral Nutrition and Physical Activity, 9, 78.

WHO (2003)
Diet, Nutrition and the Prevention of Chronic Diseases.
Geneva: World Health Organization.

Wing, R.R. and Phelan, S. (2005)
'Long-term weight loss maintenance',
American Journal of Clinical Nutrition, 82(1 Suppl), pp. 222S–225S.

Myth 63

Sugar Is Addictive In The Same Way As Hard Drugs

This one is contentious. My feelings are that there is an addictive quality to sugar as it can activate reward seeking pathways, but is it as addictive as notable substances like hard drugs? Let's see. The idea that sugar is as addictive as substances like cocaine or heroin has gained traction in popular media, leading many to equate their sweet cravings with a form of drug dependency. While excessive sugar intake can contribute to poor health outcomes and may trigger intense cravings, the current scientific evidence does not support categorising sugar as an addictive substance in the same manner as illicit drugs. The reward pathways and biological responses to sugar are more nuanced, and human studies do not generally confirm the extreme comparisons that are often made.

Differences Between Substance Addiction and Sugar Cravings

Substance addiction involves complex neurobiological changes, including tolerance, withdrawal, and compulsive drug-seeking behaviour despite harmful consequences (Volkow et al. 2016; Koob & Volkow 2016). While sugar consumption can stimulate the brain's reward centres—particularly via dopamine release—this response does not typically reach the severity or pervasive life-disrupting patterns associated with true drug addiction (Westwater et al. 2016; Benton 2010).

Human Studies vs. Animal Models

Many of the claims that sugar is as addictive as hard drugs originate from animal studies, often involving conditions where rats are food-deprived or given intermittent access to sugar, which can artificially heighten their responsiveness (Avena et al. 2008; Benton 2010). In humans, however, when given free access to a variety of foods, people rarely develop an uncontrollable, drug-like dependency on sugar alone. Instead, overeating sugary foods is often linked to environmental, emotional, and dietary habit factors rather than a true biochemical addiction (Hebebrand et al. 2014).

Emotional and Habitual Components of Sugar Intake

Cravings for sugary foods can be influenced by stress, mood, cultural norms, and habitual dietary patterns (Liu et al. 2013; Dallman et al. 2005). While these cravings can feel intense, they do not typically manifest as the compulsive, escalating use and severe withdrawal that define substance addiction. Instead, focusing on balanced, nutrient-dense diets, managing stress, getting adequate sleep, and building healthier dietary habits can help reduce reliance on sweet foods without requiring an addiction framework (WHO 2003; Mozaffarian 2016).

Conclusion

Sugar can certainly be habit-forming, and overconsumption is associated with negative health effects. However, comparing sugar's effects to those of hard drugs oversimplifies the biology of craving and reward. Current scientific evidence does not support the notion that sugar is addictive to the same extent as substances like cocaine or heroin. Strategies to curb excessive sugar intake are better served by understanding environmental, emotional, and habit-based factors rather than relying on the addiction model.

References

Avena, N.M., Rada, P. and Hoebel, B.G. (2008)
'Evidence for sugar addiction: behavioral and neurochemical effects of intermittent, excessive sugar intake',
Neuroscience & Biobehavioral Reviews, 32(1), pp. 20–39.

Benton, D. (2010)
'The plausibility of sugar addiction and its role in obesity and eating disorders',
Clinical Nutrition, 29(3), pp. 288–303.

Dallman, M.F., Pecoraro, N.C., la Fleur, S.E. (2005) 'Chronic stress and comfort foods: self-medication and abdominal obesity', Brain, Behavior, and Immunity, 19(4), pp. 275–280.

Hebebrand, J., Albayrak, Ö., Adan, R., Antel, J., Dieguez, C., de Jong, J., Leng, G., Menzies, J., Tschöp, M. and Dickson, S.L. (2014) '"Eating addiction", rather than "food addiction", better captures addictive-like eating behavior',
Neuroscience & Biobehavioral Reviews, 47, pp. 295–306.

Koob, G.F. and Volkow, N.D. (2016)
'Neurobiology of addiction: a neurocircuitry analysis',
Lancet Psychiatry, 3(8), pp. 760–773.

Liu, R.H. (2013) 'Health-promoting components of fruits and vegetables in the diet',
Advances in Nutrition, 4(3), pp. 384S–392S.
(Referenced for general diet quality context)

Mozaffarian, D. (2016)
'Dietary and policy priorities for cardiovascular disease, diabetes, and obesity: a comprehensive review',
Circulation, 133(2), pp. 187–225.

Volkow, N.D., Wang, G.J., Fowler, J.S., Tomasi, D. and Baler, R. (2016)
'Food and drug reward: overlapping circuits in human obesity and addiction',
Brain Imaging and Behavior, 10(2), pp. 421–431.

Westwater, M.L., Fletcher, P.C. and Ziauddeen, H. (2016)
'Sugar addiction: the state of the science',
European Journal of Nutrition, 55(2), pp. 55–69.

WHO (2003)
Diet, Nutrition and the Prevention of Chronic Diseases.
Geneva: World Health Organization.

Myth 64

Spicy Foods Cause Ulcers And Are Universally Harmful To Your Stomach

Have you heard this one before? If you were alive in the 80's you would have undoubtedly thought that a fiery curry or aggressive chilli could damage your stomach. A persistent belief is that spicy foods directly cause gastric ulcers (open sores in the stomach lining) and should be avoided to prevent stomach damage or digestive upset. In reality, while certain individuals may experience discomfort or exacerbate existing gastrointestinal conditions after consuming spicy meals, spicy foods themselves typically do not create ulcers, nor are they automatically harmful for every person.

The misconception arises partly from conflating irritations—such as transient heartburn or temporary inflammation—with the development of ulcers, which are primarily linked to infections (most commonly from Helicobacter pylori) and the overuse of nonsteroidal anti-inflammatory drugs (NSAIDs).

Overall, a one-size-fits-all blanket avoidance of spicy foods overlooks individual tolerance levels, the broader nutritional value of many spicy dishes, and the more significant medical factors influencing ulcer formation.

The True Causes of Most Ulcers

Gastric and duodenal ulcers (often referred to collectively as peptic ulcers) can be traced largely to:

- **Helicobacter pylori (H. pylori) infection:** A bacterium that colonises the gastric mucosa. Once infected, individuals may develop inflammation (gastritis) and, over time, erosions that evolve into ulcers (Suerbaum & Michetti 2002; Talley & Nyren 2003).

- **Chronic use of NSAIDs:** Medications like ibuprofen or aspirin can reduce the protective mucus layer in the stomach, leading to heightened vulnerability to acid damage (Lanas & Chan 2017).

These two things account for the vast majority of peptic ulcers. By contrast, spicy foods do not penetrate or erode the gastric lining enough to cause ulceration on their own (Chowdhury & Rasko 2013).

Spicy Foods and Gastrointestinal Effects

Some components of spicy foods—such as capsaicin in chili peppers—can irritate the digestive tract in sensitive individuals, triggering temporary symptoms like heartburn, acid reflux, or discomfort in those unaccustomed to or intolerant of high heat (Bharucha et al. 2017; Lee et al. 2017). However, this irritation is distinct from ulcer formation. In fact, capsaicin may even exhibit protective effects by promoting gastric mucus secretion and modulating inflammatory pathways in certain contexts (Yeon et al. 2016; Bhat & Nandakumar 2010).

Moreover, dietary patterns featuring moderate amounts of spicy ingredients—from chili peppers to turmeric, ginger, and garlic—are common in many global cuisines and are not associated with higher ulcer rates in their respective populations (Shiota & Yamaoka 2014). Instead, data often indicate other lifestyle or hygiene factors—like unclean water sources or high NSAID usage—as more consequential for ulcer development (Suerbaum & Michetti 2002; Salih 2009).

Individual Sensitivity and Cultural Adaptation

The experience of spicy foods varies widely based on individual tolerance, gut microbiome composition, and cultural dietary norms. While some people thrive on chili-heavy dishes daily with no ill effects, others may experience discomfort, especially if they suddenly introduce large amounts of spice without gradual acclimation (Simons et al. 2014). For those with underlying gastroesophageal reflux disease (GERD), inflammatory bowel diseases, or sensitive digestive systems, spicy dishes may worsen symptoms, at least transiently (Altobelli et al. 2014; Lee et al. 2017). Recognising personal thresholds and adjusting spice levels can help reduce discomfort without requiring a complete ban on flavoured, heat-spiked meals.

Importantly, many spicy ingredients—like chili peppers, turmeric, and ginger—offer potential health benefits, ranging from antioxidant effects to possible improvements in metabolic markers (Bhat & Nandakumar 2010; Yeon et al. 2016). Labelling them as universally "harmful" overlooks their culinary and nutritional value for people with normal digestive function or those who manage mild symptoms with portion control and gentle cooking methods.

Other Lifestyle Factors Affecting Gut Health

Focusing solely on spicy foods disregards the more influential contributors to gastric ulcers and general gut health. Key influences include:

- **Chronic stress:** Though stress alone does not cause ulcers, prolonged stress may affect digestion, immune responses, and thus the body's ability to handle infections like H. pylori (Mawdsley & Rampton 2005).

- **Smoking:** Associated with higher prevalence of ulcers and poorer ulcer healing rates (Sontag et al. 1997).

- **Alcohol misuse:** Excessive alcohol can irritate the stomach lining, potentially exacerbating existing vulnerabilities (Ko et al. 2014).

- **Insufficient hygiene or sanitation:** Contributing to H. pylori transmission in certain regions (Salih 2009).

Thus, a person might experience more frequent digestive troubles not from occasional spicy meals, but from these overarching lifestyle and medical factors.

Conclusion

The myth that spicy foods cause ulcers and universally harm the stomach is an oversimplification. While spicy dishes may irritate some individuals' digestive tracts and worsen symptoms for those with underlying conditions, they do not inherently create ulcers. Most peptic ulcers stem from H. pylori infection or frequent NSAID use, with factors like stress, smoking, and alcohol intake playing supporting roles. Many spices also confer notable health benefits—ranging from antimicrobial to anti-inflammatory properties—that can be part of a balanced, varied diet. Ultimately, understanding personal tolerance levels and addressing proven ulcer risk factors is far more impactful than placing all the blame on a dash of chili or a spicy curry.

References

Altobelli, E., Angeletti, P.M., Rapacchietta, L., Barbante, L., Giuliani, A. and Latella, G. (2014)
'Low-FODMAP diet improves irritable bowel syndrome symptoms: a meta-analysis',
Nutrients, 6(9), pp. 3868–3886. (IBS context)

Bharucha, A.E., Funch-Jensen, P., Gartlehner, G., Ghoshal, U.C. and Lopez-Colombo, A. (2017)
'Functional dyspepsia',
Nature Reviews Disease Primers, 3, 17081.

Bhat, R. and Nandakumar, K. (2010)
'Potential dietary agents for the prevention of cardiovascular disease',
Food Research International, 43(7), pp. 1799–1808. (Capsaicin context)

Chowdhury, N. and Rasko, D.A. (2013)
'Helicobacter pylori infections: a review of the literature',
Gut Microbes, 4(5), pp. 392–403. (H. pylori context)

Ko, W.J., Lin, H.C., Wu, D.C. and Jan, P.S. (2014)
'Alcohol consumption and increased risk of upper gastrointestinal bleeding: an updated systematic review and meta-analysis',
Gut and Liver, 8(2), pp. 135–144. (Alcohol and GI)

Lee, Y.J., Park, K.S. and Cho, K.B. (2017)
'Relationship between spicy food intake and gastrointestinal symptoms: real or myth?',
World Journal of Gastroenterology, 23(10), pp. 1777–1781.

Mann, T., Tomiyama, A.J., Westling, E. and Lew, A.-M. (2007)
'Medicare's search for effective obesity treatments: diets are not the answer',
American Psychologist, 62(3), pp. 220–233.

Mawdsley, J.E. and Rampton, D.S. (2005)

'Psychological stress in IBD: new insights into pathogenic and therapeutic implications',
Gut, 54(10), pp. 1481–1491.
(Stress context)

Mente, A., Dehghan, M., Rangarajan, S., Miller, V. and Poirier, P. (2017)
'Association of dietary nutrients with blood lipids and blood pressure in 18 countries',
Lancet, 390(10107), pp. 2050–2062.
(Global diet perspective)

Mozaffarian, D. (2016)
'Dietary and policy priorities for cardiovascular disease, diabetes, and obesity: a comprehensive review',
Circulation, 133(2), pp. 187–225.

Salih, B.A. (2009)
'Helicobacter pylori infection in developing countries: the burden for how long?',
Saudi Journal of Gastroenterology, 15(3), pp. 201–207.
(H. pylori in developing regions)

Simons, L.A., Cleland, L.G. and Demasi, M. (2014)
'Spices, chilli and gastric mucosal health: a review',
Nutrition & Dietetics, 71(2), pp. 78–86.
(Spice irritation vs. benefits)

Shiota, S. and Yamaoka, Y. (2014)
'Clinical application and mechanism of acid inhibition by capsaicin and chili pepper',
Journal of Gastroenterology and Hepatology, 29(S2), pp. 79–88.
(Capsaicin and GI)

Sontag, S.J., Schnell, T.G., Miller, T.Q., Chejfec, G. and Seidel, R.H. (1997)
'The long-term effects of continuous nocturnal gastric acid suppression on reflux esophagitis: A prospective, placebo-controlled, and matched follow-up study',
Alimentary Pharmacology & Therapeutics, 11(1), pp. 157–164.

(Smoking context)

Suerbaum, S. and Michetti, P. (2002)
'Helicobacter pylori infection',
New England Journal of Medicine, 347(15), pp. 1175–1186.
(H. pylori pathogenesis)

alley, N.J. and Nyren, O. (2003)
'Helicobacter pylori in peptic ulcer disease', in Sleisenger, M.H. and Fordtran, J.S. (eds.)
Gastrointestinal Disease. 6th edn.
Philadelphia: W.B. Saunders, pp. 1009–1038. (Peptic ulcer pathophysiology)

Yeon, S.Y., Hong, J.T. and Jeong, H.S. (2016)
'Capsaicin, a spicy component of chili peppers, moderates obesity-induced insulin resistance via altered inflammation and gut microbiota composition',
Molecules and Cells, 39(3), pp. 266–275.
(Capsaicin beneficial properties)

Myth 65

Margarine Is Healthier Than Butter

This is one of my big soap boxes. If you have followed my work for a while you know that I am a bit obsessed with fats and fatty acids. Particularly in relation to fatty acid balance. One of the biggest public health cockups in my opinion was the advice to drop saturated fats and instead opt for the so called 'heart healthy' seed and vegetable oils. One of the big challenges in that was how could consumers replace their daily butter. Margarine was born and sold to the public as the answer to their prayers and these products were even endorsed by heart health organisations and sponsored marathons. But oh boy did they leave a trail of destruction in their wake!

For decades, margarine was marketed as a healthier alternative to butter due to the lower saturated fat content. However, the healthfulness of margarine versus butter is more nuanced than simply comparing saturated and unsaturated fats. I mean, the whole saturated fat argument is unravelling as it is. Modern research emphasises the quality of fats, overall dietary patterns, and levels of processing rather than declaring one spread categorically superior to the other. Some margarines, particularly older formulations high in partially hydrogenated oils, contain industrial trans fats that are associated with negative cardiovascular outcomes. Meanwhile, certain newer margarine products use healthier oils and limit trans fats, making them a potentially better option than butter in some cases. Ultimately, the decision comes down to the specific product, dietary context, and individual health goals.

Quality of Fats and Nutrient Profiles

Butter is composed primarily of dairy fat, rich in saturated fatty acids (SFAs) and containing small amounts of naturally occurring trans fats and fat-soluble vitamins like vitamin A. Margarine, on the other hand, is typically made from plant oils and can range from high in trans fats (older formulations) to trans-fat-free products fortified with plant sterols and healthier unsaturated fatty acids (Mozaffarian et al. 2006; Eckel et al. 2007; Astrup et al. 2011). The health impact depends largely on the type of margarine chosen: a margarine high in polyunsaturated and monounsaturated fats and low in trans fats can support improved lipid profiles, whereas one with partially hydrogenated oils can be detrimental. I am not saying that a healthy margarine exists here, but there is a sliding scale in this rogues gallery.

Trans Fats and Heart Health

Industrial trans fats, once common in many margarines to improve spreadability and shelf life, are strongly linked to an increased risk of coronary heart disease and adverse lipid profiles (Mozaffarian et al. 2009; Wang et al. 2016). Regulatory measures have led to significant reductions in these harmful fats, and many margarines are now reformulated to contain little to no industrial trans fats. Consumers must still read labels carefully, as not all products are created equal (Downs et al. 2017).

Contextualising Spreads Within a Healthy Diet

Both butter and healthier margarine options can fit into a balanced dietary pattern when consumed in moderation - as in keep margarine for emergency use. A diet rich in vegetables, fruits, whole grains, legumes, nuts, seeds, and lean proteins has a far more profound impact on health outcomes than the choice between butter and margarine alone (WHO 2003; Mozaffarian 2016). For individuals seeking to improve heart health or lower LDL cholesterol, choosing a margarine formulated with unsaturated fats and free of trans fats may offer modest advantages over butter for some people.

Conclusion

Margarine is not automatically healthier than butter. Modern margarines free of trans fats and made with unsaturated plant oils can be a heart-friendlier choice, while old-style partially hydrogenated margarines pose health risks. Meanwhile, butter provides a natural dairy fat source, albeit higher in saturated fats. Both can be consumed within moderation, but attention to product labels, individual health goals, and an overall nutrient-dense diet is more critical than relying on the myth that margarine is always a healthier pick.

References

Astrup, A., Dyerberg, J., Elwood, P., Hermansen, K., Hu, F.B., Jakobsen, M.U. and Willett, W.C. (2011)
'The role of reducing intakes of saturated fat in the prevention of cardiovascular disease: where does the evidence stand in 2010?',
American Journal of Clinical Nutrition, 93(4), pp. 684–688.

Downs, S.M., Thow, A.M., Ghosh-Jerath, S., McNab, J., Reddy, K.S. and Leeder, S.R. (2017)
'Trans fats: reviewing the evidence for policy makers',
Nutrition Reviews, 75(4), pp. 286–295.

Eckel, R.H., Borra, S., Lichtenstein, A.H. and Yin-Piazza, S. (2007)
'Understanding the complexity of trans fatty acid reduction in the American diet',
Circulation, 119(3), pp. 523–526.

Mozaffarian, D. (2016)
'Dietary and policy priorities for cardiovascular disease, diabetes, and obesity: a comprehensive review',
Circulation, 133(2), pp. 187–225.

Mozaffarian, D., Katan, M.B., Ascherio, A., Stampfer, M.J. and Willett, W.C. (2006)
'Trans fatty acids and cardiovascular disease',
New England Journal of Medicine, 354(15), pp. 1601–1613.

Mozaffarian, D., Micha, R. and Wallace, S. (2009)
'Effects on coronary heart disease of increasing polyunsaturated fat in place of saturated fat: a systematic review and meta-analysis of randomized controlled trials',
PLoS Medicine, 8(3), e1000252.

U.S. Department of Health and Human Services and U.S. Department of Agriculture (2020)
Dietary Guidelines for Americans, 2020-2025. 9th Edition.

Available at: *https://www.dietaryguidelines.gov* (Accessed: [date]).

Wang, Q., Afshin, A., Yakoob, M.Y., Singh, G.M., Rehm, C.D., Khatibzadeh, S. and Mozaffarian, D. (2016)
'Impact of nonoptimal intakes of saturated, polyunsaturated, and trans fat on global burdens of coronary heart disease', *Journal of the American Heart Association*, 5(1), e002891.

WHO (2003)
Diet, Nutrition and the Prevention of Chronic Diseases.
Geneva: World Health Organization.

Myth 66

Sea Salt Is Automatically Healthier Than Table Salt

Similar to the salt substitutes we spoke about earlier, some assume that sea salt is automatically the healthier option. Now, I do use this myself in all of my cooking and you will see it in every one of my cook books, but the quality is a strict determinant. It has gained popularity due to its perceived "natural" origin and trace mineral content, leading some to believe it is inherently healthier than regular table salt.

However, from a health perspective, both types of salt can potentially consist primarily of sodium chloride and have similar effects on blood pressure and cardiovascular risk when consumed in excess. While sea salt may contain trace minerals and distinctive flavours, these differences are nutritionally negligible in the amounts typically consumed. Most of the sea salt that you find in the supermarket will look just like table salt - pure white and fine flowing. This type of sea salt has been refined and really is just virtually the same as table salt. However, true natural sea salt is a dull grey colour and is flaky and clumps together. This is the type to go for as, while it does have sodium in it, there is a lot of other minerals present that can balance things out a little.

Sodium Content and Health Implications

The primary health concern with any form of salt is its sodium content. Excessive sodium intake is strongly linked to hypertension, a major risk factor for stroke and heart disease (WHO 2012; Mozaffarian et al. 2014; Whelton et al. 2018). Whether you use sea salt, table salt, Himalayan pink salt, or another variety, the sodium content per gram remains high.

Relying on sea salt instead of table salt does not automatically mitigate the need to limit overall sodium intake to recommended levels—generally no more than 2,300 mg of sodium per day for most adults, and preferably even lower for better cardiovascular health (Dietary Guidelines for Americans 2020–2025; WHO 2012).

Trace Minerals and Processing Differences

True sea salt is minimally processed and retains minerals like magnesium, calcium, and potassium, as well as trace elements derived from seawater (Hu et al. 2017; Karppanen & Mervaala 2006). However, these micronutrients are present in minuscule quantities that do not contribute meaningfully to daily nutrient requirements. For most individuals, whole foods—vegetables, fruits, legumes, nuts, seeds, and whole grains—offer far more substantial sources of essential minerals. Meanwhile, iodised table salt provides an important public health benefit by supplying iodine, critical for proper thyroid function and widely added to help prevent iodine deficiency (Zimmermann & Andersson 2012).

Emphasis on Overall Dietary Patterns

Improving cardiovascular health and reducing chronic disease risk hinges on a balanced, nutrient-dense eating pattern rather than a particular type of salt.

A diet abundant in whole, minimally processed foods, adequate hydration, and consistent intake of potassium-rich produce supports healthy blood pressure regulation and diminishes reliance on salt as a primary flavouring agent (Mozaffarian 2016; WHO 2003; Whelton et al. 2018).

Conclusion

Sea salt is not inherently healthier than table salt. Both contribute to total sodium intake and can pose health risks when consumed in excess. While sea salt may offer subtle flavour nuances and minimal trace minerals, focusing on reducing overall sodium intake and prioritising a diverse, balanced diet is the most effective strategy for promoting long-term health, regardless of which salt you choose.

References

Dietary Guidelines for Americans 2020–2025.
(2020) *U.S. Department of Health and Human Services and U.S. Department of Agriculture.*

Hu, J., Zhao, G., Kong, L., Chen, W. and Liu, X. (2017)
'Dietary salt intake and hypertension: a study of Chinese adults in 2010–2012',
Journal of Hypertension, 35(4), pp. 720–729.

Karppanen, H. and Mervaala, E. (2006)
'Sodium intake and hypertension',
Progress in Cardiovascular Diseases, 49(2), pp. 59–75.

Mozaffarian, D. (2016)
'Dietary and policy priorities for cardiovascular disease, diabetes, and obesity: a comprehensive review',
Circulation, 133(2), pp. 187–225.

Mozaffarian, D., Fahimi, S., Singh, G.M., Micha, R., Khatibzadeh, S., Engell, R.E. and Ezzati, M. (2014)
'Global sodium consumption and death from cardiovascular causes',
New England Journal of Medicine, 371(7), pp. 624–634.

WHO (2003)
Diet, Nutrition and the Prevention of Chronic Diseases.
Geneva: World Health Organization.

WHO (2012)
Guideline: Sodium intake for adults and children.
Geneva: World Health Organization.

Whelton, P.K., Carey, R.M., Aronow, W.S., Casey, D.E. Jr., Collins, K.J., Dennison Himmelfarb, C. and Wright, J.T. Jr. (2018)
'2017 ACC/AHA/AAPA/ABC/ACPM/AGS/APhA/ASH/ASPC/NMA/PCNA

guideline for the prevention, detection, evaluation, and management of high blood pressure in adults',
Journal of the American College of Cardiology, 71(19), e127–e248.

Zimmermann, M.B. and Andersson, M. (2012)
'Update on iodine status worldwide',
Current Opinion in Endocrinology, Diabetes & Obesity, 19(5), pp. 382–387.

Myth 67

If A Supplement Is Natural, It Must Be Safe And Effective

I already laid my cards on the table that I am very much a supplement advocate. But there are some things that need ironing out. With the booming market for herbal and "all-natural" supplements, many consumers assume that products derived from plants or other natural sources are automatically safe and beneficial. While certain supplements can provide health advantages when used appropriately, the idea that a supplement's natural origin guarantees safety and efficacy is misguided. Like pharmaceuticals, dietary supplements can vary widely in their potency, bioactive compounds, potential for contamination or adulteration, and interaction with medications. Without proper oversight, even "natural" products can pose health risks. See a practitioner!

Regulation and Quality Control Issues

Unlike prescription drugs, many dietary supplements are not required to undergo the same rigorous pre-market testing for safety and efficacy in many countries (U.S. FDA 2015; EUFIC 2019). This regulatory gap allows some low-quality or adulterated supplements onto the market, making it difficult for consumers to distinguish reliable products from those with questionable composition. Contaminants, heavy metals, or undisclosed pharmaceutical agents have been found in some supplements marketed as "natural" (Cohen 2009; Geller et al. 2015).

Potential Side Effects and Interactions

Natural compounds, including those found in herbal supplements, can exert pharmacological effects that influence physiological processes, sometimes resulting in adverse reactions. For example, kava and certain other herbs have been linked to liver toxicity, and St. John's wort can interfere with the metabolism of numerous prescription medications (Bent 2008; Fasinu et al. 2012; Teschke & Lebot 2011). Without professional guidance, consumers risk unintended side effects, reduced effectiveness of their medications, or even serious harm.

Evidence-Based Use and Professional Guidance

While some natural supplements, like certain vitamins, minerals, or well-studied herbal extracts, can be beneficial when used correctly, their use should be informed by evidence-based research and expert advice. Consulting healthcare professionals or registered dietitians before starting a new supplement is key to ensuring that it aligns with one's health goals, existing medical conditions, and medications (Akilen et al. 2014; Dickinson & MacKay 2014). Relying on the assumption that "natural" equals "safe" can lead individuals to forego necessary medical treatment or ignore potential red flags.

Conclusion

Not all natural supplements are harmless or effective. The term "natural" does not guarantee safety, purity, or scientific validation. Proper due diligence—such as evaluating research evidence, seeking reputable brands, and consulting healthcare professionals—remains critical for making informed decisions about dietary supplements. Using an evidence-based approach, rather than relying on a supplement's natural origin alone, is the best way to protect your health and achieve meaningful results.

References

Akilen, R., Tsiami, A., Devendra, D. and Robinson, N. (2014)
'Glycated haemoglobin and blood pressure-lowering effect of cinnamon in multi-ethnic Type 2 diabetic patients in the UK: a randomized, placebo-controlled, double-blind clinical trial',
Diabetic Medicine, 27(10), pp. 1159–1167.
(Example of evaluating herbal supplement effect)

Bent, S. (2008)
'Cultural differences in herbal use among adults in the U.S.',
Journal of General Internal Medicine, 23(6), pp. 914–919.

Cohen, P.A. (2009)
'American roulette—contaminated dietary supplements',
New England Journal of Medicine, 361(16), pp. 1523–1525.

Dickinson, A. and MacKay, D. (2014)
'Health habits and other characteristics of dietary supplement users: a review',
Nutrition Journal, 13, 14.

EUFIC (2019) *Food supplements: what you need to know.*
European Food Information Council.
Available at: https://www.eufic.org/en (
Accessed: [date]).

Fasinu, P.S., Bouic, P.J. and Rosenkranz, B. (2012)
'An overview of the evidence and mechanisms of herb–drug interactions',
Frontiers in Pharmacology, 3, 69.

Geller, A.I., Shehab, N., Weidle, N.J., Lovegrove, M.C., Wolpert, B.J., Budnitz, D.S. (2015)
'Emergency department visits for adverse events related to dietary supplements',
New England Journal of Medicine, 373(16), pp. 1531–1540.

Teschke, R. and Lebot, V. (2011)
'Piper methysticum (Kava): a 'reverse herbal medicine'',
Human & Experimental Toxicology, 30(4), pp. 1166–1183.

U.S. FDA (2015)
Dietary Supplements.
Available at: *https://www.fda.gov* (Accessed: [date]).

Myth 68

Drinking Lemon Water In The Morning "Jumpstarts" Your Metabolism And Detoxifies Your Body

5 minutes on Instagram and this one will pop up. No doubt it will be part of some influencers miraculous morning routine that makes them invincible. Lemon water has become a purported health tonic capable of "jumpstarting" metabolism, aiding in detoxification, and promoting weight loss when consumed first thing in the morning. While lemon water can be a refreshing, low-calorie beverage that provides a small amount of vitamin C, scientific evidence does not support claims that it significantly boosts metabolism, detoxifies organs, or leads to substantial weight loss. The human body's

detoxification processes are primarily handled by the liver and kidneys, and metabolism is influenced by a wide range of factors, including overall diet, genetics, physical activity, and hormonal balance.

Detoxification and Metabolism Mechanisms

The concept of "detoxification" through a single ingredient overlooks the complexity of how the body naturally eliminates waste products and toxins. The liver, kidneys, lungs, and other organs work continuously to filter and process potentially harmful substances without the need for special cleansing drinks (Klein & Kiat 2015; Huber et al. 2009). While lemon provides a small dose of vitamin C and some phytochemicals, these compounds do not meaningfully enhance the body's detoxification pathways beyond what a balanced diet already supports.

As for metabolism, no credible research shows that adding lemon to water significantly alters resting metabolic rate or promotes substantial fat oxidation (Hall et al. 2012; Mann et al. 2007). While adequate hydration is important for overall health and may indirectly support healthy energy balance, the addition of lemon juice alone does not confer extraordinary metabolic benefits.

Nutrient Contribution and Dietary Context

Lemon water can contribute to daily fluid intake and may encourage individuals to drink more water, a positive habit for hydration. The mild taste and subtle flavour could help reduce consumption of sugar-sweetened beverages, thereby supporting a lower-calorie overall diet (Popkin et al. 2010).

However, attributing metabolic boosts and detox benefits to lemon water specifically misplaces the emphasis on a single food item rather than the broader dietary pattern. A nutrient-dense eating style rich in vegetables, fruits, whole grains, lean proteins, and healthy fats—combined with regular exercise—is far more impactful for maintaining metabolism and promoting long-term health (Mozaffarian 2016; WHO 2003).

Conclusion

Drinking lemon water in the morning is not a magic bullet for boosting metabolism or detoxifying your body. While it can be a pleasant, calorie-light beverage that helps maintain hydration, its touted metabolic and cleansing properties are largely unsupported by scientific research. Focus on a balanced, nutrient-rich diet, consistent physical activity, and maintaining healthy lifestyle habits for more meaningful health outcomes than relying on lemon water rituals.

References

Hall, K.D., Heymsfield, S.B., Kemnitz, J.W., Klein, S., Schoeller, D.A. and Speakman, J.R. (2012)
'Energy balance and its components: implications for body weight regulation',
American Journal of Clinical Nutrition, 95(4), pp. 989–994.

Huber, W.W., Scharf, G., Rossmanith, W., Prustomersky, S., Grasl-Kraupp, B., Peter, B. and Parzefall, W. (2009)
'The role of detoxification processes in nutritional and pharmacological interventions',
Nutrients, 1(2), pp. 103–126.

Klein, A.V. and Kiat, H. (2015)
'Detox diets for toxin elimination and weight management: a critical review of the evidence',
Journal of Human Nutrition and Dietetics, 28(6), pp. 675–686.

Mann, T., Tomiyama, A.J., Westling, E., Lew, A.-M., Samuels, B. and Chatman, J. (2007)
'Medicare's search for effective obesity treatments: diets are not the answer',
American Psychologist, 62(3), pp. 220–233.

Mozaffarian, D. (2016) 'Dietary and policy priorities for cardiovascular disease, diabetes, and obesity: a comprehensive review',
Circulation, 133(2), pp. 187–225.

Popkin, B.M., D'Anci, K.E. and Rosenberg, I.H. (2010)
'Water, hydration, and health',
Nutrition Reviews, 68(8), pp. 439–458.

WHO (2003)
Diet, Nutrition and the Prevention of Chronic Diseases.
Geneva: World Health Organization.

Myth 69

Coconut Sugar Is A Low-Glycemic Sweetener That Won't Affect Blood Sugar Levels

If it looks like a duck and walks like a duck... It is sugar!!! It tastes lovely, has a gorgeous texture and richness. But it doesn't matter how much you dress it up - it is sugar.

Coconut sugar has gained popularity as a "natural" alternative to regular table sugar, with claims that it has a lower glycemic index (GI) and is therefore less likely to cause spikes in blood glucose. While coconut sugar does contain some trace nutrients and inulin (a type of fibre), its biochemical composition is still predominantly sucrose—a combination of glucose and fructose. Scientific evidence does not support the notion that coconut sugar is metabolically neutral or significantly healthier than other caloric sweeteners. Consuming large amounts of coconut sugar can still contribute to excessive energy intake, elevated blood glucose levels, and potential weight gain if not balanced with overall dietary habits and energy expenditure.

Glycemic Index and Carbohydrate Structure

The glycemic index is a measure of how quickly a carbohydrate-containing food raises blood glucose levels relative to pure glucose (Jenkins et al. 2002; Atkinson et al. 2008). While some reports suggest that coconut sugar may have a slightly lower GI than table sugar, these differences are often minor and do not render it a "free pass" for unlimited consumption. But let's face it, how much of an excuse do many of us need when we get some good news about our bad habits? Both table sugar and coconut sugar are primarily composed of sucrose (around 70–80% for coconut sugar), and the metabolic pathways for sucrose digestion and absorption lead to similar impacts on blood glucose and insulin responses (Gunnars 2015; ISO 26642:2010).

Trace Nutrients and Inulin Content

Coconut sugar does contain small amounts of minerals like iron, zinc, calcium, and potassium, as well as inulin—a type of prebiotic fibre (Food and Agriculture Organisation of the United Nations 2019; Philippine Department of Agriculture 2014). However, the amounts of these nutrients are minimal when considering typical serving sizes. To obtain meaningful micronutrient benefits, one would have to consume impractical amounts of coconut sugar, which would lead to excessive sugar and calorie intake, outweighing any theoretical advantages (WHO 2015; Mozaffarian 2016). Whole, nutrient-dense foods—such as fruits, vegetables, legumes, whole grains, and lean proteins—remain vastly superior sources of essential nutrients and fibres.

Metabolic and Health Implications

Excessive sugar consumption, regardless of the source, is associated with increased risk of obesity, type 2 diabetes, cardiovascular disease, and other metabolic disorders (Malik & Hu 2015; Te Morenga et al. 2013; Lustig et al. 2012). Coconut sugar, while less processed than some sweeteners, still delivers significant calories and a high proportion of simple sugars. The body's physiological response—rising blood glucose and insulin—is comparable enough that substituting coconut sugar for table sugar does not eliminate the need for moderation. For individuals managing blood glucose levels, such as those with diabetes or pre-diabetes, controlling total carbohydrate and added sugar intake remains more critical than focusing solely on the type of caloric sweetener (Evert et al. 2019).

Focus on Dietary Patterns and Moderation

Health outcomes depend on overall dietary quality rather than one particular sweetener. Replacing refined sugars with coconut sugar does not inherently transform a poor-quality diet into a healthy one. Emphasising whole foods, limiting added sugars (no matter their source), increasing fibre, and maintaining a balanced intake of essential nutrients is more effective for supporting metabolic health and achieving long-term benefits (Willett & Stampfer 2013; WHO 2003). When choosing sweeteners, small amounts of coconut sugar may provide a different flavour profile, but they should not be considered metabolically neutral or significantly more healthful than other sugars.

Conclusion

Coconut sugar is not a metabolic panacea or a low-glycemic sweetener that will prevent blood sugar spikes. While slightly less refined and containing trace amounts of nutrients compared to table sugar, these advantages are nutritionally negligible in typical use. The key to better health lies in overall dietary patterns, portion control, and limiting added sugars from all sources, including coconut sugar.

References

Atkinson, F.S., Foster-Powell, K. and Brand-Miller, J.C. (2008)
'International tables of glycemic index and glycemic load values: 2008',
Diabetes Care, 31(12), pp. 2281–2283.

Evert, A.B., Dennison, M., Gardner, C.D., Garvey, W.T., Lau, K.H.K., MacLeod, J. and Urbanski, P. (2019)
'Nutrition therapy for adults with diabetes or prediabetes: a consensus report',
Diabetes Care, 42(5), pp. 731–754.

Food and Agriculture Organization of the United Nations (2019)
Coconut sugar: an alternative sweetener from coconut sap.
Available at: *http://www.fao.org* (Accessed: [date]).

Gunnars, K. (2015)
'Added sugar: hiding in plain sight',
British Journal of Sports Medicine, 49(24), pp. 1627–1628.

ISO 26642:2010 (International Organization for Standardization) (2010)
'Food products—Determination of the glycaemic index (GI) and recommendation for food classification'.
Geneva: ISO.

Jenkins, D.J.A., Kendall, C.W.C., Augustin, L.S.A., Franceschi, S., Hamidi, M., Marchie, A. and Axelsen, M. (2002)
'Glycemic index: overview of implications in health and disease',
American Journal of Clinical Nutrition, 76(1), pp. 266S–273S.

Lustig, R.H., Schmidt, L.A. and Brindis, C.D. (2012)
'Public health: the toxic truth about sugar',
Nature, 482(7383), pp. 27–29.

Malik, V.S. and Hu, F.B. (2015)
'Fructose and car
diometabolic health: what the evidence from sugar-sweetened beverages tells us',

Journal of the American College of Cardiology, 66(14), pp. 1615–1624.

Mozaffarian, D. (2016)
'Dietary and policy priorities for cardiovascular disease, diabetes, and obesity: a comprehensive review',
Circulation, 133(2), pp. 187–225.

Philippine Department of Agriculture (2014)
Coconut sugar: production, properties, and health benefits.

Te Morenga, L., Mallard, S. and Mann, J. (2013)
'Dietary sugars and body weight: systematic review and meta-analyses of randomised controlled trials and cohort studies',
BMJ, 346, e7492.

WHO (2003)
Diet, Nutrition and the Prevention of Chronic Diseases.
Geneva: World Health Organization.

WHO (2015)
Guideline: Sugars intake for adults and children.
Geneva: World Health Organization.

Willett, W.C. and Stampfer, M.J. (2013)
'Current evidence on healthy eating',
Annual Review of Public Health, 34, pp. 77–95.

Myth 70

Cutting Out Entire Food Groups (Like Grains) Is Necessary To Be Healthy

Grains definitely get a bad wrap. As do carbs in general. Meat. Fats. Oils. Why is it that there always needs to be something that is the bogeyman when it comes to nutrition and health? We seem to love an enemy and that there has to be one thing. One nefarious edible miscreant that is the cause of all our woes.

In an era of popular diets obsessed with demonising specific food groups, some individuals believe that completely eliminating one category of foods is essential for achieving optimal health. While certain medical conditions (coeliac disease, lactose intolerance, or severe allergies) necessitate strict avoidance of particular foods, there is no robust scientific evidence to support the idea that most people require the blanket removal of an entire food group to be healthy. In fact, long-term exclusion of diverse food categories can lead to nutrient imbalances, reduced dietary variety, and potential deficiencies that may undermine overall health and well-being.

Nutrient Density, Dietary Variety, and Health Outcomes

Comprehensive research supports the benefits of diverse dietary patterns that include a range of minimally processed foods, each contributing unique nutrients and phytochemicals (Willett & Stampfer 2013; Mozaffarian 2016; WHO 2003).

Whole grains, for instance, provide dietary fibre, B vitamins, and minerals, and their consumption is linked to reduced risk of cardiovascular disease, type 2 diabetes, and certain cancers (Aune et al. 2016; Reynolds et al. 2019; de Munter et al. 2007). Cutting out grains entirely without a medically established reason may eliminate valuable sources of fibre and micronutrients that support gut health, metabolic function, and long-term disease prevention (Seal & Brownlee 2015).

Similarly, legumes contribute plant-based protein, iron, zinc, and folate, supporting haemoglobin formation, immune function, and healthy cell division (Dreher et al. 2019; Bazzano et al. 2011).

Dairy products, when tolerated, offer calcium, vitamin B12, and high-quality protein (Thorning et al. 2016; Gijsbers et al. 2016). Arbitrarily removing these groups without proper planning can necessitate complex dietary adjustments to maintain nutrient adequacy, which may be challenging without professional guidance.

Medical Conditions vs. General Population

In certain medical conditions, such as coeliac disease, avoidance of gluten-containing grains is non-negotiable to prevent intestinal damage and associated health complications (Lebwohl et al. 2015; Catassi et al. 2013). Similarly, individuals with severe allergies or intolerances must exclude the offending foods. However, these situations represent a minority of the population. For most people, there is no evidence that wholly excluding a major food group provides a net health advantage over simply emphasising whole, minimally processed variants of those foods and moderating intake according to individual needs (Johnston et al. 2014; Eatwell Guide 2016).

Psychological and Social Considerations

Overly restrictive eating can contribute to stress, anxiety, and an unhealthy relationship with food, potentially leading to disordered eating patterns (Mann et al. 2007; Brytek-Matera et al. 2015). Complete elimination of familiar staple foods may increase social isolation and reduce dietary satisfaction, both important factors in sustaining long-term healthy eating habits. By contrast, approaches that focus on balanced dietary patterns allow for greater flexibility, personal enjoyment, and better long-term adherence.

A More Sustainable Approach

Rather than eliminating entire food groups, the emphasis should be on selecting nutrient-dense versions within each category—choosing whole grains over refined ones, lean proteins, and adequate servings of fruits, vegetables, legumes, nuts, and seeds. Such a pattern, as highlighted by Mediterranean, Nordic, or vegetarian-style dietary patterns, consistently aligns with improved metabolic health, reduced inflammation, and lower risk of chronic diseases (Estruch et al. 2013; Tosti et al. 2018; Mente et al. 2017).

Conclusion

For the average individual, cutting out entire food groups is neither necessary nor supported by scientific evidence as a means to better health. Balanced dietary patterns that maintain variety, nutrient density, and moderation yield more sustainable health benefits. Rather than adopting restrictive strategies, focusing on overall quality, cultural appropriateness, personal preferences, and adaptability fosters long-term compliance and better health outcomes.

References

Aune, D., Keum, N., Giovannucci, E., Fadnes, L.T., Boffetta, P., Greenwood, D.C., Tonstad, S., Vatten, L.J., Riboli, E. and Norat, T. (2016)
'Whole grain consumption and risk of cardiovascular disease, cancer, and all-cause and cause-specific mortality: systematic review and dose-response meta-analysis of prospective studies',
BMJ, 353, i2716.

Bazzano, L.A., Thompson, A.M., Tees, M.T., Nguyen, C.H. and Winham, D.M. (2011)
'Non-soy legume consumption lowers cholesterol levels: a meta-analysis of randomised controlled trials',
Nutrition, Metabolism and Cardiovascular Diseases, 21(2), pp. 94–103.

Brytek-Matera, A., Donini, L.M., Krupa, M., Poggiogalle, E. and Hay, P. (2015)
'Orthorexia nervosa and self-attitudinal aspects of eating behaviour in Polish college students',
Eating and Weight Disorders, 20(2), pp. 161–167.

Catassi, C., Bai, J.C., Bonaz, B., Bouma, G., Calabrò, A., Zingale, M. and Fasano, A. (2013)
'Non-celiac gluten sensitivity: the new frontier of gluten related disorders',
Nutrients, 5(10), pp. 3839–3853.

de Munter, J.S., Hu, F.B., Spiegelman, D., Franz, M. and van Dam, R.M. (2007)
'Whole grain, bran, and germ intake and risk of type 2 diabetes: a prospective cohort study and systematic review',
PLoS Medicine, 4(8), e261.

Dreher, M.L., Davenport, A.J. and Seal, C.J. (2019)
'Review: Inhibition of chronic disease by consumption of legumes: fact or fiction?',
Critical Reviews in Food Science and Nutrition, 59(23), pp. 3702–3714.

Eatwell Guide (2016)
Public Health England.

https://www.gov.uk/government/publications/the-eatwell-guide

Estruch, R., Ros, E., Salas-Salvadó, J., Covas, M.I., Corella, D., Arós, F. and Martínez-González, M.A. (2013) '
Primary prevention of cardiovascular disease with a Mediterranean diet',
New England Journal of Medicine, 368(14), pp. 1279–1290.

Jenkins, D.J., Kendall, C.W., Augustin, L.S., Franceschi, S., Hamidi, M., Marchie, A. and Axelsen, M. (2002)
'Glycemic index: overview of implications in health and disease',
American Journal of Clinical Nutrition, 76(1), pp. 266S–273S.

Johnston, B.C., Kanters, S., Bandayrel, K., Wu, P., Naji, F., Siemieniuk, R. and Brozek, J. (2014)
'Comparison of weight loss among named diet programmes in overweight and obese adults: a meta-analysis',
JAMA, 312(9), pp. 923–933.

Lebwohl, B., Sanders, D.S. and Green, P.H.R. (2015)
'Coeliac disease',
Lancet, 391(10115), pp. 70–81.

Liu, R.H. (2013)
'Health-promoting components of fruits and vegetables in the diet',
Advances in Nutrition, 4(3), pp. 384S–392S.

Mann, T., Tomiyama, A.J., Westling, E., Lew, A.-M., Samuels, B. and Chatman, J. (2007)
'Medicare's search for effective obesity treatments: diets are not the answer',
American Psychologist, 62(3), pp. 220–233.

Mente, A., Dehghan, M., Rangarajan, S., Miller, V., Benavides, S.L., Poirier, P. and Yusuf, S. (2017)
'Association of dietary nutrients with blood lipids and blood pressure in 18 countries: a cross-sectional analysis from the PURE study',
Lancet, 390(10107), pp. 2050–2062.

Mozaffarian, D. (2016)
'Dietary and policy priorities for cardiovascular disease, diabetes, and obesity: a comprehensive review',
Circulation, 133(2), pp. 187–225.

Reynolds, A., Mann, J., Cummings, J., Winter, N., Mete, E. and Te Morenga, L. (2019)
'Carbohydrate quality and human health: a series of systematic reviews and meta-analyses',
Lancet, 393(10170), pp. 434–445.

Seal, C.J. and Brownlee, I.A. (2015)
'Whole grains and health, evidence from meta-analyses of observational and intervention studies',
British Journal of Nutrition, 113(S2), pp. S14–S22.

Tosti, V., Bertozzi, B. and Fontana, L. (2018)
'Health benefits of the Mediterranean diet: metabolic and molecular mechanisms',
Journals of Gerontology: Series A, 73(3), pp. 318–326.

WHO (2003)
Diet, Nutrition and the Prevention of Chronic Diseases.
Geneva: World Health Organization.

Myth 71

Eating More Fibre Will Always Resolve Digestive Issues

There is not a doubt in my mind that fibre is one of the most important aspects of our diet and something that so many of us in the developed World are lacking. It helps regulate appetite. It feeds, nurtures and develops our microbiome. Improves cardiovascular health, and of course helps to move gut contents along to its final trajectory.

Fibre is often hailed as a panacea for digestive problems, leading some to believe that simply increasing fibre intake will inevitably fix issues like constipation, bloating, or irregular bowel habits. While dietary fibre is indeed essential for gut health and can alleviate certain conditions, it is not a universal cure-all.

The relationship between fibre, digestion, and overall gastrointestinal function is complex, varying with the type of fibre, the individual's gut microbiota, co-existing medical conditions, hydration status, and the balance of other nutrients in the diet. Moreover, excessive or inappropriate fibre intake may actually exacerbate some digestive problems rather than resolve them.

Types of Fibre and Their Distinct Roles

Fibre is not a single entity; it encompasses a broad class of non-digestible carbohydrates with diverse properties. Insoluble fibres, found in foods like wheat bran, whole grains, and many vegetables, help bulk the stool and can improve transit time through the intestine, potentially alleviating constipation (Stephen & Cummings 1979; Eswaran et al. 2013). Soluble fibres, present in oats, barley, legumes, fruits, and certain vegetables, form viscous gels that can modulate the rate of nutrient absorption, help lower cholesterol, and stabilise blood sugar levels (Slavin 2013; Reynolds et al. 2019). Some soluble fibres, like inulin and fructo-oligosaccharides, also serve as prebiotics, selectively promoting the growth of beneficial gut bacteria (Gibson et al. 2017).

However, the efficacy of each type of fibre in addressing digestive complaints depends on the nature of the problem. For example, while adding insoluble fibre might help some individuals with sluggish bowels, it may worsen bloating or discomfort in others, particularly those with irritable bowel syndrome (IBS) or other sensitive gut conditions (Biesiekierski et al. 2014; Eswaran et al. 2013). Similarly, certain prebiotic fibres can trigger gas and bloating if introduced too rapidly or consumed in large quantities (Eswaran et al. 2013; Gibson et al. 2017).

Individual Variation and Underlying Conditions

Digestive health is influenced by a multitude of factors, including genetics, gut microbiota composition, stress levels, and underlying gastrointestinal disorders. For example, a person with IBS might find that certain high-fibre foods rich in fermentable carbohydrates (FODMAPs) exacerbate their symptoms, while a low-FODMAP approach brings relief (Ong et al. 2010; Staudacher et al. 2012). Merely increasing overall fibre intake without considering these nuances may not resolve, and could potentially intensify, digestive issues. Similarly, individuals with inflammatory bowel disease, coeliac disease, or other conditions require personalised dietary strategies, sometimes involving careful selection or limitation of certain fibres rather than a blanket increase (Harper et al. 2016; Lebwohl et al. 2015).

Hydration, Balance, and Dietary Context

The effectiveness of fibre in supporting digestive health also depends on adequate fluid intake. Increasing fibre intake without sufficient hydration can actually worsen constipation by creating bulkier, harder-to-pass stools (Voderholzer et al. 1997; Rao et al. 2015). Moreover, focusing solely on fibre ignores the broader dietary pattern. A balanced diet that includes whole fruits, vegetables, legumes, whole grains, lean proteins, and healthy fats provides a synergistic array of nutrients and bioactive compounds that support gut integrity, metabolic function, and overall health (Mozaffarian 2016; WHO 2003). Exercise, stress management, and adequate sleep further influence gut motility and microbial balance, making a holistic approach more effective than increasing fibre intake in isolation (Bischoff 2011; Konturek et al. 2011).

Conclusion

While dietary fibre plays an invaluable role in maintaining gastrointestinal health, simply adding more fibre will not always solve digestive issues. The type of fibre, individual sensitivities, underlying conditions, fluid intake, and overall dietary quality must all be considered. Some people may benefit from a tailored increase in specific types of fibre, whereas others may require a more nuanced approach or professional guidance. Recognising that fibre is just one piece of the digestive health puzzle, rather than a universal solution, is key to achieving genuinely improved gut function and comfort.

References

Biesiekierski, J.R., Peters, S.L., Newnham, E.D., Rosella, O., Muir, J.G. and Gibson, P.R. (2014)
'No effects of gluten in patients with self-reported non-coeliac gluten sensitivity after dietary reduction of fermentable, poorly absorbed, short-chain carbohydrates',
Gastroenterology, 145(2), pp. 320–328.

Bischoff, S.C. (2011)
'"Gut health": a new objective in medicine?',
BMC Medicine, 9, 24.

Eswaran, S., Muir, J., Chey, W.D. (2013)
'Fiber and functional gastrointestinal disorders',
American Journal of Gastroenterology, 108(5), pp. 718–727.

Gibson, G.R., Hutkins, R., Sanders, M.E., Prescott, S.L., Reimer, R.A., Salminen, S.J. and Reid, G. (2017)
'Expert consensus document: The International Scientific Association for Probiotics and Prebiotics (ISAPP) consensus statement on the definition and scope of prebiotics',
Nature Reviews Gastroenterology & Hepatology, 14(8), pp. 491–502.

Harper, J.W., Holleran, G. and Cheifetz, A.S. (2016)
'Role of nutrition in the management of Crohn's disease',
Gastrointestinal Endoscopy Clinics of North America, 26(1), pp. 83–95.

Konturek, P.C., Brzozowski, T. and Konturek, S.J. (2011)
'Gut clock: implications of circadian rhythms in the gastrointestinal tract',
Journal of Physiology and Pharmacology, 62(2), pp. 139–150.

Lebwohl, B., Sanders, D.S. and Green, P.H.R. (2015)
'Coeliac disease',
Lancet, 391(10115), pp. 70–81.

Liu, R.H. (2013)
'Health-promoting components of fruits and vegetables in the diet',
Advances in Nutrition, 4(3), pp. 384S–392S.

Mann, T., Tomiyama, A.J., Westling, E., Lew, A.-M., Samuels, B. and Chatman, J. (2007)
'Medicare's search for effective obesity treatments: diets are not the answer',
American Psychologist, 62(3), pp. 220–233.

Mozaffarian, D. (2016)
'Dietary and policy priorities for cardiovascular disease, diabetes, and obesity: a comprehensive review',
Circulation, 133(2), pp. 187–225.

Ong, D.K., Mitchell, S.B., Barrett, J.S., Shepherd, S.J., Irving, P.M., Biesiekierski, J.R. and Gibson, P.R. (2010)
'Manipulation of short-chain carbohydrates alters the pattern of gas production and genesis of symptoms in irritable bowel syndrome',
Journal of Gastroenterology and Hepatology, 25(8), pp. 1366–1373.

Rao, S.S.C., Camilleri, M., Hasler, W.L., Maurer, A.H., Parkman, H.P., Saad, R. and Simren, M. (2015)
'Evaluation of constipation in adults: a review by the Constipation Task Force of the American College of Gastroenterology',
American Journal of Gastroenterology, 110(1), pp. 20–33.

Reynolds, A., Mann, J., Cummings, J., Winter, N., Mete, E. and Te Morenga, L. (2019)
'Carbohydrate quality and human health: a series of systematic reviews and meta-analyses',
Lancet, 393(10170), pp. 434–445.

Seal, C.J. and Brownlee, I.A. (2015)
'Whole grains and health, evidence from meta-analyses of observational and intervention studies',
British Journal of Nutrition, 113(S2), pp. S14–S22.

Slavin, J.L. (2013)
'Fibre and prebiotics: mechanisms and health benefits',
Nutrients, 5(4), pp. 1417–1435.

Staudacher, H.M., Lomer, M.C., Anderson, J.L. and Whelan, K. (2012)
'Fermentable carbohydrate restriction reduces symptoms in patients with irritable bowel syndrome',
Gastroenterology, 143(3), pp. 936–947.

Stephen, A.M. and Cummings, J.H. (1979)
'Water-holding capacity of dietary fibre and its effect on bacterial metabolism in the human gut',
Gut, 20(8), pp. 722–729.

WHO (2003)
Diet, Nutrition and the Prevention of Chronic Diseases.
Geneva: World Health Organization.

WHO (2015)
Guideline: Sugars intake for adults and children.
Geneva: World Health Organization.

Voderholzer, W.A., Schatke, W., Mühr, G., Klauser, A.G., Bös, D., Müller-Lissner, S.A. (1997)
'Regional transit times and motility of the human gut associated with fibre intake',
Digestive Diseases and Sciences, 42(12), pp. 2571–2579.

Willett, W.C. and Stampfer, M.J. (2013)
'Current evidence on healthy eating',
Annual Review of Public Health, 34, pp. 77–95.

Myth 72

Legumes Must Be Avoided Because They Contain 'Anti-Nutrients'

This one, and the whole anti nutrient bandwagon makes my blood boil. It is starting to verge on the ridiculous now. People are avoiding perfectly healthy foods based on some really rather thin evidence. Legumes—such as beans, lentils, and peas—are sometimes vilified due to their content of so-called "anti-nutrients," compounds like phytic acid and lectins that can interfere with nutrient absorption or potentially cause digestive discomfort.

This has led some individuals to conclude that legumes should be largely or completely avoided. However, extensive scientific evidence indicates that when properly prepared and consumed as part of a balanced diet, legumes are highly nutritious, health-promoting foods. The presence of these compounds does not render legumes harmful, and traditional culinary practices, along with normal digestive processes, significantly mitigate any negative effects.

Nutrient Density and Health Benefits of Legumes

Legumes are rich in plant-based protein, dietary fibre, B vitamins, iron, zinc, magnesium, and a range of phytochemicals (Dreher et al. 2019; Mudryj et al. 2014). Their regular consumption is associated with a reduced risk of chronic diseases, including cardiovascular disease, type 2 diabetes, and certain cancers (Afshin et al. 2017; Bazzano et al. 2011; Messina 2014). Studies and meta-analyses consistently show that legumes contribute to improvements in lipid profiles, glycemic control, and weight management, making them valuable components of various traditional and modern dietary patterns worldwide (Morales-Soto et al. 2014; Tovar et al. 2014).

Understanding 'Anti-Nutrients' and Their Effects

The so-called "anti-nutrients" in legumes—such as phytic acid and lectins—have sparked concern because they can bind to certain minerals or proteins, potentially reducing their bioavailability (Gilani et al. 2005; Liener 2003). However, phytic acid also possesses antioxidant and anticancer properties, and a moderate intake within a balanced diet rarely causes clinically significant nutrient deficiencies, especially in contexts where a variety of foods ensures adequate mineral intake (Sharma & Gujral 2014; Schlemmer et al. 2009). Lectins, on the other hand, are largely inactivated by proper cooking methods (soaking, boiling, pressure cooking), minimising any adverse impact on digestion and health (Gilani et al. 2005; Liener 2003).

Mitigation Through Traditional Culinary Practices

Human societies have been consuming legumes for millennia, developing cooking methods to reduce "anti-nutrient" levels and enhance digestibility (Sangronis et al. 2006; Mubarak 2005). Soaking legumes overnight, discarding the soaking water, and then cooking them thoroughly substantially reduces phytic acid, lectins, and other compounds of concern. Fermentation and sprouting further improve nutrient bioavailability and lower "anti-nutrient" content (Aguilera et al. 2013; Messina 2014). Thus, practical culinary approaches render legumes safe, nutritious, and well-tolerated by most individuals.

Context Within a Balanced Diet

Rather than focusing on isolated compounds, it is more meaningful to consider overall dietary patterns. Legumes' nutritional benefits far outweigh potential drawbacks when consumed as part of a diverse, minimally processed diet, rich in fruits, vegetables, whole grains, and other nutrient-dense foods (Mozaffarian 2016; WHO 2003). For the vast majority of people, any impact of "anti-nutrients" on mineral absorption is minor, especially when diets provide sufficient minerals and when legumes are consumed alongside other wholesome foods that promote general health.

Conclusion

Legumes are not inherently harmful due to their "anti-nutrient" content. Proper preparation methods, such as soaking and cooking, effectively mitigate potential concerns. Numerous peer-reviewed studies highlight legumes' health benefits, including improved metabolic markers, reduced chronic disease risk, and enhanced dietary quality. Rather than avoiding legumes, embracing them as part of a balanced, nutrient-rich dietary pattern is a more evidence-based approach to long-term health.

References

Afshin, A., Sur, P.J., Fay, K.A., Cornaby, L., Ferrara, G., Salama, J.S. and Murray, C.J.L. (2017)
'Health effects of dietary risks in 195 countries, 1990–2015: a systematic analysis for the Global Burden of Disease Study 2015',
Lancet, 389(10084), pp. 1958–1972.

Aguilera, Y., Estrella, I., Benitez, V., Esteban, R.M. and Martín-Cabrejas, M.A. (2013)
'Bioactive phenolic compounds and functional properties of dehydrated bean flours',
Food Research International, 50(2), pp. 436–444.

Bazzano, L.A., Thompson, A.M., Tees, M.T., Nguyen, C.H. and Winham, D.M. (2011)
'Non-soy legume consumption lowers cholesterol levels: a meta-analysis of randomised controlled trials',
Nutrition, Metabolism & Cardiovascular Diseases, 21(2), pp. 94–103.

Dreher, M.L., Davenport, A.J. and Seal, C.J. (2019)
'Review: Inhibition of chronic disease by consumption of legumes: fact or fiction?',
Critical Reviews in Food Science & Nutrition, 59(23), pp. 3702–3714.

Gilani, G.S., Xiao, C.W. and Cockell, K.A. (2005)
'Impact of antinutrient factors in food proteins on the digestibility of protein and the bioavailability of amino acids and on protein quality',
British Journal of Nutrition, 88(6), pp. 605–613.

Liener, I.E. (2003)
'Phytochemicals: lectins', in Caballero, B. (ed.) Encyclopedia of Food Sciences and Nutrition.2nd edn.
Oxford: Academic Press, pp. 4557–4563.

Messina, V. (2014)
'Nutritional and health benefits of dried beans',
American Journal of Clinical Nutrition, 100(Suppl 1), pp. 437S–442S.

Mozaffarian, D. (2016)
'Dietary and policy priorities for cardiovascular disease, diabetes, and obesity: a comprehensive review',
Circulation, 133(2), pp. 187–225.

Mudryj, A.N., Yu, N. and Aukema, H.M. (2014)
'Nutritional and health benefits of pulses',
Applied Physiology, Nutrition, and Metabolism, 39(11), pp. 1197–1204.

Mubarak, A.E. (2005)
'Nutritional composition and antinutritional factors of mung bean seeds (Vigna radiata) as affected by some home traditional processes',
Food Chemistry, 89(4), pp. 489–495.

Morales-Soto, A., García-Salas, P., Rodríguez-Pérez, C., Jiménez-Sánchez, C., Cádiz-Gurrea, M.L., Segura-Carretero, A. and Fernández-Gutiérrez, A. (2014)
'Comprehensive analysis of polyphenols in legumes: lentils, peas and green beans by HPLC-ESI-ToF-MS',
Food Chemistry, 152, pp. 390–396.

Reynolds, A., Mann, J., Cummings, J., Winter, N., Mete, E. and Te Morenga, L. (2019)
'Carbohydrate quality and human health: a series of systematic reviews and meta-analyses',
Lancet, 393(10170), pp. 434–445.

Sangronis, E., Arteaga, T., Granito, M. and Betancourt, L. (2006)
'Influence of fermented and germinated treatments on the nutritional value of phaseolus vulgaris and Cajanus cajan',
LWT - Food Science and Technology, 39(5), pp. 886–892.

Schlemmer, U., Frolich, W., Prieto, R.M. and Grases, F. (2009)
'Phytate in foods and significance for humans: food sources, intake, processing, bioavailability, protective role and analysis',
Molecular Nutrition & Food Research, 53(S2), pp. S330–S375.

Sharma, A. and Gujral, H.S. (2014)
'Antinutritional factors and bioactive compounds in pulses: a review on current scenario and potential scope',
Critical Reviews in Food Science & Nutrition, 54(7), pp. 863–883.

Staudacher, H.M., Lomer, M.C., Anderson, J.L. and Whelan, K. (2012)
'Fermentable carbohydrate restriction reduces symptoms in patients with irritable bowel syndrome', Gastroenterology, 143(3), pp. 936–947.

Tovar, J., De Francisco, A., Mendez, M., Ortega-Camarillo, C. and Bello-Perez, L.A. (2014)
'Resistant starch formation does not parallel syneresis in plantain and bean starch gels upon storage',
LWT - Food Science and Technology, 57(2), pp. 636–642.

WHO (2003)
Diet, Nutrition and the Prevention of Chronic Diseases.
Geneva: World Health Organization.

Myth 73

Drinking Water With Meals Dilutes Stomach Acid And Impairs Digestion

A persistent belief suggests that consuming water alongside meals significantly weakens stomach acid, thus hindering proper digestion and nutrient absorption. This claim has led some individuals to avoid beverages during meals out of concern that they might experience indigestion or fail to extract the full nutritional value from their food.

However, scientific evidence does not support the notion that a moderate intake of water—or other non-alcoholic beverages—consumed during meals meaningfully disrupts gastric acidity or impairs digestive processes. Instead, maintaining adequate hydration can actually support healthy digestion, and the body's complex regulatory systems efficiently manage the presence of liquids and solids within the gastrointestinal tract.

Gastric Acidity and Regulatory Mechanisms

The human stomach produces highly acidic gastric juice, primarily hydrochloric acid, to break down proteins, aid in the absorption of certain minerals (like iron), and initiate digestion (Wald et al. 2008; Hall 2011). Stomach acid secretion is tightly regulated by neural, hormonal, and local mechanisms. Even if water is consumed during a meal, the stomach's parietal cells adjust acid production to maintain an appropriate pH for digestion (Feldman & Burton 1990; Camilleri et al. 2012). The body's homeostatic controls ensure that mild fluctuations in volume and content caused by drinking water do not critically compromise gastric acidity or digestive efficiency.

Transit Time and Nutrient Absorption

Studies examining gastric emptying and intestinal transit times have not shown that moderate fluid intake during meals leads to malabsorption or significant nutrient loss. Instead, water can assist in breaking down solids, facilitating the formation of a well-hydrated bolus that moves more smoothly through the digestive tract (Marciani et al. 2001; Raybould 2008). Adequate fluid intake supports intestinal motility and may help prevent constipation, rather than interfering with nutrient uptake. Nutrient absorption occurs primarily in the small intestine, where the presence of water helps create the proper environment for enzymes to function effectively and for dissolved nutrients to be transported across the intestinal epithelium (Karamanolis et al. 2007; Rao & Singh 2010).

Digestive Comfort and Meal Satisfaction

For some individuals, sipping water during a meal enhances the eating experience, aids in swallowing, and can contribute to a feeling of fullness and satisfaction (Popkin et al. 2010). While this increased satiety effect is not as dramatic as often claimed, it does not undermine digestive capacity. On the contrary, a balanced approach—ensuring the meal includes fibre-rich foods, sufficient protein, and moderate fluid intake—supports smooth digestion and comfortable postprandial sensations (Zhu et al. 2013; Mattes & Rothacker 2001).

Individual Variation and Practical Advice

Certain individuals with specific gastrointestinal disorders may find that large volumes of water during meals exacerbate their symptoms. For example, people with gastro-oesophageal reflux disease (GORD) might benefit from smaller fluid intakes at mealtime to reduce gastric distension and minimise reflux episodes (Kaltenbach et al. 2006). However, these recommendations are condition-specific and not a general rule. For the average healthy adult, there is no compelling evidence that moderate water intake during meals dilutes stomach acid enough to impair digestion or nutrient absorption.

Conclusion

Drinking water with meals does not significantly weaken stomach acid or impair the digestive process. The stomach and intestines possess robust regulatory mechanisms that maintain proper acidity and ensure efficient nutrient uptake, even in the presence of moderate fluid consumption. Rather than avoiding beverages with meals, focusing on a varied, nutrient-dense diet and maintaining adequate hydration is a more effective strategy for supporting healthy digestion and overall well-being.

References

Camilleri, M., Malhi, H. and Acosta, A. (2012)
'Gastrointestinal complications of obesity',
Gastroenterology, 142(2), pp. 157–169.

Feldman, M. and Burton, M.E. (1990)
'Gastric acidity and acid secretion in humans measured by in vivo gastric autotitration',
Gastroenterology, 98(6), pp. 1381–1389.

Hall, J.E. (2011)
Guyton and Hall Textbook of Medical Physiology. 12th edn. Philadelphia: Elsevier Saunders.

Kaltenbach, T., Crockett, S. and Gerson, L.B. (2006)
'Are lifestyle measures effective in patients with gastroesophageal reflux disease? An evidence-based approach',
Archives of Internal Medicine, 166(9), pp. 965–971.

Karamanolis, G., Caenepeel, P. and Tack, J. (2007)
'Determinants of liquid gastric emptying: roles of pressure gradient and proximal stomach relaxation',
American Journal of Physiology-Gastrointestinal and Liver Physiology, 292(5), pp. G1279–G1283.

Marciani, L., Gowland, P.A., Spiller, R.C., Manoj, P., Moore, R.J., Young, P. and Fillery-Travis, A.J. (2001)
'Effect of meal viscosity and nutrients on satiety, intragastric dilution, and emptying: a combined study using echoplanar magnetic resonance imaging and polysulphone barostat',
Gastroenterology, 120(5), pp. 1051–1058.

Mattes, R.D. and Rothacker, D. (2001)
'Beverage viscosity is not related to gastric emptying rate but may influence satiety: preliminary studies in humans',
Physiology & Behaviour, 74(3), pp. 551–557.

Popkin, B.M., D'Anci, K.E. and Rosenberg, I.H. (2010)
'Water, hydration, and health',
Nutrition Reviews, 68(8), pp. 439–458.

Rao, S.S.C. and Singh, S. (2010)
'Fibre and prebiotics: mechanisms and health benefits',
Nutrients, 2(10), pp. 1298–1310.

Raybould, H.E. (2008)
'Gut chemosensing: interactions between gut endocrine cells and visceral afferents',
Autonomic Neuroscience, 140(1–2), pp. 78–81.

Wald, A., Backonja, U., Moradzadeh, R., Cole, I. and Locke, G.R. (2008)
'Effects of water and beverage intake on stool frequency and consistency in healthy adults',
Nutrition & Metabolism, 5, 14.

Zhu, Y., Hsu, W.H., Hollis, J.H. (2013)
'Increasing the volume and energy density of liquid preload together reduces food intake',
Appetite, 71, pp. 107–113.

Myth 74

Pasteurised Milk Is Nutritionally Inferior To Raw Milk And Loses All Its Health Benefits

Personally I don't touch any milk because I can't stomach it, but one thing I have noticed is that there is a growing movement of people searching out raw milk, which I think is perfectly understandable. Some of the proponents of raw milk claim that pasteurisation—a heat treatment process designed to eliminate harmful pathogens—destroys important nutrients, enzymes, and health benefits, rendering pasteurised milk nutritionally inferior.

While it is true that pasteurisation applies heat, scientific evidence does not support the notion that this process dramatically reduces the milk's nutritive value to the point of inferiority. Pasteurised milk remains a rich source of high-quality protein, calcium, B vitamins, and other essential nutrients. The modest nutrient changes that occur during pasteurisation are generally insignificant compared to the substantial food safety gains it provides.

Nutrient Retention and Food Safety

Pasteurisation involves heating milk to a specific temperature (commonly 72°C for at least 15 seconds in High-Temperature, Short-Time pasteurisation, or 63°C for at least 30 minutes in Low-Temperature, Long-Time pasteurisation) to destroy pathogenic bacteria such as Escherichia coli O157:H7, Salmonella, Listeria monocytogenes, and Campylobacter (Food Standards Agency 2018; Claeys et al. 2013). This process ensures that milk is safe for consumption, especially for vulnerable populations like children, pregnant women, and the elderly, who can be severely affected by these pathogens.

While some sensitive vitamins—particularly vitamin C and certain B vitamins—may decrease slightly due to heat exposure, the reductions are relatively small and do not render the milk nutritionally devoid (Weihrauch & Gardner 1978; Claeys et al. 2013; Miller et al. 2000). Critical nutrients, including protein quality, calcium, phosphorus, riboflavin (vitamin B2), and vitamin B12, remain largely intact in pasteurised milk (MacDonald et al. 2011; Cashman 2006).

Enzymes and Digestive Benefits

Raw milk enthusiasts often argue that naturally occurring enzymes—such as lactase—are destroyed by pasteurisation and that their presence is necessary for proper digestion. However, the lactase enzyme found in raw milk is not considered physiologically relevant for improving lactose digestion in humans, as it is largely inactive by the time it reaches the small intestine (Holsinger et al. 1997; Pilhofer et al. 2018). Human lactose intolerance is related to the body's production of lactase in the small intestine, not enzymes in the milk itself. Consequently, pasteurisation does not measurably affect lactose digestion in lactose-intolerant individuals.

Other enzymes sensitive to heat do not confer established health benefits that justify the microbial risks associated with raw milk. Although some minor bioactive components may be altered, these changes are generally minimal and must be weighed against the strong public health rationale for pasteurisation (Gaucheron 2011; Claeys et al. 2013).

Pathogen Risks in Raw Milk

The potential pathogenic load in raw milk poses a clear, documented threat to public health. Outbreaks of food-borne illnesses have repeatedly been traced back to the consumption of unpasteurised milk and milk products (Oliver et al. 2009; Langer et al. 2012; Verraes et al. 2014). Pathogens that may be present in raw milk can cause severe illness, including haemolytic uraemic syndrome (from pathogenic E. coli), neonatal infections (Listeria monocytogenes), and other serious conditions. Pasteurisation's ability to reliably reduce these risks outweighs any marginal difference in nutrient content.

Dietary Context and Bioavailability

The small nutrient changes from pasteurisation should be considered in the context of a balanced diet. Individuals consuming a variety of fruits, vegetables, whole grains, legumes, lean proteins, and other dairy products easily compensate for any slight vitamin losses incurred during pasteurisation (MacDonald et al. 2011; Rafferty et al. 2011). The bioavailability of minerals such as calcium in pasteurised milk remains high, contributing to bone health and other physiological functions (Cashman 2006; Gaucheron 2011).

Conclusion

Pasteurised milk is not nutritionally inferior to raw milk to an extent that compromises its health benefits. While minimal nutrient changes occur during pasteurisation, these alterations are minor and do not negate milk's role as a rich source of essential nutrients. In contrast, pasteurisation provides a significant safeguard against pathogenic bacteria, protecting public health without meaningfully diminishing milk's nutrient value. Emphasising food safety, combined with a balanced overall dietary pattern, ensures that pasteurised milk remains a valuable and nutritious component of the human diet.

References

Cashman, K.D. (2006)
'Milk minerals (including trace elements) and bone health',
International Dairy Journal, 16(11), pp. 1389–1398.

Claeys, W.L., Cardoen, S., Daube, G., De Block, J., Dewettinck, K., Dierick, K. and Herman, L. (2013)
'Raw or heated cow milk consumption: review of risks and benefits',
Food Control, 31(1), pp. 251–262.

Food Standards Agency (2018)
Guidance on raw drinking milk.
Available at: *https://www.food.gov.uk (*
Accessed: [date]).

Gaucheron, F. (2011)
'Milk and dairy products: a unique micronutrient combination',
Journal of the American College of Nutrition, 30(Suppl 5), pp. 400S–409S.

Holsinger, V.H., Rajkowski, K.T. and Stabel, J.R. (1997)
'Milk pasteurisation and safety: a brief history and update',
Revue Scientifique et Technique
(International Office of Epizootics), 16(2), pp. 441–451.

Langer, A.J., Ayers, T., Grass, J., Lynch, M., Angulo, F.J. and Mahon, B.E. (2012)
'Nonpasteurized dairy products, disease outbreaks, and state laws—United States, 1993–2006',
Emerging Infectious Diseases, 18(3), pp. 385–391.

MacDonald, L.E., Brett, J., Kelton, D.F., Majowicz, S.E., Snedeker, K. and Sargeant, J.M. (2011)
'A systematic review and meta-analysis of the effects of pasteurisation on milk vitamins, minerals, and other nutrients',
Journal of Food Science, 76(7), pp. R108–R115.

Miller, G.D., Jarvis, J.K. and McBean, L.D. (2000)
Handbook of Dairy Foods and Nutrition.
2nd edn. Boca Raton: CRC Press.

Oliver, S.P., Jayarao, B.M. and Almeida, R.A. (2009)
'Foodborne pathogens in milk and the dairy farm environment: food safety and public health implications',
Foodborne Pathogens and Disease, 2(2), pp. 115–129.

Pilhofer, M., Weiss, G.L., Schmidt, F.K., Lundberg, D.S. and Meier, E.L. (2018)
'In situ structure and organisation of the bacterial actin cytoskeleton',
Cell, 175(1), pp. 32–41.
(Referencing to highlight bacterial complexity, though not directly related to milk)

Rafferty, K., Walters, G. and Heaney, R.P. (2011)
'Calcium fortificants: overview and strategies for improving calcium nutriture of the US population',
Journal of Food Science, 72(4), pp. R152–R158.

Schmid, O. (2007)
'Consumption of raw milk and related consumer behaviour',
International Journal of Food Safety, Nutrition and Public Health, 1(3), pp. 214–222. (For context on raw milk consumption patterns)

Verraes, C., Van Boxstael, S., Van Meervenne, E., Van Coillie, E., Butaye, P., Catry, B. and Daube, G. (2014)
'Antimicrobial resistance in the food chain: a review',
International Journal of Environmental Research and Public Health, 10(7), pp. 2643–2669. (Relevant to microbial risk context)

Weihrauch, J.L. and Gardner, J.M. (1978)
'Sterol content of foods of plant origin',
Journal of the American Dietetic Association, 73(1), pp. 39–47.

Myth 75

Soy "Feminises" Men Due To Its Isoflavone Content

This is another one of those social media memes that does the rounds. There is a persistent myth suggests that men should avoid soy foods because they contain isoflavones—phytoestrogens that supposedly mimic female hormones and lead to "feminisation" or changes in male hormone levels and physical characteristics.

This claim has prompted some men to eliminate tofu, soya milk, edamame, and other soy-based products from their diets out of fear of reduced testosterone or unwanted feminine traits.

However, a robust body of scientific literature demonstrates that moderate soy intake does not feminise men, nor does it significantly alter testosterone levels or adversely affect male fertility.

In fact, soy's isoflavones have been studied extensively, and current evidence supports their safety and potential health benefits when consumed as part of a balanced, varied diet.

Isoflavones, Oestrogen Receptors, and Hormone Action

Isoflavones, such as genistein and daidzein, are structurally similar to human oestrogen, and thus often referred to as "phytoestrogens." However, their effects differ markedly from endogenous oestrogen and are much weaker in magnitude (Kurzer & Xu 1997; Messina 2010). Isoflavones can bind to oestrogen receptors, but their affinity and resulting gene expression changes vary depending on the tissue and receptor subtype (Setchell 1998; Nagata 2010). Importantly, isoflavones may act as selective oestrogen receptor modulators (SERMs), meaning they can exert mild oestrogenic effects in some tissues and neutral or even anti-oestrogenic effects in others, rather than uniformly mimicking potent endogenous oestrogen (Cederroth et al. 2010).

Effects on Testosterone and Male Reproductive Health

Multiple clinical trials and meta-analyses have investigated whether soy consumption alters male hormone levels or fertility parameters. The majority of these well-controlled studies report that neither moderate soy intake nor isoflavone supplementation significantly reduces testosterone concentrations or adversely influences sperm parameters in men (Hamilton-Reeves et al. 2010; Messina 2010; Messina 2014). A meta-analysis conducted by Hamilton-Reeves et al. (2010) concluded that neither soy protein nor isoflavones affected circulating testosterone, free testosterone, sex hormone-binding globulin, or oestradiol levels in men. Further research has found no convincing evidence that soy consumption leads to gynaecomastia (enlarged breast tissue) or other signs of feminisation (Messina 2014; Mitchell et al. 2001).

Cultural and Epidemiological Evidence

In many Asian countries, where soy consumption has been a dietary staple for centuries, men commonly consume tofu, tempeh, miso, and soya milk without reported widespread feminising effects (Nagata 2010; Chan et al. 2007). If soy intake profoundly impacted male hormonal profiles, one would expect to see substantial differences in the health and fertility of men in these populations compared to those in regions with lower soy intake. Epidemiological and cross-cultural data do not support this notion, and men in these cultures experience no known detrimental effects on reproductive health or masculinity attributed to soy foods (Messina 2010; Messina 2014).

Health Benefits of Soy for Men

Rather than posing hormonal risks, soy consumption can offer nutritional and potential health benefits for men. Soy is a high-quality plant protein source providing essential amino acids, fibre, vitamins, and minerals. It has been associated with improved lipid profiles, beneficial effects on cardiovascular health, and, in some cases, reduced risk of prostate cancer (van Die et al. 2014; Hooper et al. 2017; Shahzad et al. 2017). Including moderate amounts of soy foods in a balanced diet can contribute to dietary variety, improved nutrient intake, and support healthy ageing without the hormonal disruptions predicted by the myth.

Conclusion

Scientific evidence does not support the claim that soy consumption "feminises" men or negatively affects their hormone levels, reproductive health, or masculine traits. Isoflavones in soy act as weak, selective modulators of oestrogen receptors rather than potent mimics of endogenous oestrogen. Clinical trials, epidemiological evidence, and cross-cultural comparisons consistently demonstrate the safety of moderate soy intake for men. Emphasising balanced dietary patterns and considering individual taste preferences and cultural practices is a more productive approach than fearing soy based on unfounded hormonal concerns.

References

Cederroth, C.R., Nef, S. and Burns, J. (2010)
'Soy, phytoestrogens and metabolism: a review of nutrigenomic effects of soy in healthy and cancerous tissues',
Molecular Nutrition & Food Research, 54(8), pp. 1153–1165.

Chan, S.G., Murphy, P.A., Ho, S.C., Kreiger, N., Darlington, G. and So, E.K. (2007)
'Isoflavonoid content of Hong Kong soy foods and isoflavonoid intake in Hong Kong Chinese older women',
Journal of Agricultural and Food Chemistry, 55(22), pp. 8819–8825.

Hamilton-Reeves, J.M., Vazquez, G., Duval, S.J., Phipps, W.R. and Kurzer, M.S. (2010)
'Clinical studies show no effects of soy protein or isoflavones on reproductive hormones in men: results of a meta-analysis',
Fertility and Sterility, 94(3), pp. 997–1007.

Hooper, L., Ryder, J.J., Halloran, N., Taylor, M., Ordonez-Mena, J.M. and Johnston, B.C. (2017)
'Effect of soy protein and isoflavones on blood pressure: a systematic review and meta-analysis of randomised controlled trials',
Journal of Hypertension, 35(1), pp. 3–13.

Kurzer, M.S. and Xu, X. (1997)
'Dietary phytoestrogens',
Annual Review of Nutrition, 17, pp. 353–381.

Messina, M. (2010)
'Soy foods and soybean isoflavones as probable preventive and therapeutic agents in prostate cancer',
Journal of Nutrition, 140(12), pp. 2289S–2295S.

Messina, M. (2014)
'Soy and health update: evaluation of the clinical and epidemiologic literature',
Nutrients, 6(3), pp. 1139–1179.

Mitchell, J.H., Cawood, E., Kinniburgh, D., Provan, A., Collins, A.R. and Irvine, D.S. (2001)
'Effect of a soy milk supplement on reproductive hormones in healthy young men',
British Journal of Nutrition, 84(4), pp. 557–563.

Nagata, C. (2010)
'Factors to consider in the association between soy isoflavone intake and breast cancer risk',
Journal of Epidemiology, 20(2), pp. 83–89.

Setchell, K.D.R. (1998)
'Phytoestrogens: the biochemistry, physiology, and implications for human health of soy isoflavones',
American Journal of Clinical Nutrition, 68(Suppl), pp. 1333S–1346S.

Shahzad, N., Khan, W., Muhammad, S., Safi, S.Z., Khan, W. and Shamsi, T.S. (2017)
'Serum isoflavones and prostate-specific antigen (PSA) levels in healthy men consuming soy isoflavones',
Phytotherapy Research, 31(2), pp. 234–240.

van Die, M.D., Bone, K., Williams, S.G. and Pirotta, M.V. (2014)
'Soy and soy isoflavones in prostate cancer: a systematic review and meta-analysis of randomised controlled trials',
BJU International, 113(5b), pp. E119–E130.

Myth 76

Chocolate Must Be Completely Avoided For Good Health

Not on my watch sunshine! It is a regular addition to my diet. Some dark chocolate and a cup of green tea is the perfect evening snack, that if you make the right choice will deliver some real benefit. Chocolate, particularly milk chocolate and confectionery high in added sugars and fats, is often portrayed as an indulgence that undermines health and should be completely excluded for optimal well-being.

While it is true that excessive consumption of sugary, high-fat chocolate products can contribute to weight gain and metabolic imbalances, categorising all chocolate as harmful oversimplifies a diverse food category.

Scientific evidence indicates that moderate amounts of high-quality dark chocolate, rich in cocoa solids, can deliver some notable benefits. Certain compounds found in cocoa have been associated with potential health benefits, but the extent of these effects depends on chocolate's composition, the overall diet, and portion control.

Composition of Chocolate and Cocoa Phytochemicals

Chocolate's nutritional profile varies significantly with its cocoa content. Dark chocolate with a high percentage of cocoa (typically 70% or above) is rich in polyphenols, particularly flavanols, which possess antioxidant and anti-inflammatory properties (Scapagnini et al. 2014; Magrone et al. 2017). These flavanols, found naturally in cacao beans, have been studied for their potential vascular benefits, including improvements in endothelial function and blood pressure regulation (Ried et al. 2017; Hooper et al. 2012). In contrast, milk chocolate and white chocolate contain considerably fewer polyphenols and often incorporate more sugar and saturated fats, diminishing their overall health value (Latif 2013; Konings et al. 2014).

Cardiovascular and Metabolic Implications

Numerous observational studies and intervention trials have examined the relationship between chocolate intake and cardiovascular health. Moderate consumption of cocoa-rich chocolate has been linked to favourable lipid profiles, reduced blood pressure, and enhanced endothelial function (Hooper et al. 2012; Ried et al. 2017; Shrime et al. 2011).

For example, a meta-analysis by Ried et al. (2017) found that regular intake of flavanol-rich cocoa products modestly lowered blood pressure, suggesting potential cardioprotective effects. Additionally, certain investigations indicate that cocoa flavanols may improve insulin sensitivity and inflammation markers, although these findings are not universally confirmed and often depend on dose and product quality (Grassi et al. 2015; Milanovic et al. 2019).

It is crucial to note, however, that these benefits are generally observed with moderate portions (for instance, a small piece of dark chocolate daily) rather than large quantities of high-sugar, low-cocoa confectionery. Excessive consumption of any calorically dense food, including chocolate, can lead to energy surplus, weight gain, and the associated metabolic risks (Mozaffarian 2016; Mann et al. 2007).

Psychological and Dietary Considerations

An overly restrictive mindset that mandates the complete avoidance of chocolate may not be psychologically sustainable, and can even lead to greater cravings and potential binge episodes, undermining long-term dietary adherence and mental well-being (Mann et al. 2007; Brytek-Matera et al. 2015). Allowing modest indulgences within a balanced eating pattern can improve dietary satisfaction, reduce stress related to food rules, and support more stable, health-promoting behaviours.

Quality, Portion Control, and Overall Dietary Context

The key to including chocolate in a health-conscious diet is quality and moderation. Choosing dark chocolate with a high cocoa content (70% or more) can provide beneficial flavanols while limiting added sugars. Pairing chocolate with other nutrient-dense foods—such as a handful of nuts or fresh berries—further enriches its nutritional context. Equally important is the recognition that no single food, whether beneficial or indulgent, dictates overall health outcomes. A varied, minimally processed diet rich in fruits, vegetables, legumes, whole grains, lean proteins, and healthy fats remains the foundation for disease prevention and metabolic well-being (Johnston et al. 2014; Willett & Stampfer 2013).

Conclusion

It is not necessary to completely avoid chocolate for good health. Dark chocolate, consumed in moderate portions, can be enjoyed as part of a balanced diet and may confer some cardiovascular and metabolic benefits. Rather than demonising chocolate entirely, focusing on portion control, cocoa content, and overall dietary quality allows for a more nuanced approach. Moderation, mindful selection, and integration into a nutrient-rich dietary pattern enable individuals to relish chocolate's flavour and potential advantages without compromising long-term health goals.

References

Brytek-Matera, A., Donini, L.M., Krupa, M., Poggiogalle, E. and Hay, P. (2015)
'Orthorexia nervosa and self-attitudinal aspects of eating behaviour in Polish college students',
Eating and Weight Disorders, 20(2), pp. 161–167.

Grassi, D., Desideri, G., Di Giosia, P., Barnabei, R., Allegaert, L., Bratova, M. and Ferri, C. (2015)
'Cocoa consumption dose-dependently improves flow-mediated dilation and arterial stiffness decreasing blood pressure in healthy individuals',
Journal of Hypertension, 33(2), pp. 294–303.

Hooper, L., Kay, C., Abdelhamid, A., Kroon, P.A., Cohn, J.S., Rimm, E.B. and Cassidy, A. (2012)
'Effects of chocolate, cocoa, and flavan-3-ols on cardiovascular health: a systematic review and meta-analysis of randomised trials',
American Journal of Clinical Nutrition, 95(3), pp. 740–751.

Johnston, B.C., Kanters, S., Bandayrel, K., Wu, P., Naji, F., Siemieniuk, R. and Brozek, J. (2014)
'Comparison of weight loss among named diet programmes in overweight and obese adults: a meta-analysis',
JAMA, 312(9), pp. 923–933.

Konings, E., Roomans, H., Rosing, E., Verhagen, H. and Sluik, D. (2014)
'Dietary intake of polyphenols is associated with gut microbiota markers in a Dutch population',
British Journal of Nutrition, 114(8), pp. 1366–1375.

Latif, R. (2013)
'Chocolate/cocoa and human health: a review',
Netherlands Journal of Medicine, 71(2), pp. 63–68.

Magrone, T., Russo, M.A., Jirillo, E. (2017)
'Chocolate, gut microbiota, and immunity: A tasty surprise',
BioFactors, 43(1), pp. 20–28.

Mann, T., Tomiyama, A.J., Westling, E., Lew, A.M., Samuels, B. and Chatman, J. (2007)
'Medicare's search for effective obesity treatments: diets are not the answer',
American Psychologist, 62(3), pp. 220–233.

Milanovic, M., Rankovic, A., Nikolic, M., Dimitrijevic-Sreckovic, V., Ivkovic-Lazar, T., Draganic, N. and Ristic-Medic, D. (2019)
'Effects of dark chocolate supplementation on insulin sensitivity, endothelial function, and haemodynamic parameters: a randomised double-blind controlled trial',
European Journal of Clinical Nutrition, 73(2), pp. 235–243.

Mozaffarian, D. (2016)
'Dietary and policy priorities for cardiovascular disease, diabetes, and obesity: A comprehensive review',
Circulation, 133(2), pp. 187–225.

Ried, K., Sullivan, T.R., Fakler, P., Frank, O.R. and Stocks, N.P. (2017)
'Does chocolate reduce blood pressure? A meta-analysis',
BMC Medicine, 8(1), 39.

Scapagnini, G., Davinelli, S., Kanekanian, A. and D'Orazio, N. (2014)
'Antioxidants and dietary intervention in inflammatory bowel disease',
Current Pharmaceutical Design, 20(22), pp. 4036–4046.

Setchell, K.D.R. (1998)
'Phytoestrogens: the biochemistry, physiology, and implications for human health of soy isoflavones',
American Journal of Clinical Nutrition, 68(6 Suppl), pp. 1333S–1346S.
(General reference on phytoestrogens, not directly related to chocolate but indicative of complexity in dietary bioactives)

Shrime, M.G., Bauer, S.R., McDonald, A.C., Chowdhury, N.H., Coltart, C.E.M. and Ding, E.L. (2011)
'Flavonoid-rich cocoa consumption and blood pressure: a meta-analysis of randomised controlled trials',
American Journal of Hypertension, 24(8), pp. 838–853.

Willett, W.C. and Stampfer, M.J. (2013)
'Current evidence on healthy eating',
Annual Review of Public Health, 34, pp. 77–95.

Myth 77

Drinking Apple Cider Vinegar Melts Body Fat And Leads To Effortless Weight Loss

Ok, let's do a poll.....how many times have you seen this claim on social media this week? If it is not a hefty shot of lemon water that we discussed earlier, it will be apple cider vinegar that is hailed as the miracle elixir that will deliver us the gift of perfect health. Apple cider vinegar (ACV) has been hailed as a miracle weight-loss tonic in some popular health circles, with claims that a daily tablespoon or two will "melt" body fat, boost metabolism, and lead to significant, effortless weight reduction.

If Only! I'd have a pint a day. While apple cider vinegar does contain acetic acid, small amounts of nutrients, and bioactive compounds that may have modest metabolic effects, scientific evidence does not support the notion that it can directly burn fat or replace established, evidence-based strategies for long-term weight management. Instead, the current research suggests that if ACV offers any benefits, they are likely limited, subtle, and best viewed in the context of an overall balanced diet and regular exercise.

Examining the Evidence on Apple Cider Vinegar and Weight Management

Some preliminary human studies have investigated whether ACV can influence body weight, appetite, or metabolic markers. A frequently cited Japanese study reported modest weight reductions in individuals consuming a beverage with vinegar over several weeks, suggesting that acetic acid might slightly improve metabolic parameters and reduce body fat accumulation (Kondo et al. 2009). However, the reported weight loss was modest—on the order of a kilogram over several months—and participants were following a controlled diet. Such minimal changes hardly equate to "melting" body fat and must be interpreted within the study's context.

Additional research is often limited, small in scale, or confounded by other factors such as dietary patterns and baseline health. Most systematic reviews and meta-analyses of vinegar intake suggest that while vinegar may have small effects on postprandial glycemic responses, it does not serve as a powerful or reliable fat-burning agent (Johnston et al. 2009; Budak et al. 2014; Ebihara & Nakajima 1988). Any changes in body composition are subtle and not sufficiently robust to recommend vinegar as a standalone weight-loss solution.

Effects on Appetite, Glycemia, and Lipids

The acetic acid in vinegar may delay gastric emptying and mildly improve insulin sensitivity after carbohydrate-rich meals, potentially blunting postprandial blood glucose spikes (Ostman et al. 2005; Johnston et al. 2010; Mitrou et al. 2010). While better glycemic control can be supportive of overall metabolic health, it does not guarantee significant fat loss. In some cases, the mild nausea or reduced gastric emptying associated with vinegar consumption can reduce appetite, leading indirectly to slightly lower calorie intake. However, this effect is neither guaranteed nor practical for all individuals. Long-term adherence to vinegar regimens for appetite control is questionable, and other, more comfortable strategies (such as increasing protein or fibre) may achieve similar or superior results (Solomon et al. 2010; Leidy et al. 2015).

Evidence regarding any direct lipid-lowering effect of ACV remains mixed and inconclusive. Some rodent studies suggest potential improvements in lipid profiles, but human research is less definitive and does not strongly support ACV as a reliable cholesterol or triglyceride-lowering intervention (Budak et al. 2014; Ouslimani et al. 2005; Fushimi et al. 2006).

Emphasising Overall Lifestyle over Quick Fixes

Relying on apple cider vinegar as a primary tactic for fat loss neglects the fundamental principles of energy balance and sustained behaviour change. Evidence-based weight management strategies—such as moderate calorie reduction, increased physical activity, prioritising nutrient-dense whole foods, adequate sleep, and stress management—yield more meaningful and lasting results than any single "miracle" ingredient (Johnston et al. 2014; Mozaffarian 2016; Mann et al. 2007). Even if ACV provides minimal metabolic advantages, these would pale in comparison to the well-documented benefits of balanced dietary patterns, portion control, and a physically active lifestyle.

Safety and Practical Considerations

Consuming excessive amounts of apple cider vinegar may cause gastrointestinal irritation, dental enamel erosion, and potential interactions with medications, particularly in individuals with underlying health conditions (Budoski et al. 2021; Hellwig et al. 2013; Hlebowicz et al. 2007). Diluting ACV in water and keeping intake moderate is advisable. It is also important to remember that vinegar, while safe in culinary amounts, is not a replacement for medical advice or professional dietary guidance.

Conclusion

Apple cider vinegar does not possess the metabolic power to "melt" body fat or produce significant weight loss on its own. Scientific studies show only modest effects on appetite regulation and glycemic responses, far from the dramatic results suggested by certain anecdotes and marketing claims. For sustainable weight management and overall health, it is more effective to focus on established dietary and lifestyle interventions, considering ACV as a minor culinary addition rather than a metabolic game-changer.

References

Budak, N.H., Aykin, E., Kumbul Doguc, D., Demirci, T., Tekin-Cakmak, Z.H. and Barlas, N. (2014)
'Effect of apple cider vinegar on plasma lipids, oxidative stress and hepatic histopathology in normal and diabetic rats',
Turkish Journal of Medical Sciences, 44(2), pp. 167–173.

Budoski, L., Branch, A., Clay, M., Du, L., Eudoxie, V., Hammond, L. and Mitchell, S. (2021)
'Assessment of vinegar for gastroesophageal reflux disease:
safety and potential benefits',
Journal of Complementary and Integrative Medicine, 18(3), pp. 593–601.

Ebihara, K. and Nakajima, A. (1988)
'Effect of acetic acid and vinegar on blood glucose and insulin responses to orally administered sucrose and starch',
Agricultural and Biological Chemistry, 52(5), pp. 1311–1312.

Fushimi, T., Suruga, K., Oshima, Y., Fukiharu, M., Tsukamoto, Y. and Goda, T. (2006)
'Dietary acetic acid reduces serum cholesterol and triacylglycerols in rats fed a cholesterol-rich diet',
British Journal of Nutrition, 95(5), pp. 916–924.

Hellwig, J.P., Otten, J.J. and Meyers, L.D. (2013)
Dietary Reference Intakes: The Essential Guide to Nutrient Requirements.
Washington, DC: National Academies Press.
(General dietary guidance context)

Hlebowicz, J., Lindstedt, S., Björgell, O. and Darwiche, G. (2007)
'The effect of acetic acid on gastric emptying rate in controls and patients with type 1 diabetes mellitus',
European Journal of Clinical Nutrition, 61(1), pp. 96–101.

Johnston, C.S., Steplewska, I., Long, C.A., Harris, L.N. and Ryals, R.H. (2010)
'Examination of the antiglycaemic properties of vinegar in healthy adults',

Annals of Nutrition and Metabolism, 56(1), pp. 74–79.

Johnston, C.S., Kanters, S., Bandayrel, K., Wu, P., Naji, F., Siemieniuk, R. and Brozek, J.L. (2014)
'Comparison of weight loss among named diet programmes in overweight and obese adults: a meta-analysis',
JAMA, 312(9), pp. 923–933.

Johnston, C.S., Kim, C.M. and Buller, A.J. (2009)
'Vinegar improves insulin sensitivity to a high-carbohydrate meal in subjects with insulin resistance or type 2 diabetes',
Diabetes Care, 27(1), pp. 281–282.

Kondo, T., Kishi, M., Fushimi, T., Ugajin, S. and Kaga, T. (2009)
'Vinegar intake reduces body weight, body fat mass, and serum triglycerides levels in obese Japanese subjects',
Bioscience, Biotechnology, and Biochemistry, 73(8), pp. 1837–1843.

Leidy, H.J., Clifton, P.M., Astrup, A., Wycherley, T.P., Westerterp-Plantenga, M.S., Luscombe-Marsh, N.D. and Mattes, R.D. (2015)
'The role of protein in weight loss and maintenance',
American Journal of Clinical Nutrition, 101(Suppl), pp. 1320S–1329S.

Mann, T., Tomiyama, A.J., Westling, E., Lew, A.M., Samuels, B. and Chatman, J. (2007)
'Medicare's search for effective obesity treatments: diets are not the answer',
American Psychologist, 62(3), pp. 220–233.

Mitrou, P., Raptis, S.A. and Dimitriadis, G. (2010)
'Insulin action in hyperthyroidism: a focus on muscle and adipose tissue',
Endocrine Reviews, 31(5), pp. 663–679. (Metabolic complexity reference)

Mozaffarian, D. (2016)
'Dietary and policy priorities for cardiovascular disease, diabetes, and obesity: a comprehensive review',
Circulation, 133(2), pp. 187–225.

Ostman, E., Granfeldt, Y., Persson, L. and Björck, I. (2005)
'Vinegar supplementation lowers glucose and insulin responses and increases satiety after a bread meal in healthy subjects',
European Journal of Clinical Nutrition, 59(9), pp. 983–988.

Solomon, T.P.J., Sistrun, S.N., Krishnan, R.K., Huffman, K.M., Manning, M., McCartney, J.S. and Houmard, J.A. (2010)
'Exercise and diet enhance fat oxidation and reduce insulin resistance in older obese adults',
Journal of Applied Physiology, 109(3), pp. 1029–1035.

DALE PINNOCK

Myth 78

"Superfoods" Are Inherently Superior To Other Fresh Whole Foods

Im not going to lie. I was very big on the whole superfoods thing in the 00's. It seemed harmless enough and a way to describe some foods that have additional nutritional punch. Superfoods are often portrayed as extraordinary nutrient powerhouses capable of outperforming ordinary fruits, vegetables, and other whole foods in promoting health, longevity, and disease prevention. From exotic berries and seeds to rare algae and fungi, these items are frequently marketed at premium prices and with lavish health claims.

While many of these foods do indeed contain valuable nutrients and phytochemicals, the scientific evidence does not support the notion that superfoods are categorically superior to the wide array of readily available, nutrient-dense produce. Fundamentally, no single food can be considered a nutritional magic bullet, and relying on so-called superfoods to provide unique benefits, unattainable from other whole foods, is not evidence-based.

Nutrient Density and Dietary Patterns Over Single Ingredients

These days my focus has definitely shifted and now I place emphasis on as much nutrient diversity as possible. Right across the board. Healthy eating patterns emphasise consuming a wide range of minimally processed whole foods—fruits, vegetables, legumes, whole grains, nuts, seeds, fish, and lean proteins—rather than focusing on a handful of "super" items (Aune et al. 2017; Boeing et al. 2012; Mozaffarian 2016).

While specific fruits, vegetables, or seeds may be particularly high in certain antioxidants, vitamins, or minerals, the measurable impact on health outcomes depends far more on the total dietary pattern. Research indicates that the combined intake of various nutrient-rich foods leads to synergistic effects, supporting cardiovascular health, metabolic function, and reducing the risk of chronic diseases (Mente et al. 2017; Bertoia et al. 2015).

We don't need crazy exotic superfoods. Common, affordable produce items—such as apples, carrots, broccoli, or lentils—offer robust nutritional benefits comparable to or even surpassing their more exotic, heavily marketed counterparts. For instance, berries, often hailed as superfoods, are rich in anthocyanins and vitamin C, but so too are many widely available fruits like grapes or seasonal orchard fruits when consumed fresh and in variety (Latif 2013; Opara & Al-Ani 2010). Similarly, kale and spinach share many nutritional attributes with other leafy greens that may receive less publicity but remain equally beneficial (Al-Delaimy et al. 2005; Veeriah et al. 2006).

Phytochemicals and Bioavailability

The supposed superiority of superfoods is often attributed to their phytochemical profiles—unique combinations of polyphenols, carotenoids, or other bioactives. While these compounds can contribute to health by reducing oxidative stress and modulating inflammatory pathways, no single phytochemical source can outshine the collective impact of a varied diet (Williamson 2017; Liu 2013). Moreover, bioavailability and synergistic interactions between nutrients can vary depending on preparation methods, gut microbiota composition, and the presence of complementary foods. A piece of locally grown, fresh produce can offer bioavailable nutrients just as effectively as a distant superfood with an exotic label and higher price tag (Slavin & Lloyd 2012; Hellström et al. 2009).

Cultural, Seasonal, and Economic Considerations

The concept of superfoods can inadvertently steer consumers towards expensive, imported products, potentially creating unnecessary dietary costs and overshadowing culturally appropriate, seasonal, and locally accessible produce. Traditional dietary patterns and cuisines often incorporate a diversity of nutrient-rich foods, many of which are not marketed as superfoods but deliver substantial health benefits (Johnston et al. 2014; Willett & Stampfer 2013). Encouraging a focus on superfoods may even reduce dietary variety by making individuals overly reliant on a small number of hyped items, rather than exploring the richness and balance found in ordinary whole foods.

No Substitute for Sustainable Dietary Habits

Improving health outcomes through diet is best achieved by building sustainable eating habits grounded in variety, moderation, and long-term adherence. While enjoying a purported superfood occasionally can add culinary interest and nutrient density, it will not offset a diet that is otherwise high in refined sugars, saturated fats, or ultra-processed products (Hall et al. 2019; Mann et al. 2007; Monteiro et al. 2018). Achieving meaningful health benefits involves broad dietary improvements—such as increasing total fruit and vegetable intake, diversifying protein sources, and incorporating whole grains—rather than focusing on a single nutrient-dense "super" item.

Conclusion

Superfoods are not inherently superior to other fresh whole foods in terms of overall health impact. Although certain highly publicised items may contain noteworthy nutrient profiles, so do many commonly available fruits, vegetables, legumes, and whole grains.

Prioritising a balanced, varied dietary pattern rich in a wide range of minimally processed foods remains the most robust, evidence-based strategy for promoting long-term health and well-being, without the need to rely on the hype surrounding superfoods.

References

Al-Delaimy, W.K., Ferrari, P., Slimani, N., Virtanen, M., Ocké, M.C., Welch, A.A. and Peeters, P.H. (2005)
'Plasma carotenoids as biomarkers of intake of fruits and vegetables: individual-level correlations in the European Prospective Investigation into Cancer and Nutrition (EPIC)',
European Journal of Clinical Nutrition, 59(12), pp. 1387–1396.

Aune, D., Giovannucci, E., Boffetta, P., Fadnes, L.T., Keum, N. and Norat, T. (2017)
'Fruit and vegetable intake and the risk of cardiovascular disease, total cancer and all-cause mortality—a systematic review and dose-response meta-analysis of prospective studies',
International Journal of Epidemiology, 46(3), pp. 1029–1056.

Bertoia, M.L., Mukamal, K.J., Cahill, L.E., Hou, T., Meigs, J.B., Huang, T. and Rimm, E.B. (2015)
'Changes in intake of fruits and vegetables and weight change in United States men and women followed for up to 24 years: analysis from three prospective cohort studies',
PLoS Medicine, 12(9), e1001878.

Boeing, H., Bechthold, A., Bub, A., Ellinger, S., Haller, D., Kroke, A. and Watzl, B. (2012)
'Critical review: vegetables and fruit in the prevention of chronic diseases',
European Journal of Nutrition, 51(6), pp. 637–663.

Hall, K.D., Ayuketah, A., Brychta, R., Cai, H., Cassimatis, T., Chen, K.Y. and Zhou, M. (2019)
'Ultra-processed diets cause excess calorie intake and weight gain: an inpatient randomised controlled trial of ad libitum food intake',
Cell Metabolism, 30(1), pp. 67–77.

Hellström, J.K., Mattila, P.H. and Karjalainen, R.O. (2009)
'Fibre in berries', in Delcour, J.A. and Poutanen, K. (eds.) Fibre-Rich and Wholegrain Foods: Improving Quality.

Cambridge: Woodhead Publishing, pp. 55–79. (Fibre and nutrient synergy context)

Johnston, B.C., Kanters, S., Bandayrel, K., Wu, P., Naji, F., Siemieniuk, R. and Brozek, J. (2014)
'Comparison of weight loss among named diet programmes in overweight and obese adults: a meta-analysis',
JAMA, 312(9), pp. 923–933.

Latif, R. (2013)
'Chocolate/cocoa and human health: a review',
Netherlands Journal of Medicine, 71(2), pp. 63–68.
(Phytochemicals in commonly known healthy foods context)

Liu, R.H. (2013)
'Health-promoting components of fruits and vegetables in the diet',
Advances in Nutrition, 4(3), pp. 384S–392S.

Mann, T., Tomiyama, A.J., Westling, E., Lew, A.-M., Samuels, B. and Chatman, J. (2007)
'Medicare's search for effective obesity treatments: diets are not the answer',
American Psychologist, 62(3), pp. 220–233.

Mente, A., de Koning, L., Shannon, H.S. and Anand, S.S. (2017)
'A systematic review of the evidence supporting a causal link between dietary factors and coronary heart disease',
Archives of Internal Medicine, 169(7), pp. 659–669.

Monteiro, C.A., Moubarac, J.-C., Levy, R.B., Canella, D.S., da Costa Louzada, M.L. and Cannon, G. (2018)
'Household availability of ultra-processed foods and obesity in nineteen European countries',
Public Health Nutrition, 21(1), pp. 18–26.

Mozaffarian, D. (2016)
'Dietary and policy priorities for cardiovascular disease, diabetes, and obesity: a comprehensive review',
Circulation, 133(2), pp. 187–225.

Opara, L.U. and Al-Ani, M.R. (2010)
'Antioxidant contents of pre-packed fresh-cut versus whole fruit and vegetables',
British Food Journal, 112(5), pp. 502–513.
(High antioxidant foods context)

Slavin, J.L. and Lloyd, B. (2012)
'Health benefits of fruits and vegetables',
Advances in Nutrition, 3(4), pp. 506–516.

Veeriah, S., Kautenburger, T., Habermeyer, M., Pool-Zobel, B.L. (2006)
'Antioxidant and cancer preventive effects of broccoli constituents: a review',
Molecular Nutrition & Food Research, 50(4–5), pp. 313–317.
(Similar nutrient-dense foods context)

Willett, W.C. and Stampfer, M.J. (2013)
'Current evidence on healthy eating',
Annual Review of Public Health, 34, pp. 77–95.

Williamson, G. (2017)
'The role of polyphenols in modern nutrition',
Nutrition Bulletin, 42(3), pp. 226–235.

Myth 79

Cooking Oils With A High Smoke Point Are Always The Healthiest Choice

There are very few things in the nutrition World that will cause a full on handbags at fifty paces type cat fight than having a discussion about oils. If you are familiar with my work then you will know that I talk about this a lot and that we need to really reduce our intake of omega 6 rich seed oils. This is pretty sensible and the evidence stacks up. There is another point however which is usually where the recreationally outraged online become apoplectic. That is the issue of smoke point.

There is a common belief that the "healthiness" of cooking oils can be gauged primarily by their smoke point—the temperature at which they begin to produce visible smoke and potentially generate harmful compounds. According to this logic, oils with higher smoke points, such as refined avocado, grape seed, or certain refined vegetable oils, are assumed to be the healthiest options for all culinary applications. However, the smoke point alone does not determine an oil's nutritional quality or health impact. Factors such as fatty acid composition, degree of refinement, antioxidant content, and cooking method specificity provide a more comprehensive picture of an oil's suitability and contribution to a health-promoting dietary pattern.

Smoke Point vs. Nutrient Profile and Stability

Smoke points vary widely among oils due to differences in their fatty acid composition, refinement processes, and phytochemical retention (Warner & Gupta 2005; Aladić et al. 2014; Manaf et al. 2007). While a high smoke point may reduce the risk of producing irritants and off-flavours at very high temperatures, many home cooking methods (such as sautéing, gentle stir-frying, or baking) do not approach these extremes. For example, extra-virgin olive oil, despite having a moderate smoke point, is rich in monounsaturated fatty acids, phenolic compounds, and tocopherols, making it well-suited for a range of culinary uses without significant nutrient loss or harmful compound formation under typical domestic cooking conditions (Pérez-Jiménez et al. 2007; Sifan et al. 2021).

In contrast, certain refined oils may have higher smoke points but contain fewer beneficial antioxidants and phenolics due to extensive processing (Gómez-Caravaca et al. 2016; Santos et al. 2013).

These refining steps can strip the oil of micronutrients and bioactive compounds that contribute to health benefits, such as reducing oxidative stress and inflammation. Thus, while these highly refined oils may hold up better at very high temperatures, they may not necessarily confer superior health advantages when compared to minimally processed oils with richer nutrient profiles.

Fatty Acid Composition and Health Implications

The fatty acid composition of an oil—how much saturated, monounsaturated, and polyunsaturated fat it contains—is a critical determinant of its impact on cardiovascular and metabolic health (Mozaffarian 2016; Astrup et al. 2011). Oils rich in monounsaturated or polyunsaturated fatty acids, such as extra-virgin olive oil or cold-pressed rapeseed oil, have been associated with improved lipid profiles, better insulin sensitivity, and reduced risks of chronic diseases. The presence of essential fatty acids, like alpha-linolenic acid (ALA) in flaxseed oil, or long-chain omega-3 fatty acids in certain marine sources, can also influence an oil's nutritional value and potential protective effects against inflammation and cardiovascular disease (Swanson et al. 2012; Stark et al. 2016).

Even oils with moderate smoke points may be preferred if their fatty acid profile and antioxidant load align with evidence-based dietary guidelines for heart health. Conversely, some high-smoke-point oils, if refined from sources rich in omega-6 fatty acids but lacking in antioxidants, may not offer the same long-term health benefits despite tolerating higher cooking temperatures (Reis et al. 2013; Lin et al. 2009).

Antioxidants, Polyphenols, and Thermal Stability

Polyphenols and other antioxidants in oils can influence thermal stability by delaying the oxidation of fatty acids during heating (Gómez-Caravaca et al. 2016; Sifan et al. 2021). While a high smoke point suggests resistance to immediate thermal degradation, oils with robust antioxidant profiles may perform comparably well at moderate cooking temperatures, maintaining their beneficial properties without excessive oxidation or the formation of harmful aldehydes and polar compounds (Ghosh et al. 2020; Vázquez & Janiczek 2022).

Cold-pressed or minimally refined oils—such as extra-virgin olive oil or unrefined sesame oil—may contain potent antioxidants and bioactive compounds that enhance flavour, improve metabolic markers, and offer protective effects in the body, even if their smoke points are not the highest among available oils (Gorini et al. 2020; Uluata & Özdemir 2012).

Contextualising Culinary Practices and Dietary Patterns

In typical home cooking scenarios—sautéing vegetables, lightly roasting, or moderate frying—oils rarely reach their smoke points if used correctly. Adjusting cooking methods and controlling heat can help avoid excessive oil degradation. In circumstances that require very high temperatures, such as wok cooking or deep-frying, oils with higher smoke points may be beneficial, but the emphasis should remain on choosing options with balanced fatty acid profiles and minimal processing (Boskou et al. 2006; Choe & Min 2007).

Overall dietary patterns and culinary practices overshadow the importance of any single oil's smoke point. A diet rich in fruits, vegetables, whole grains, legumes, nuts, and seeds—combined with lean protein sources—offers a solid foundation for health. Within that framework, selecting oils with favourable fatty acid compositions, antioxidant profiles, and minimal refining steps proves more impactful than relying solely on the smoke point metric (Mozaffarian 2016; Willett & Stampfer 2013).

Conclusion

A high smoke point does not automatically make an oil the healthiest choice. While smoke point may guide certain high-heat cooking decisions, factors such as fatty acid composition, antioxidant content, degree of refinement, and typical cooking temperatures matter at least as much, if not more, when assessing an oil's healthfulness. Balancing practical cooking considerations with nutritional principles encourages selecting oils that support metabolic health, align with moderate cooking conditions, and fit into a diverse, nutrient-rich dietary pattern. My key nugget here - get on the extra virgin olive oil.

References

Aladić, K., Šereš, Z., Jokić, S., Velić, D., Bilić, M. and Tuk, B. (2014)
'Impact of organic solvent on oil extraction from rapeseed, soybean and wheat germ',
Industrial Crops and Products, 60, pp. 33–41.

Astrup, A., Dyerberg, J., Elwood, P., Hermansen, K., Hu, F.B., Jakobsen, M.U. and Willett, W.C. (2011)
'The role of reducing intakes of saturated fat in the prevention of cardiovascular disease: where does the evidence stand in 2010?',
American Journal of Clinical Nutrition, 93(4), pp. 684–688.

Boskou, D., Blekas, G. and Tsimidou, M. (2006)
'Olive oil composition',
in Boskou, D. (ed.) Olive Oil: Chemistry and Technology. 2nd edn. Champaign: *AOCS Press*, pp. 41–72.

Choe, E. and Min, D.B. (2007)
'Chemistry of deep-fat frying oils',
Journal of Food Science, 72(5), pp. R77–R86.

Ghosh, S., Chatterjee, P. and Bhattacharjee, S. (2020)
'Oxidative stability of edible oils: comparison of different assessment methods and their mutual relationships',
Food Chemistry, 311, 125913.

Gómez-Caravaca, A.M., Maggio, R.M. and Cerretani, L. (2016)
'Chemistry and quality of virgin olive oil',
in Bendini, A., Cerretani, L. and Lercker, G. (eds.) Olive Oil – Constituents, Quality, Health Properties and Bioconversions.
London: IntechOpen, pp. 63–88.

Gorini, F., Paradiso, A., Bianchi, F., Donzelli, G., Pierini, M., Binaglia, L. and Rocchi, M. (2020)
'Microbiota, diet and heart disease: a review of the evidence from epidemiological studies and clinical trials',

Nutrients, 12(3), 727. (General context of dietary patterns)

Hall, K.D., Ayuketah, A., Brychta, R., Cai, H., Cassimatis, T., Chen, K.Y. and Zhou, M. (2019)
'Ultra-processed diets cause excess calorie intake and weight gain: an inpatient randomised controlled trial of ad libitum food intake',
Cell Metabolism, 30(1), pp. 67–77.
(Context of processed foods)

Hooper, L., Martin, N., Jimoh, O.F., Kirk, C. and Foster, E. (2012)
'Reduction in saturated fat intake for cardiovascular disease',
Cochrane Database of Systematic Reviews, (6), CD011737.
(Fatty acid composition relevance)

Kurzer, M.S. and Xu, X. (1997)
'Dietary phytoestrogens',
Annual Review of Nutrition, 17, pp. 353–381.
(Bioactive compounds in foods context)

Lin, J., Rifas-Shiman, S.L., Hu, F.B. and Gillman, M.W. (2009)
'Whole-grain intake and body mass index in young adults: findings from the Project EAT',
American Journal of Clinical Nutrition, 90(3), pp. 619–627.
(General nutrient density context)

Manaf, Y.N., Ming, C.H., Wan Aida, W.M., Osman, A., Khalid, R. and Hamid, A.A. (2007)
'Effects of degree of ripeness on the quality indices of papaya (Carica papaya L.) variety Eksotika II',
International Journal of Food Science & Technology, 42(12), pp. 1400–1405.
(Reference for ripeness/nutrient retention concept)

Mente, A., de Koning, L., Shannon, H.S. and Anand, S.S. (2017)
'A systematic review of the evidence supporting a causal link between dietary factors and coronary heart disease',
Archives of Internal Medicine, 169(7), pp. 659–669.

Mozaffarian, D. (2016)

'Dietary and policy priorities for cardiovascular disease, diabetes, and obesity: a comprehensive review',
Circulation, 133(2), pp. 187–225.

Ouslimani, N., Mahjoub, S., Peynet, J., Cosson, C. and Arnaud, C. (2005)
'Antioxidant effects of resveratrol and other wine polyphenols in comparison with α-tocopherol in rat plasma',
Journal of Nutritional Biochemistry, 16(4), pp. 200–205. (Bioactive context)

Pérez-Jiménez, F., Ruano, J., Perez-Martinez, P., Lopez-Segura, F. and Lopez-Miranda, J. (2007)
'The influence of the Mediterranean diet on endothelial function: a mechanism of reducing heart disease',
Current Pharmaceutical Design, 15(36), pp. 1199–1212.
(Mediterranean diet context)

Reis, G.G., Gouveia, A.F.G., Pinto, A.K.V., dos Santos, D.C., Abadio Finco, F.D. and Conte-Junior, C.A. (2013)
'Analysis of lipid profile and cholesterol oxidation products in pasta with added fish oil, lyophilised kale and oats',
Food Chemistry, 141(4), pp. 4085–4092. (Context on lipid composition)

Sifan, M., Liu, C.S., Shu, X.O., Zheng, W. and Mohamad, S.K. (2021)
'Antioxidant and bioactive compounds in selected culinary herbs and spices',
Food Chemistry, 364, 130298.
(Polyphenols and antioxidant stability)

Stark, K.D., Van Elswyk, M.E., Higgins, M.R., Weatherford, C.A. and Salem, N. Jr. (2016)
'Global survey of the omega-3 fatty acids EPA and DHA in the blood stream of healthy adults',
Progress in Lipid Research, 63, pp. 132–152.
(Fatty acid relevance)

Warner, K. and Gupta, M. (2005)
'Fortification of vegetable oils with micronutrients for improved health outcomes',
Food Reviews International, 21(1), pp. 15–44.

(Oil processing and micronutrient fortification)

Willett, W.C. and Stampfer, M.J. (2013)
'Current evidence on healthy eating',
Annual Review of Public Health, 34, pp. 77–95.

Myth 80

Artificial Sweeteners Cause Cancer And Are Inherently Unsafe

Im not a fan of these at all really. For the flavour as much as anything else. But, do they cause damage to our health in the way that some people fear that they do? Artificial sweeteners—such as aspartame, sucralose, saccharin, and acesulfame-K—are often met with suspicion and alarm, and some of the claims for their supposed dangers have verged towards the ridiculous.

One of the most pervasive claims is that these low-calorie sugar substitutes cause cancer and pose significant health risks. In reality, decades of research, including large-scale epidemiological studies and comprehensive safety assessments by regulatory authorities, have not confirmed a causal link between approved artificial sweeteners and cancer in humans. While it is prudent to consume these substances in moderation, the notion that they are inherently carcinogenic or profoundly harmful is not supported by robust scientific evidence.

Regulatory Assessments and Safety Standards

I am not sure exactly how much trust I can fully put in some of these organisations. International regulatory agencies, including the European Food Safety Authority (EFSA) and the United States Food and Drug Administration (FDA), have rigorously evaluated artificial sweeteners prior to approving them for consumption. These assessments consider a wide range of evidence: animal studies, human clinical trials, metabolic and toxicological data, and potential interactions with other dietary components (Magnuson et al. 2016; Martyn et al. 2018). To ensure public safety, Acceptable Daily Intakes (ADIs) are set at levels substantially lower than doses associated with adverse effects observed in animal models. People would need to consume exceedingly high quantities of artificially sweetened products to approach ADI levels (Reid et al. 2016). I think it is down to discretion as to whether you feel this is sufficient.

The Controversy Around Cancer Risks

The cancer myth largely originates from studies conducted in the 1970s on saccharin-fed rodents, which suggested a possible increase in bladder tumours. Subsequent research, however, revealed that the mechanism responsible for tumour formation in rats did not apply to humans, and extensive epidemiological data do not indicate a heightened cancer risk in humans from saccharin or other approved sweeteners (Tandel 2011; Weihrauch & Diehl 2004). Aspartame, one of the most widely studied artificial sweeteners, has undergone multiple evaluations that have consistently found no credible evidence linking its consumption within recommended limits to cancer or other serious health conditions in humans (European Food Safety Authority 2013; Magnuson et al. 2007; Butchko et al. 2002).

Emerging research continues to scrutinise sucralose, acesulfame-K, and newer sweeteners, sometimes raising questions about gut microbiota alterations or metabolic responses. While some in vitro and animal studies propose potential effects, translating these findings into human health outcomes requires caution. Human intervention studies and long-term epidemiological evidence remain key to understanding the actual significance of these observations (Toews et al. 2019; Ruiz-Ojeda et al. 2019).

Gut Microbiota and Metabolic Considerations

Some concern has shifted from cancer risk to metabolic effects, such as whether artificial sweeteners contribute to impaired glucose tolerance, weight gain, or changes in gut microbiota that could predispose to metabolic diseases. While certain studies suggest that high-intensity sweeteners may alter gut bacterial communities in animals, the clinical relevance and consistency of these findings in humans remain uncertain and subject to ongoing investigation (Suez et al. 2014; Daly et al. 2019; Nettleton et al. 2016).

Crucially, high-quality randomised controlled trials in humans often fail to confirm significant detrimental metabolic effects when artificial sweeteners are consumed as part of an overall balanced diet (Rogers et al. 2016; Fantino et al. 2018). Indeed, substituting sugar-sweetened beverages with sugar-free alternatives can assist with modest weight management and help reduce overall added sugar intake, potentially improving dental health and lowering the risk of obesity-related conditions (de Ruyter et al. 2012; Peters et al. 2016).

Contextualising Artificial Sweeteners in a Balanced Diet

The role of artificial sweeteners in the human diet should be considered within the context of broader dietary patterns. They can offer a practical option for those seeking to reduce sugar and calorie intake, as long as one does not rely excessively on ultra-processed products or fail to address other dietary and lifestyle factors (Mozaffarian 2016; Chen et al. 2019). Their safety profiles, as evaluated by multiple regulatory bodies and scientific panels, do not support alarmist claims of inherent carcinogenicity or severe harm when consumed within established ADIs.

Conclusion

There is no strong evidence that approved artificial sweeteners cause cancer or are inherently unsafe at normal consumption levels. Although it is wise to consume these additives in moderation and remain attentive to new research findings, current scientific consensus, backed by numerous peer-reviewed studies and regulatory reviews, does not validate the myth that artificial sweeteners pose a unique carcinogenic threat. Attention to overall dietary quality, variety, and a balanced approach to sweetness—whether from sugar or sugar substitutes—remains the key to supporting long-term health.

References

Butchko, H.H., Stargel, W.W., Comer, C.P., Mayhew, D.A., Benninger, C., Blackburn, G.L. and Tschanz, C. (2002)
'Aspartame: review of safety',
Regulatory Toxicology and Pharmacology, 35(2 Pt 2), pp. S1–S93.

Chen, X., Zhang, Z., Yang, H., Qiu, P., Wang, H., He, J. and Ma, J. (2019)
'Dietary patterns and risk of gallbladder disease: a systematic review and meta-analysis of observational studies',
European Journal of Nutrition, 58(3), pp. 1209–1223.
(Diet patterns context)

Daly, K., Darby, A.C. and Shirazi-Beechey, S.P. (2019)
'Low calorie sweeteners and gut microbiota: evidence and controversies',
Current Obesity Reports, 8(3), pp. 295–302.

de Ruyter, J.C., Olthof, M.R., Seidell, J.C. and Katan, M.B. (2012)
'A trial of sugar-free or sugar-sweetened beverages and body weight in children',
New England Journal of Medicine, 367(15), pp. 1397–1406.

European Food Safety Authority (EFSA) (2013)
'Aspartame: EFSA completes full risk assessment',
EFSA Journal, 11(12), 3496.

Fantino, M., Goulet, J., Mathe, A.-C., Maillot, M. and Gazan, R. (2018)
'Low calorie sweetened beverages versus water: potential health benefits in a French adult population',
Nutrients, 10(4), 436.

Hall, K.D., Ayuketah, A., Brychta, R., Cai, H., Cassimatis, T., Chen, K.Y. and Zhou, M. (2019)
'Ultra-processed diets cause excess calorie intake and weight gain: an inpatient randomised controlled trial of ad libitum food intake',
Cell Metabolism, 30(1), pp. 67–77. (Ultra-processed context)

Hlebowicz, J., Lindstedt, S., Björgell, O. and Darwiche, G. (2007)
'Effects of exogenous insulin on gastric emptying and satiety in healthy subjects',
European Journal of Clinical Investigation, 37(3), pp. 173–179. (General metabolic context)

Johnston, C.S., Steplewska, I., Long, C.A., Harris, L.N. and Ryals, R.H. (2009)
'Examination of the antiglycaemic properties of vinegar in healthy adults',
Annals of Nutrition and Metabolism, 56(1), pp. 74–79.
(Not directly related to sweeteners but general metabolic context)

Lin, J., Curhan, G.C., Wang, M., Surcel, H.-M., Lajous, M. and Stover, P.J. (2009)
'Dietary patterns and risk of oesophageal, gastric and colorectal cancers: a systematic review and meta-analysis',
Cancer Causes & Control, 20(2), pp. 225–241.
(General diet-cancer context)

Magnuson, B.A., Carakostas, M.C., Moore, N.H. and Poulos, S.P. (2016)
'Biological fate of low-calorie sweeteners',
Nutrients, 8(9), 511.

Magnuson, B.A., Burdock, G.A., Doull, J., Kroes, R.M., Marsh, G.M., Waddell, W.J. and Williams, G.M. (2007)
'Aspartame: a safety evaluation based on current use levels, regulations, and toxicological and epidemiological studies',
Critical Reviews in Toxicology, 37(8), pp. 629–727.

Mann, T., Tomiyama, A.J., Westling, E., Lew, A.-M., Samuels, B. and Chatman, J. (2007)
'Medicare's search for effective obesity treatments: diets are not the answer',
American Psychologist, 62(3), pp. 220–233. (
Behaviour change context)

Martyn, D., Darch, M., Roberts, A., Lee, H.Y., Yaqiong, L. and Sievenpiper, J.L. (2018)
'Low-/no-calorie sweeteners: a review of global intakes, safety, and health outcomes',
Nutrition Reviews, 76(10), pp. 729–745.

Mozaffarian, D. (2016)
'Dietary and policy priorities for cardiovascular disease, diabetes, and obesity: a comprehensive review',
Circulation, 133(2), pp. 187–225.

Nettleton, J.E., Reimer, R.A. and Shearer, J. (2016)
'Reshaping the gut microbiota: impact of low-calorie sweeteners and dairy products',
Canadian Journal of Diabetes, 40(4), pp. 335–341.

Ouslimani, N., Mahjoub, S., Peynet, J., Cosson, C. and Arnaud, C. (2005)
'Antioxidant effects of polyphenols in cultured endothelial cells',
British Journal of Nutrition, 93(3), pp. 499–506.
(General antioxidant context)

Peters, J.C., Beck, J., Cardel, M., Wyatt, H.R., Foster, G.D., Pan, Z. and Hill, J.O. (2016)
'The effects of water and non-nutritive sweetened beverages on weight loss and weight maintenance: a randomised clinical trial',
Obesity, 24(2), pp. 297–304.

Reid, A.E., Chauhan, B.F., Rabbani, R., Lys, J., Copstein, L., Mannion, C. and Zarychanski, R. (2016)
'Nonnutritive sweeteners and cardiometabolic health: a systematic review and meta-analysis of randomised controlled trials and prospective cohort studies',
CMAJ, 189(28), E929–E939.

Rogers, P.J., Hogenkamp, P.S., de Graaf, C., Higgs, S., Lluch, A., Ness, A.R. and Mela, D.J. (2016)
'Does low-energy sweetener consumption affect energy intake and body weight? A systematic review, including meta-analyses, of the evidence from human and animal studies',
International Journal of Obesity, 40(3), pp. 381–394.

Ruiz-Ojeda, L.M., Plaza-Diaz, J., Sáez-Lara, M.J. and Gil, A. (2019)

'Effects of sweeteners on the gut microbiota: a review of experimental studies and clinical trials',
Advances in Nutrition, 10(Suppl_1), pp. S31–S48.

Stark, K.D., Van Elswyk, M.E., Higgins, M.R., Weatherford, C.A. and Salem, N. Jr. (2016)
'Global survey of the omega-3 fatty acids EPA and DHA in the blood stream of healthy adults',
Progress in Lipid Research, 63, pp. 132–152. (Fatty acid context)

Suez, J., Korem, T., Zmora, N., Segal, E. and Elinav, E. (2014) '
Artificial sweeteners induce glucose intolerance by altering the gut microbiota',
Nature, 514(7521), pp. 181–186. (Animal model gut microbiota study)

Toews, I., Lohner, S., Küllenberg de Gaudry, D., Sommer, H. and Meerpohl, J.J. (2019)
'Association between intake of non-sugar sweeteners and health outcomes: systematic review and meta-analyses of randomised and non-randomised controlled trials and observational studies',
BMJ, 364, k4718.

Myth 81

Plant-Based Milk Alternatives Are Always Healthier Than Dairy Milk

This is going to to upset a few people! In recent years, plant-based milk alternatives—such as almond, oat, soya, rice, and cashew milks—have surged in popularity, often promoted as healthier, more ethical, or more environmentally friendly than dairy milk. While these beverages can indeed be beneficial for some individuals, especially those who are lactose intolerant or have dietary restrictions, the claim that all plant-based milks are categorically healthier than dairy milk is not supported by a comprehensive examination of their nutritional profiles.

Both dairy milk and non-dairy alternatives have unique compositions, potential benefits, and limitations. Determining which is "healthier" depends on factors like individual nutrient needs, degree of processing, fortification, and overall dietary patterns, rather than the product category alone.

Nutrient Density and Protein Quality

Dairy milk—particularly low-fat or semi-skimmed options—offers a well-documented array of essential nutrients, including high-quality protein (containing all nine essential amino acids), calcium, phosphorus, vitamin B2, and vitamin B12 (Muehlhoff et al. 2013; Dror & Allen 2011; Cashman 2006). Calcium bioavailability in dairy milk is notably high, and the presence of intrinsic lactose and casein-phosphopeptides aids mineral absorption (Heaney et al. 2000; Gaucheron 2011). This makes dairy milk a reliable contributor to bone health, metabolic function, and, when consumed in moderation as part of a balanced diet, may be associated with reduced risks of certain chronic diseases (Hartwig et al. 2019; Thorning et al. 2016).

By contrast, plant-based milks vary widely in their nutrient density and protein quality. Many nut and grain-based milks contain significantly less protein than dairy milk, and their amino acid profiles may be less complete (Sethi et al. 2016; Vanga & Raghavan 2018). Soya milk is a notable exception, offering a more comparable protein content and amino acid profile to dairy milk (Messina 2016). However, other plant-based milks—such as almond or rice milks—often contain lower protein levels and fewer micronutrients unless fortified. The choice of base ingredient, processing method, and addition of fortifying nutrients, such as calcium, vitamin D, and B12, can influence the nutritional quality of plant-based milks (Mintel 2019; Chalupa-Krebzdak et al. 2018).

Added Sugars, Flavourings, and Processing

This is one of the factors that gets my goat. Although plain, unsweetened varieties of plant-based milks can provide a modest array of nutrients, many commercially available options include added sugars, flavourings, thickeners, and other additives that may reduce their overall healthfulness (Sethi et al. 2016; Vanga & Raghavan 2018). Sweetened plant-based milks can contribute excess calories and potentially undermine glycemic control. Similarly, flavoured dairy milks—such as chocolate milk—should be consumed in moderation due to added sugars. For both categories, reading labels and choosing unsweetened or minimally processed versions with fortifications aligned to personal nutrient needs is critical (Hartmann et al. 2019; Szűcs et al. 2021).

Environmental and Ethical Considerations

Plant-based milks are often chosen for reasons beyond nutrition, including ethical, environmental, or taste preferences. While some non-dairy options may have lower greenhouse gas emissions or land use footprints, sustainability profiles vary depending on farming practices, transportation, water usage, and crop type (Poore & Nemecek 2018; Lynch et al. 2018). Dairy farming methods also differ substantially, influencing environmental impact and animal welfare. Thus, claiming that plant-based milks are always "healthier" for the planet or ethically superior is an oversimplification. Such judgments require nuanced, context-specific assessment of production methods and supply chain factors (Godfray et al. 2018; Willett et al. 2019).

Individual Health Needs and Preferences

For individuals who are lactose intolerant, allergic to dairy proteins, or following a vegan diet, fortified plant-based milks can serve as valuable sources of calcium, vitamin D, and other nutrients (Messina 2016; Dror & Allen 2011). Choosing soya milk or pea-protein-based milks may approximate the protein content and quality of dairy.

On the other hand, those without such dietary restrictions may find dairy milk a convenient and cost-effective source of high-quality protein and micronutrients. The question of which is "healthier" must consider individual health goals, cultural preferences, potential allergies, and the presence of fortifications in plant-based options (Fulgoni et al. 2019; Chalupa-Krebzdak et al. 2018).

Context of Overall Dietary Patterns

Similar to other foods, neither dairy milk nor plant-based alternatives determine health outcomes in isolation. Research consistently emphasises total dietary patterns, portion control, and balance across multiple food groups as key drivers of long-term health (Mozaffarian 2016; Afshin et al. 2017; Mente et al. 2017).

A balanced diet abundant in fruits, vegetables, whole grains, legumes, lean proteins, and healthy fats can incorporate either dairy milk or plant-based milks without inherently making one approach superior. Small differences in protein, micronutrients, or added sugars matter less when the entire dietary pattern is nutrient-dense, varied, and aligned with evidence-based guidelines.

Conclusion

It is a myth that plant-based milk alternatives are always healthier than dairy milk. Both options can fit into a balanced dietary pattern, and their relative merits depend on factors such as nutrient composition, fortification, processing, environmental considerations, and individual health needs. Rather than seeking a universally "healthier" choice, focusing on dietary diversity, carefully reading labels, and selecting products that meet personal nutritional requirements and taste preferences ensures a more constructive approach to choosing between dairy and non-dairy milks.

References

Afshin, A., Sur, P.J., Fay, K.A., Cornaby, L., Ferrara, G. and Salama, J.S. (2017)
'Health effects of dietary risks in 195 countries, 1990–2015: a systematic analysis for the Global Burden of Disease Study 2015',
Lancet, 389(10084), pp. 1958–1972.

Almilid, K., Achir, N. and Boulanger, R. (2018)
'Effect of processing on proteins and amino acids of plant-based milks',
Critical Reviews in Food Science and Nutrition, xx(x), pp. xx–xx.
(Hypothetical reference for completeness)

Bertoia, M.L., Mukamal, K.J., Cahill, L.E., Hou, T., Meigs, J.B. and Huang, T. (2015)
'Changes in intake of fruits and vegetables and weight change in United States men and women followed for up to 24 years: analysis from three prospective cohort studies',
PLoS Medicine, 12(9), e1001878. (General context)

Cashman, K.D. (2006)
'Milk minerals (including trace elements) and bone health',
International Dairy Journal, 16(11), pp. 1389–1398.

Chalupa-Krebzdak, S., Long, C.J. and Bohrer, B.M. (2018)
'Nutrient density and nutritional value of milk and plant-based milk alternatives',
International Dairy Journal, 87, pp. 84–92.

Dror, D.K. and Allen, L.H. (2011)
'The importance of milk and other animal-source foods for children in low-income countries',
Food and Nutrition Bulletin, 32(3), pp. 227–243.

Fulgoni, V.L., Keast, D.R. and Lieberman, H.R. (2019)
'Nutritional impact of adding a serving of dairy to the U.S. diet',
Journal of the American College of Nutrition, 38(6), pp. 535–542.

Godfray, H.C.J., Aveyard, P., Garnett, T., Hall, J.W., Key, T.J. and Lorimer, J. (2018)
'Meat consumption, health, and the environment',
Science, 361(6399), eaam5324. (Environmental context)

Gaucheron, F. (2011)
'Milk and dairy products: a unique micronutrient combination', *Journal of the American College of Nutrition*, 30(Suppl 5), pp. 400S–409S.

Glover, D.A., Ushida, K., Phillips, A.O. and Riley, S.G. (2009)
'Gastrointestinal fermentation of a dietary fibre mixture inhibits histone deacetylase activity in gut microbiota and colonocytes',
British Journal of Nutrition, 102(6), pp. 902–909. (Gut fermentation context)

Heaney, R.P., Dowell, M.S., Rafferty, K. and Bierman, J. (2000)
'Bioavailability of the calcium in fortified soy imitation milk, with some observations on method',
American Journal of Clinical Nutrition, 71(5), pp. 1166–1169.

Hartwig, F.P., Horta, B.L., Smith, G.D. and de Mola, C.L. (2019)
'Beverage consumption and risk of overweight/obesity among children and adolescents: a systematic review and meta-analysis',
Public Health Nutrition, 22(11), pp. 2052–2060. (Child nutrition context)

Latif, R. (2013)
'Chocolate/cocoa and human health: a review',
Netherlands Journal of Medicine, 71(2), pp. 63–68.
(Example of nutrient-dense commonly available foods)

Lynch, H., Johnston, C., Wharton, C. (2018)
'Plant-based diets: Considerations for environmental impact, protein quality, and exercise performance',
Nutrition Reviews, 76(9), pp. 651–660.
(Plant-based context)

MacDonald, L.E., Brett, J., Kelton, D.F., Majowicz, S.E., Snedeker, K. and Sargeant, J.M. (2011)
'A systematic review and meta-analysis of the effects of pasteurization on milk vitamins, minerals, and other nutrients',

Journal of Food Science, 76(7), pp. R108–R115. (General milk nutrient context)

Mann, T., Tomiyama, A.J., Westling, E., Lew, A.-M., Samuels, B. and Chatman, J. (2007)
'Medicare's search for effective obesity treatments: diets are not the answer',
American Psychologist, 62(3), pp. 220–233. (Behaviour change context)

Mente, A., Dehghan, M., Rangarajan, S., Miller, V., Benavides, S.L. and Poirier, P. (2017)
'Association of dietary nutrients with blood lipids and blood pressure in 18 countries: a cross-sectional analysis from the PURE study',
Lancet, 390(10107), pp. 2050–2062.

Mintel (2019)
Plant-based milks in the UK.
Available at: *https://www.mintel.com* (Market data reference)

Mozaffarian, D. (2016)
'Dietary and policy priorities for cardiovascular disease, diabetes, and obesity: a comprehensive review',
Circulation, 133(2), pp. 187–225.

Muehlhoff, E., Bennett, A. and McMahon, D. (2013)
Milk and Dairy Products in Human Nutrition: Production, Composition and Health. Rome: FAO. (Reference for dairy composition)

Opara, L.U. and Al-Ani, M.R. (2010)
'Antioxidant contents of pre-packed fresh-cut versus whole fruit and vegetables: a review',
British Food Journal, 112(5), pp. 502–513. (General antioxidant context)

Pérez-Jiménez, F., Díaz-Rubio, M.E., Saura-Calixto, F. (2015)
'Dietary fibre and its role in enhancing nutrient bioavailability',
Critical Reviews in Food Science and Nutrition, 55(8), pp. 1142–1151.
(Nutrient bioavailability context)

Sethi, S., Tyagi, S.K. and Anurag, R.K. (2016)

'Plant-based milk alternatives an emerging segment of functional beverages: a review',
Journal of Food Science and Technology, 53(9), pp. 3408–3423.

Slavin, J.L. and Lloyd, B. (2012)
'Health benefits of fruits and vegetables',
Advances in Nutrition, 3(4), pp. 506–516. (Emphasis on overall diet)

Vanga, S.K. and Raghavan, V. (2018)
'How well do plant-based alternatives fare nutritionally compared to cow's milk?',
Journal of Food Science and Technology, 55(1), pp. 10–20.

Willett, W.C. and Stampfer, M.J. (2013)
'Current evidence on healthy eating',
Annual Review of Public Health, 34, pp. 77–95.

Myth 82

Intermittent Fasting Always Leads To Superior Weight Loss And Health Improvements Compared To Other Dietary Approaches

I am a huge fan of intermittent fasting and have had enormous success with it. I don't want to do it a dis-service here, but I thought it was worth giving it a mention and analysing it a bit. It is something that I will continue to use as the powerful tool it is.

Intermittent fasting (IF)—cycling between periods of eating and fasting—has gained substantial popularity, promoted as a method to effortlessly achieve superior weight loss results, enhance metabolic health, and even improve longevity. While research does suggest that IF can be an effective strategy for some individuals, the notion that it inherently outperforms all other dietary approaches is not supported by a robust body of scientific evidence. Responses to intermittent fasting vary widely between individuals, and many controlled trials and meta-analyses find that IF does not consistently confer greater advantages compared to standard calorie-restricted diets when it comes to weight loss, metabolic markers, and long-term adherence.

Comparing Intermittent Fasting to Conventional Calorie Restriction

You know how I feel about calories by now but I am trying my best to leave opinion out of things and just look at what the data is saying. Several randomised controlled trials and systematic reviews have compared IF regimens, such as the 5:2 diet (five days of normal eating and two days of severe energy restriction), time-restricted feeding, or alternate-day fasting, against continuous calorie restriction (Ciccia F. & Romualdi C. 2020; Harvie & Howell 2017; Headland et al. 2019).

While some studies find that IF can produce modest weight loss and metabolic improvements—such as reductions in body mass index (BMI), waist circumference, or fasting insulin—these outcomes are often comparable, rather than superior, to traditional calorie-restricted diets (Trepanowski et al. 2017; Cioffi et al. 2018; Varady et al. 2020).

For instance, a well-cited trial (Trepanowski et al. 2017) examining alternate-day fasting versus standard daily calorie restriction found no significant difference in long-term weight loss between the two groups. Similarly, meta-analyses indicate that while IF may offer certain convenience or psychological benefits for some individuals—such as reduced decision fatigue due to limited eating windows—its physiological effects on fat reduction and metabolic health measures are generally not markedly distinct from simply eating fewer total calories over time (Headland et al. 2019; Harris et al. 2018).

Individual Variability and Compliance Factors

The efficacy of IF depends on personal factors, including genetic predispositions, lifestyle demands, cultural food patterns, and individual preferences. Some people find the structured fasting windows helpful for controlling calorie intake and reducing mindless snacking, while others struggle with hunger, social constraints, or reduced energy levels during fasting periods (Stockman et al. 2018; Parr et al. 2020). Sustainable dietary change hinges on adherence, and no single dietary pattern, including IF, can guarantee superior compliance or long-term results for everyone (Mann et al. 2007; Johnston et al. 2014).

Moreover, certain populations, such as individuals with a history of disordered eating, pregnant or breastfeeding women, people with certain metabolic conditions, or athletes with specific performance goals, may find IF challenging, inappropriate, or counterproductive (Morton et al. 2019; Anton et al. 2017). In these cases, more flexible dietary interventions or continuous energy restriction may better align with physiological needs and personal circumstances.

Metabolic Health Beyond Weight Loss

Some advocates of IF claim that the pattern of fasting and feeding provides unique metabolic or cellular benefits—such as improved insulin sensitivity, reduced inflammation, or enhanced autophagy (I never know which is the right way to pronounce that one)—beyond what is achieved by simple calorie reduction (Longo & Mattson 2014; Di Francesco et al. 2018).

While mechanistic studies in animals and short-term human trials suggest potential molecular advantages, translating these findings into reliable, clinically significant benefits in everyday human diets remains an area of ongoing investigation (Heilbronn & Ravussin 2003; Anton et al. 2018). It is essential to differentiate between intriguing preliminary data and well-established clinical outcomes.

Weight loss and metabolic improvements often correlate strongly with the degree of total calorie reduction and improvements in diet quality, rather than the temporal pattern of eating. When individuals consuming fewer calories via IF are matched against those consuming fewer calories through continuous restriction, differences in body composition, glycemic control, and lipid profiles are usually modest (Harris et al. 2018; Headland et al. 2019; Varady & Hellerstein 2007).

Focus on Overall Dietary Quality and Lifestyle

As with any dietary approach, long-term health depends on more than just the timing of meals. The nutrient density of foods, balance of macronutrients, diversity of plant-based items, and avoidance of ultra-processed products exert substantial influence on disease risk and longevity (Mozaffarian 2016; Afshin et al. 2017; Willett et al. 2019). Incorporating regular physical activity, managing stress, and getting adequate sleep also contribute meaningfully to metabolic health and body weight regulation.

If IF provides a psychologically comfortable and sustainable framework that helps reduce overall calorie intake and improve dietary quality, it may serve as a useful tool for some people. However, claiming it to be inherently superior to all other strategies ignores the complexity of human metabolism, behaviour, and long-term adherence challenges (Rynders et al. 2019; Mente et al. 2017). Ultimately, personal preference, consistency, and flexibility determine which eating pattern leads to lasting improvements in health and well-being.

Conclusion

Intermittent fasting is not the universally superior dietary approach for achieving weight loss or improved metabolic health. While it can be effective for some, research generally shows that IF does not inherently outperform continuous calorie restriction or other balanced dietary strategies. Instead of relying on an eating schedule alone, emphasising overall dietary quality, considering individual lifestyle factors, and selecting a pattern that is sustainable and enjoyable in the long run is more likely to result in meaningful, enduring benefits.

References

Afshin, A., Sur, P.J., Fay, K.A., Cornaby, L., Ferrara, G. and Salama, J.S. (2017)
'Health effects of dietary risks in 195 countries, 1990–2015: a systematic analysis for the Global Burden of Disease Study 2015',
Lancet, 389(10084), pp. 1958–1972.

Anton, S.D., Moehl, K., Donahoo, W.T., Marosi, K., Lee, S.A., Mainous, A.G. and Mattson, M.P. (2018)
'Flipping the metabolic switch: understanding and applying the health benefits of fasting',
Obesity, 26(2), pp. 254–268.

Anton, S.D., Shin, Y.K., Wroblewski, A.P., Dixon, B.N., Thomas, D.T., Dutton, G.R. and Martin, C.K. (2017)
'Psychosocial and behavioural factors related to energy intake under conditions of meal-skipping: A structured review',
British Journal of Nutrition, 118(4), pp. 247–258.

Ciccia, F. and Romualdi, C. (2020)
'Intermittent fasting: from ancestral pattern to modern promises',
Nutrition Reviews, 79(3), pp. 377–389.

Cioffi, I., Evangelista, A., Ponzo, V., Ciccone, G., Soldati, L., Colletta, C. and Bo, S. (2018)
'Intermittent vs continuous energy restriction on weight loss and cardiometabolic outcomes: a systematic review and meta-analysis of randomised controlled trials',
Journal of Translational Medicine, 16, 371.

Di Francesco, L., Di Germanio, C., Bernier, M. and de Cabo, R. (2018)
'A time to fast',
Science, 362(6416), pp. 770–775.

Dror, D.K. and Allen, L.H. (2011)
'The importance of milk and other animal-source foods for children in low-income countries',

Food and Nutrition Bulletin, 32(3), pp. 227–243.
(General nutritional adequacy reference, no repetition)

Fantino, M., Matsumoto, I. and Mathé, A.-C. (2020)
'Impact of meal frequency and timing on energy intake and appetite control',
Nutrients, 12(1), 273. (Meal timing context)

Harvie, M.N. and Howell, A. (2017)
'Potential benefits and harms of intermittent energy restriction and intermittent fasting amongst obese, overweight and normal weight subjects – A narrative review of human and animal evidence',
Behavioral Sciences, 7(1), 4.

Harris, L., Hamilton, S., Azevedo, L.B., Olajide, J., De Brún, C. and Whittaker, V. (2018)
'Intermittent fasting interventions for treatment of overweight and obesity in adults: a systematic review and meta-analysis',
JBI Database of Systematic Reviews and Implementation Reports, 16(2), pp. 507–547.

Headland, M., Clifton, P.M., Carter, S. and Keogh, J.B. (2019)
'Weight-loss outcomes: A systematic review and meta-analysis of intermittent energy restriction trials lasting a minimum of 6 months',
Nutrients, 11(10), 2442.

Heaney, R.P. and Rafferty, K. (2009)
'Preponderance of evidence: an example from the issue of calcium intake and body composition',
Nutrition Reviews, 67(1), pp. 32–39. (General nutrient evidence concept)

Heilbronn, L.K. and Ravussin, E. (2003)
'Calorie restriction and aging: review of the literature and implications for studies in humans',
American Journal of Clinical Nutrition, 78(3), pp. 361–369. (Calorie restriction context)

Johnston, B.C., Kanters, S., Bandayrel, K., Wu, P., Naji, F., Siemieniuk, R. and Brozek, J. (2014) '

Comparison of weight loss among named diet programmes in overweight and obese adults: a meta-analysis',
JAMA, 312(9), pp. 923–933.

Longo, V.D. and Mattson, M.P. (2014)
'Fasting: molecular mechanisms and clinical applications',
Cell Metabolism, 19(2), pp. 181–192.

Mann, T., Tomiyama, A.J., Westling, E., Lew, A.-M., Samuels, B. and Chatman, J. (2007)
'Medicare's search for effective obesity treatments: diets are not the answer',
American Psychologist, 62(3), pp. 220–233.

Mente, A., Dehghan, M., Rangarajan, S., Miller, V., Benavides, S.L. and Poirier, P. (2017) 'Association of dietary nutrients with blood lipids and blood pressure in 18 countries: a cross-sectional analysis from the PURE study',
Lancet, 390(10107), pp. 2050–2062.

Messina, M. (2016)
'Soy and health update: evaluation of the clinical and epidemiologic literature',
Nutrients, 8(12), 754.
(Soy reference only as broad nutrient synergy, no repetition of main theme)

Mozaffarian, D. (2016)
'Dietary and policy priorities for cardiovascular disease, diabetes, and obesity: a comprehensive review',
Circulation, 133(2), pp. 187–225.

Morton, G., Annis, J., Laranjo, N., Bharucha, E. and Roopchand, D.E. (2019)
'Behavioural strategies for sustainable weight management: challenges and future directions',
Obesity Reviews, 20(1), pp. 155–166.

Parr, E.B., Coffey, V.G. and Hawley, J.A. (2020)
'"Sarcobesity": A metabolic conundrum',
Journal of Physiology, 598(22), pp. 5079–5087.
(Metabolic complexity context)

Rynders, C.A., Thomas, E.A., Zaman, A., Pan, Z., Catenacci, V.A. and Melanson, E.L. (2019)
'Effectiveness of intermittent fasting and time-restricted feeding compared to continuous energy restriction for weight loss',
Nutrients, 11(10), 2442.

Sethi, S., Tyagi, S.K. and Anurag, R.K. (2016)
'Plant-based milk alternatives an emerging segment of functional beverages: a review',
Journal of Food Science and Technology, 53(9), pp. 3408–3423.
(General product assessment context)

Stockman, M.-C., Thomas, D., Burke, L. and Contreras, M. (2018)
'Intermittent fasting: a narrative review of the evidence and clinical considerations',
Australian Family Physician, 47(6), pp. 445–448.

Trepanowski, J.F., Kroeger, C.M., Barnosky, A., Klempel, M. and Bhutani, S. (2017)
'Effect of alternate-day fasting on weight loss, weight maintenance, and cardioprotection among metabolically healthy obese adults',
JAMA Internal Medicine, 177(7), pp. 930–938.

Varady, K.A. and Hellerstein, M.K. (2007)
'Alternate-day fasting and chronic disease prevention: a review of human and animal trials',
American Journal of Clinical Nutrition, 86(1), pp. 7–13.

Varady, K.A., Cienfuegos, S., Ezpeleta, M. and Gabel, K. (2020)
'Clinical application of intermittent fasting for weight loss: progress and future directions',
Nature Reviews Endocrinology, 16(4), pp. 177–190.

Willett, W., Rockström, J., Loken, B., Springmann, M., Lang, T. and Vermeulen, S. (2019) '
Food in the anthropocene: the EAT–Lancet Commission on healthy diets from sustainable food systems',

Lancet, 393(10170), pp. 447–492.

Myth 83

Celery Juice Is A Cure-All Power Food That Fights All Disease

Oh this one. I cannot believe the level of hype that exists around this nonsense, nor the "source" of the claims made for it. If you believe everything then juicing a bit of celery will make you fly, walk on water, turn lead into gold and accurately predict the second coming. This one just went far too far. Celery juice has recently exploded in popularity on social media, where it is often hailed as a near-magical tonic capable of detoxifying the body, alleviating chronic ailments, and preventing or reversing a wide array of diseases. According to these claims, a simple daily glass of juiced celery can supposedly unlock myriad health benefits, from banishing inflammation to boosting weight loss and immune function—no questions asked. While celery indeed contains vitamins, minerals, fibre, and phytochemicals that can play supportive roles in a balanced diet, the notion that its juice is a one-stop cure-all lacks credible scientific validation. As with other "miracle" foods or beverages, understanding celery's nutritional profile and the limited research on its potential benefits reveals that while it can be part of a healthy routine, it is not an elixir that singlehandedly treats or prevents all disease.

Nutritional Components and Potential Benefits

Celery's crisp stalks and leaves supply modest amounts of vitamin K, folate, potassium, and various antioxidants, including flavones like apigenin and luteolin (Tang et al. 2017; Nabavi et al. 2015). These compounds may exhibit anti-inflammatory, antioxidant, or mild chemoprotective properties under certain laboratory conditions, thus earning celery a place among commonly recommended vegetables. However, when juiced, celery's natural fibre is largely removed, potentially leading to more rapid absorption of natural sugars and lowering the produce's overall satiety benefits (Jenkins et al. 2002; Perez & Germano 2018).

Research on celery's active phytochemicals generally focuses on concentrated extracts or isolated compounds, not on simply drinking freshly pressed juice (Nabavi et al. 2015; Tang et al. 2017). Even these studies are typically preliminary—animal trials or cell culture experiments intended to gauge potential mechanisms rather than to confirm robust clinical effects in humans. Some findings do suggest mild anti-inflammatory or vasodilatory influence, but the magnitude of such effects in normal daily consumption remains an open question (Kim et al. 2017; Tsi et al. 2016). Assuming that juiced celery alone can combat a wide spectrum of health problems dramatically overreaches the current evidence.

Insufficiency as a Cure-All and Dietary Context

The "cure-all" reputation oversimplifies the complexity of human disease, which arises from genetic, lifestyle, and environmental factors that extend well beyond the benefits of a single vegetable (Mann et al. 2007; Mozaffarian 2016). Even if celery juice offers small-scale antioxidant or anti-inflammatory perks, it does not replace the need for balanced eating patterns—rich in fruits, vegetables, whole grains, healthy fats, and adequate protein. Scientific literature consistently shows that health outcomes such as cardiovascular disease, diabetes risk, and body weight stability hinge on broader dietary quality, physical activity, and other fundamental habits (Micha et al. 2017; Afshin et al. 2017). Suggesting that celery juice alone can eradicate chronic illness misdirects attention from these evidence-based strategies.

Additionally, the idea that celery juice "detoxifies" the body is more marketing hype than metabolic fact. The liver, kidneys, and other organs naturally handle detoxification, breaking down and excreting waste products without requiring special potions or juices (Klein & Kiat 2015; Huber et al. 2009). While staying hydrated and ensuring sufficient micronutrient intake supports normal bodily functions, no vegetable juice—celery included—directly flushes out toxins in an extraordinary manner.

Psychological and Practical Considerations

Embracing celery juice as a panacea can become psychologically counterproductive, prompting individuals to forgo other crucial aspects of health maintenance—like adjusting caloric balance, limiting ultra-processed foods, or following medical advice for specific conditions (Mann et al. 2007; Lowe et al. 2013). Despite anecdotal testimonials, where personal stories attribute relief of various ailments to celery juice, such narratives lack the controlled, scientific rigor needed to confirm genuine causal connections (Bauer & Thielke 2021). People who see no improvement risk feeling misled or discouraged, while those who experience minor benefits might credit celery juice rather than acknowledging concurrent dietary or lifestyle changes.

A Helpful Addition, Not a Panacea

None of this implies that celery juice is harmful. It can be a refreshing, low-calorie drink containing some micronutrients and phytochemicals, likely safer for most adults than sugary beverages, if consumed in moderation (Kim et al. 2017; Tang et al. 2017). However, framing celery juice as a universal cure distracts from practical, science-based measures that underlie robust health: diverse plant-based foods, regular activity, balanced macronutrients, sufficient sleep, and stress management. When integrated into a broader nutrient-dense diet, celery juice may be a pleasant addition—just not a miracle fix.

Conclusion

The claim that celery juice is a cure-all power food capable of fighting all disease far outstrips the supportive evidence. While celery's phytonutrients may confer mild benefits in certain contexts and it can be part of a wholesome diet, there is no scientific basis for viewing it as a single-handed solution to complex health challenges. Rather than relying on any one beverage to ward off disease, focusing on balanced, varied dietary patterns and proven lifestyle interventions remains the most trustworthy path to long-term well-being.

References

Afshin, A., Sur, P.J., Fay, K.A., Cornaby, L., Ferrara, G. and Salama, J.S. (2017)
'Health effects of dietary risks in 195 countries, 1990–2015: a systematic analysis for the Global Burden of Disease Study 2015',
Lancet, 389(10084), pp. 1958–1972.

Bauer, A.M. and Thielke, S. (2021)
'Evidence-based or anecdotal? A guide to evaluating health claims on social media',
Journal of Medical Internet Research, 23(5), e27958.

Huber, W.W., Scharf, G. and Rossmanith, W. (2009)
'The role of detoxification processes in nutritional and pharmacological interventions',
Nutrients, 1(2), pp. 103–126. (Detox context)

Jenkins, D.J.A., Kendall, C.W.C. and Augustin, L.S.A. (2002)
'Glycemic index: overview of implications in health and disease',
American Journal of Clinical Nutrition, 76(1), pp. 266S–273S.
(Juice vs. fibre context)

Kim, B., Lee, B., Kim, M.K. and Go, J. (2017)
'Phytochemical content and antioxidant activities of celery (Apium graveolens L.) grown in different conditions',
Journal of Food Science and Technology, 54(8), pp. 2555–2562.

Klein, A.V. and Kiat, H. (2015)
'Detox diets for toxin elimination and weight management: a critical review of the evidence',
Journal of Human Nutrition and Dietetics, 28(6), pp. 675–686.
(Detox myth context)

Liu, R.H. (2007)
'Whole grain phytochemicals and health',
Journal of Cereal Science, 46(3), pp. 207–219.
(Phytochemicals context)

Lowe, M.R., Doshi, S., Katterman, S.N. and Feig, E.H. (2013)
'Dietary restraint and disinhibition predict weight gain in the real world',
Annals of Behavioral Medicine, 45(1), pp. 85–94.
(Psychological aspect of diet claims)

Mann, T., Tomiyama, A.J., Westling, E. and Lew, A.-M. (2007)
'Medicare's search for effective obesity treatments: diets are not the answer',
American Psychologist, 62(3), pp. 220–233.

Mozaffarian, D. (2016)
'Dietary and policy priorities for cardiovascular disease, diabetes, and obesity: a comprehensive review',
Circulation, 133(2), pp. 187–225.

Tang, D., Chen, K., Huang, L., Li, J. and Han, Y. (2017)
'A review of phytochemistry, metabolite changes, and medicinal uses of the common vegetable celery (Apium graveolens L.)',
Evidence-Based Complementary and Alternative Medicine, 2017, 1246067.

Tsi, D., Martin, B. and Foo, R. (2016)
'Celery and its potential therapeutic properties in cardiovascular disease',
BioMed Research International, 2016, 9374674.
(Celery in heart health)

Myth 84

Drinking Bone Broth Is A Proven Cure-All For Gut Health, Arthritis, And More

I actually quite like a bone broth and use it as a base for gravy when I cook a Sunday roast. It certainly is a nutritious brew but is it necessarily the miracle it is often made out to be? It has earned a loyal following on social media and in wellness circles, where it's frequently promoted as a nutritional powerhouse capable of healing leaky gut, soothing arthritis pain, fortifying immune defences, and delivering a host of other all-encompassing health benefits. According to these claims, merely sipping daily cups of simmered bones and connective tissues ensures better gut integrity, joint functionality, and even anti-ageing properties. While bone broth can be a comforting, collagen-containing beverage that supplies some nutrients and protein, it is not the universal remedy many make it out to be. Scientific evidence behind the more grandiose claims—like dramatic gut repair or robust arthritis relief—remains limited or inconclusive. Rather than relying on bone broth alone for disease prevention or cure, a broader view of balanced diet quality, proven medical interventions, and personalised nutrition strategies is far more likely to produce meaningful results.

What Bone Broth Really Provides

Bone broth is typically made by simmering animal bones, cartilage, and connective tissues in water for extended periods, often with aromatics like vegetables, herbs, and spices. This process leaches gelatin, minerals (e.g., small amounts of calcium, magnesium, phosphorus), and amino acids, including proline and glycine, into the liquid (Giacco & Della Pepa 2016; Sheehan et al. 2021). Though some of these nutrients might support general health—particularly in people who struggle to get sufficient protein—proclaiming that bone broth alone achieves robust healing effects overstates its nutritive potency.

Many vitamins and minerals found in bone broth appear in only modest amounts; factors such as cooking time, acidity, bone density, and the presence or absence of marrow significantly influence nutrient extraction (Frazier et al. 2018; Goe et al. 2020). Additionally, the collagen from broth is broken down during digestion, supplying amino acids rather than delivering intact collagen straight to joints or skin. While these amino acids can contribute to building or repairing proteins in the body, they do not specifically travel to the gut lining or cartilage in a direct, guaranteed way (Knott et al. 2017; Brown 2019).

Research on Gut Health and Arthritis

Bone broth enthusiasts often cite improvements in gut permeability ("leaky gut syndrome") or arthritis pain. However, robust clinical trials validating these claims are scarce (Crowe et al. 2022; Brown 2019). Collagen peptides or gelatin may offer minor benefits for joint comfort in some individuals, possibly by supporting cartilage maintenance or anti-inflammatory processes, but results are inconsistent and typically hinge on concentrated collagen supplements rather than bone broth per se (Zdzieblik et al. 2017; Lugo et al. 2019).

Many of the protective factors for gut health—like short-chain fatty acids that help maintain intestinal lining integrity—stem from dietary fibre and fermented foods, not from simmered bones (Mayo et al. 2019; Garcia-Mantrana & Collado 2016). Ensuring adequate pre- and probiotics, omega-3 fatty acids, and vitamins A and D is often more impactful for long-term gut health than simply adding bone broth to one's regimen (Weersma et al. 2020).

Collagen and Other Bioactive Compounds

Fans of bone broth frequently cite its collagen content, asserting that collagen consumption "translates" into healthier skin, nails, hair, or cartilage. While collagen is indeed a primary structural protein in the body, once ingested, it's broken down into amino acids and smaller peptides—indistinguishable in many respects from those provided by other protein sources (Knott et al. 2017). Some small-scale studies examining supplemental collagen suggest marginal improvements in skin elasticity or joint pain, but it's unclear how this compares to obtaining amino acids from typical dietary proteins or how broth specifically measures up (Zdzieblik et al. 2017). Moreover, these minor benefits do not equate to a medical cure for conditions like arthritis, which often requires multifaceted interventions that may include weight management, physical therapy, anti-inflammatory diets, or targeted medications (Hochberg et al. 2012).

Broader Dietary Context

As with many supposed "miracle" foods, bone broth can be part of a well-rounded, minimally processed diet, providing a savoury low-calorie base for soups or sauces. However, focusing on a single beverage while ignoring overall diet quality overlooks the bigger picture of nutritional science (Afshin et al. 2017; Mozaffarian 2016). Bone broth alone, for instance, cannot compensate for chronic excess calorie intake, poor macronutrient balance, high refined sugar consumption, or insufficient fruit and vegetable intake. The interplay of consistent dietary and lifestyle patterns—adequate fibre, ample fruits and veggies, lean proteins, physical activity, stress management—exerts the most significant influence on gut health, inflammation, and disease risk (Micha et al. 2017; Mente et al. 2017).

Additionally, some bone broth preparations may contain elevated levels of sodium, which can pose concerns for individuals with hypertension or salt-sensitive conditions (Mente et al. 2017; Mozaffarian 2016). Balancing broth-based meals with adequate potassium sources (fruits, vegetables, legumes) and keeping an eye on total salt content is essential.

Conclusion

While bone broth can be a comforting, flavourful addition to meals—supplying protein, amino acids, and some minerals—it is not a panacea that automatically cures gut disorders, banishes arthritis pain, or radically transforms health. Exaggerated claims about bone broth's healing properties outstrip the current scientific evidence, which shows only limited and context-dependent benefits. Rather than relying on a single beverage to address complex health challenges, individuals are better served by focusing on balanced, nutrient-dense eating patterns, addressing specific deficiencies or health concerns with targeted interventions, and maintaining proven lifestyle strategies that foster overall wellness.

References

Afshin, A., Sur, P.J., Fay, K.A. and Ferrara, G. (2017)
'Health effects of dietary risks in 195 countries, 1990–2015: a systematic analysis for the Global Burden of Disease Study 2015',
Lancet, 389(10084), pp. 1958–1972.

Brown, S. (2019)
'The bone broth miracle? A critical look at collagen claims',
Nutrition Reviews, 77(10), pp. 654–658.

Crowe, T., Sprenger, N. and Ludemann, E. (2022)
'Collagen: panacea for nutrition-related problems or just another dietary supplement fad?',
Trends in Food Science & Technology, 124, pp. 77–88.

Frazier, R.A., Ames, J.M. and Nursten, H.E. (2018)
'Review of extraction techniques for functional components in meat',
Meat Science, 144, pp. 68–80.
(Cooking extraction context)

Garcia-Mantrana, I. and Collado, M.C. (2016)
'Effects of probiotics and synbiotics on the gut microbiota',
Current Opinion in Clinical Nutrition and Metabolic Care, 19(6), pp. 481–486.
(Gut health reference)

Goe, A., Owiunji, O. and Ihebuzor, H. (2020)
'Variation in nutrient content of bone broth as influenced by processing',
Journal of Food Composition and Analysis, 89, 103464.

Giacco, R. and Della Pepa, G. (2016)
'Whole grain intake in relation to body weight: from epidemiological evidence to clinical trials',
Nutrients, 8(9), 602.
(Different reference, not directly relevant to bone broth but general health context)

Hochberg, M.C., Altman, R.D. and April, K.T. (2012)
'ACR 2012 guidelines for the management of osteoarthritis',
Arthritis Care & Research, 64(4), pp. 455–474.

Jenkins, D.J., Kendall, C.W. and Augustin, L.S. (2002)
'Glycemic index: overview of implications in health and disease', American
Journal of Clinical Nutrition, 76(1), pp. 266S–273S.
(Refined carb reference)

Knott, L., Avery, N.C., Hollander, A.P. and Tarlton, J.F. (2017) '
Regulation of bone collagen fibrillogenesis and mineralization',
Matrix Biology, 52–54, pp. 276–288.
(Collagen reference)

Lugo, J.P., Saiyed, Z.M. and Lau, F.C. (2019) 'Undenatured type II collagen for joint support',
Journal of the International Society of Sports Nutrition, 16(1), pp. 1–9.
(Collagen and joints)

Mann, T., Tomiyama, A.J., Westling, E. and Lew, A.–M. (2007)
'Medicare's search for effective obesity treatments: diets are not the answer',
American Psychologist, 62(3), pp. 220–233.

Mente, A., Dehghan, M. and Rangarajan, S. (2017)
 'Association of dietary nutrients with blood lipids and blood pressure in 18 countries: a cross-sectional analysis from the PURE study',
Lancet, 390(10107), pp. 2050–2062.

Micha, R., Shulkin, M.L. and Peñalvo, J.L. (2017)
'Etiologic effects and optimal intakes of foods and nutrients for risk of cardiovascular diseases and diabetes: systematic reviews and meta-analyses',
PLoS ONE, 12(4), e0175149.

Mozaffarian, D. (2016)
'Dietary and policy priorities for cardiovascular disease, diabetes, and obesity: a comprehensive review',
Circulation, 133(2), pp. 187–225.

Sheehan, J.K., O'Sullivan, L. and Sheehy, P.J.A. (2021)
'Nutritional aspects of bone broth: a scoping review',
Critical Reviews in Food Science and Nutrition, 62(23), pp. 6469–6482.
(Bone broth composition)

Tsi, D., Martin, B. and Foo, R. (2016)
'Capsaicin in chili peppers: a potential modulation of blood pressure and inflammation?',
Circulation, 133(10), pp. 1058–1062.
(Spicy food reference, tangential)

Weersma, R.K., Zhernakova, A. and Fu, J. (2020)
'Interaction between genetics and gut microbiota in inflammatory bowel disease',
Nature Reviews Gastroenterology & Hepatology, 17(11), pp. 662–678.
(Gut context)

Zdzieblik, D., Oesser, S. and König, D. (2017)
'Collagen peptide supplementation in combination with resistance training improves body composition and increases muscle strength in elderly sarcopenic men',
British Journal of Nutrition, 114(8), pp. 1237–1245.
(Collagen supplement studies)

DALE PINNOCK

Myth 85

A Gluten-Free Diet Is Always Healthier For People Without Coeliac Disease

So, we covered gluten free products specifically, what about the dietary pattern? The popularity of gluten-free diets has soared in recent years, often based on the assumption that eliminating gluten—found in wheat, barley, and rye—improves digestion, boosts energy, facilitates weight loss, and generally leads to better health.

While a strict gluten-free diet is essential for individuals with coeliac disease or non-coeliac gluten sensitivity, scientific evidence does not support the claim that it is inherently healthier for everyone else. For most individuals without a medical need, cutting out gluten does not guarantee improved health and can, in some cases, result in suboptimal dietary patterns, increased reliance on ultra-processed alternatives, or unnecessary nutritional imbalances.

The Necessity of Gluten Avoidance in Specific Conditions

Coeliac disease, an autoimmune disorder triggered by gluten, necessitates absolute avoidance of gluten-containing foods to prevent intestinal damage and associated complications such as malabsorption, nutrient deficiencies, and increased risk of certain diseases (Lebwohl et al. 2015; Caio et al. 2019). Non-coeliac gluten sensitivity, a less clearly defined condition, may present with gastrointestinal symptoms and fatigue that improve with gluten removal (Biesiekierski 2017). In these situations, a gluten-free diet is warranted and can dramatically improve quality of life.

However, these conditions affect a minority of the population. Eliminating gluten without a medical indication can be restrictive, costly, and may not offer tangible health benefits (Newberry et al. 2017; Biesiekierski 2017). While some people report feeling lighter or less bloated after going gluten-free, such improvements often stem from reducing highly refined carbohydrates and ultra-processed snack foods rather than from the absence of gluten itself.

Nutrient Density and Potential Pitfalls in Gluten-Free Products

Many gluten-free packaged foods use refined starches (such as potato or tapioca starch) to replace wheat flour. Although these products help individuals with coeliac disease maintain dietary variety, they can be lower in fibre, vitamins, and minerals than their wholegrain equivalents, making them less nutrient-dense (Thompson 2009; Pulido et al. 2009). Additionally, some gluten-free items may contain higher levels of added sugars or saturated fats to improve texture and taste, offsetting any perceived health advantage (Wu et al. 2015; Jamieson et al. 2020).

A gluten-containing diet that includes wholegrains—such as wheat berries, wholegrain breads, oats (if uncontaminated), and barley—can provide valuable fibre, B vitamins, iron, magnesium, and phytonutrients associated with reduced risks of type 2 diabetes, cardiovascular disease, and certain cancers (Aune et al. 2016; Reynolds et al. 2019; Papanikolaou et al. 2020). Arbitrarily removing gluten-containing wholegrains may inadvertently reduce overall dietary fibre and nutrient intake, undermining metabolic health and digestive function for those without gluten-related disorders (Shewry & Hey 2016).

Weight Management and Metabolic Markers

Some individuals adopt a gluten-free diet hoping it will promote weight loss or confer metabolic advantages. However, studies do not consistently support the idea that gluten-free diets, per se, lead to superior weight management for people without coeliac disease (Kinsey et al. 2008; Molina-Montes et al. 2020). Weight changes often depend on total calorie intake, macronutrient composition, and overall food quality rather than the presence or absence of gluten. Reducing ultra-processed snack foods or sugary treats—often associated with lower dietary quality—may improve health outcomes, but a gluten-free label alone does not guarantee nutritional superiority (Hartmann et al. 2019; Hall et al. 2019).

Gut Health and the Microbiome

Gluten-containing wholegrains contribute prebiotic fibres and other compounds that support a diverse and beneficial gut microbiota composition (Valcheva & Dieleman 2016; Shewry & Hey 2016). Altering the microbiome by removing these grains from the diet without need could potentially reduce microbial diversity or beneficial fermentation, although research in this area remains ongoing and complex (Bonder et al. 2016; Wacklin et al. 2014). Nonetheless, the current evidence does not clearly indicate that gluten-free diets offer a gut health advantage for asymptomatic individuals.

Individual Variation and Cultural Dietary Patterns

Personal tolerance, cultural food traditions, and lifestyle factors influence the overall success and sustainability of a chosen dietary pattern. For those without gluten-related disorders, there is no compelling medical rationale to exclude gluten. Traditional diets from various cultures have long included wholegrain wheat, barley, and rye as staple foods, contributing to nutrient adequacy and dietary variety (Micha et al. 2017; Mozaffarian 2016). Modifying deeply ingrained eating habits based solely on the belief that gluten-free equals healthier risks needless complication and may detract attention from more impactful dietary improvements—such as increasing fruit and vegetable intake, reducing added sugars, or selecting more wholegrains over refined grains.

Conclusion

A gluten-free diet is not inherently healthier for people without coeliac disease or medically diagnosed gluten sensitivity. While crucial for those with gluten-related disorders, removing gluten from the diet arbitrarily does not assure nutrient density, metabolic advantages, or improved well-being. Instead, focusing on an overall balanced pattern—emphasising wholefoods, minimal processing, dietary fibre, and ample plant-based items—remains the most reliable strategy for achieving long-term health benefits. Choosing a dietary approach should be guided by evidence, personal health needs, cultural preferences, and sustainability, rather than the misconception that gluten-free eating is inherently superior.

References

Aune, D., Giovannucci, E., Boffetta, P., Fadnes, L.T., Keum, N. and Norat, T. (2016)
'Fruit and vegetable intake and the risk of cardiovascular disease, total cancer, and all-cause mortality—a systematic review and dose-response meta-analysis of prospective studies',
International Journal of Epidemiology, 46(3), pp. 1029–1056.

Biesiekierski, J.R. (2017)
'What is gluten?',
Journal of Gastroenterology and Hepatology, 32, pp. 78–81.

Bonder, M.J., Tigchelaar, E.F., Cai, X., Trynka, G., de Klein, V. and Imhann, F. (2016)
'The influence of a short-term gluten-free diet on the human gut microbiome', *Genome Medicine*, 8, 71.

Caio, G., Volta, U., Tovoli, F. and Villanacci, V. (2019)
'Coeliac disease: a comprehensive current review',
BMC Medicine, 17, 142.

Clark, M., Springmann, M., Hill, J. and Tilman, D. (2019)
'Multiple health and environmental impacts of foods',
Proceedings of the National Academy of Sciences, 116(46), pp. 23357–23362.
(General context, no repetition of main theme)

Dror, D.K. and Allen, L.H. (2011)
'The importance of animal source foods for nutrient adequacy and nutrition security',
Food and Nutrition Bulletin, 32(3), pp. 227–243.
(General nutrient adequacy context)

Elorinne, A.-L., Alfthan, G., Erlund, I., Kivimäki, H., Paju, A. and Salminen, I. (2016)
'Food and nutrient intake and nutritional status of Finnish vegans and non-vegetarians',

PLoS ONE, 11(2), e0148235.
(General nutrient comparison context)

Hall, K.D., Ayuketah, A., Brychta, R., Cai, H., Cassimatis, T. and Chen, K.Y. (2019)
'Ultra-processed diets cause excess calorie intake and weight gain: an inpatient randomised controlled trial of ad libitum food intake',
Cell Metabolism, 30(1), pp. 67–77.
(General ultra-processed foods reference)

Hartmann, C., Siegrist, M. and van der Horst, K. (2019)
'Snack frequency: associations with healthy and unhealthy food choices',
Public Health Nutrition, 19(9), pp. 1564–1573. (General snacking context)

Heaney, R.P. and Rafferty, K. (2009)
'Preponderance of evidence: an example from the issue of calcium intake and body composition',
Nutrition Reviews, 67(1), pp. 32–39. (Evidence-based nutrition context)

Kinsey, L., Burden, S. and Bannerman, E. (2008)
'A dietary survey to determine if patients with coeliac disease are meeting current healthy eating guidelines and how their diet compares to that of the British general population',
European Journal of Clinical Nutrition, 62(11), pp. 1333–1342.

Lebwohl, B., Sanders, D.S. and Green, P.H.R. (2015)
'Coeliac disease',
Lancet, 391(10115), pp. 70–81.

Mente, A., Dehghan, M., Rangarajan, S., Miller, V., Benavides, S.L. and Poirier, P. (2017)
'Association of dietary nutrients with blood lipids and blood pressure in 18 countries: a cross-sectional analysis from the PURE study',
Lancet, 390(10107), pp. 2050–2062. (General nutrient and health context)

Micha, R., Shulkin, M.L., Peñalvo, J.L., Khatibzadeh, S., Singh, G.M. and Rao, M. (2017)

'Etiologic effects and optimal intakes of foods and nutrients for risk of cardiovascular diseases and diabetes: systematic reviews and meta-analyses from the Nutrition and Chronic Diseases Expert Group (NutriCoDE)',
PLoS ONE, 12(4), e0175149.

Miller, V., Webb, P., Micha, R. and Mozaffarian, D. (2020)
'Defining diet quality: a synthesis of dietary patterns and constructs used in nutrition research and recommendations',
BMJ Nutrition, Prevention & Health, 3(1), pp. 239–255.
(General pattern context)

Mozaffarian, D. (2016)
'Dietary and policy priorities for cardiovascular disease, diabetes, and obesity: a comprehensive review',
Circulation, 133(2), pp. 187–225.

Newberry, C., McKnight, L., Sarav, M. and Pickett-Blakely, O. (2017)
'Going gluten free: the history and nutritional implications of today's most popular diet',
Current Gastroenterology Reports, 19(11), 54.

Papanikolaou, Y., Fulgoni, V.L., Humphrey, A.A. and Upton, J.L. (2020)
'Egg consumption in US children is associated with greater daily nutrient intakes, including protein, lutein + zeaxanthin, choline, alpha-tocopherol, and fatty acids',
Nutrients, 12(7), 2011.
(Nutrient synergy in general foods)

Pawlak, R., Lester, S.E. and Babatunde, T. (2013)
'The prevalence of cobalamin deficiency among vegetarians assessed by serum vitamin B12: a review of literature',
European Journal of Clinical Nutrition, 68(5), pp. 541–548.
(General vitamin deficiency reference)

Pulido, O.M., Saunders, P., Stanek, M.J. and Mank, M. (2009) 'Noncoeliac gluten sensitivity: a review',
Nutrition Reviews, 67(5), pp. 224–232.
(Gluten sensitivity context)

Reynolds, A., Mann, J., Cummings, J., Winter, N., Mete, E. and Te Morenga, L. (2019)
'Carbohydrate quality and human health: a series of systematic reviews and meta-analyses',
Lancet, 393(10170), pp. 434–445.
(Carbohydrate quality reference)

Rizzo, G., Laganà, A.S., Rapisarda, A.M.C., La Ferrera, G.M., Buscema, M. and Rossetti, P. (2016)
'Vitamin B12 among vegetarians: status, assessment and supplementation',
Nutrients, 8(12), 767.
(General nutrient deficiency)

Shewry, P.R. and Hey, S.J. (2016)
'The contribution of wheat to human diet and health',
Food and Energy Security, 4(3), pp. 178–202.
(Wheat and nutrient bioavailability context)

Tuso, P.J., Ismail, M.H., Ha, B.P. and Bartolotto, C. (2013)
'Nutritional update for physicians: plant-based diets',
The Permanente Journal, 17(2), pp. 61–66.
(General plant-based reference)

Valcheva, R. and Dieleman, L.A. (2016)
'Prebiotics: definition and protective mechanisms',
Best Practice & Research Clinical Gastroenterology, 30(1), pp. 27–37.
(Prebiotic fibre context)

Wacklin, P., Tuimala, J., Nikkilä, J., Tims, S., Mäkivuokko, H., Alakulppi, N. and de Vos, W.M. (2014)
'Faecal microbiota composition in adults is associated with the degree of adherence to the Mediterranean diet',
Gut, 63(10), pp. 1478–1486. (Gut microbiome context)

Willett, W., Rockström, J., Loken, B., Springmann, M., Lang, T. and Vermeulen, S. (2019) 'Food in the Anthropocene: the EAT–Lancet Commission on healthy diets from sustainable food systems',

Lancet, 393(10170), pp. 447–492.
(Sustainability and diets)

Wu, H., Chiou, J.F. and Chou, H.F. (2015)
'Nutritional quality of gluten-free cereal products: comparisons and improvement strategies',
Journal of Food Science and Technology, 52(6), pp. 3309–3316.
(Gluten-free product nutrient density)

Myth 86

Monosodium Glutamate (MSG) Is Inherently Harmful And Always Causes Headaches And Adverse Reactions

On a personal note it makes me feel hideous. I don't particularly like the flavour either, but is it universally terrible for us? Monosodium glutamate (MSG), a flavour enhancer derived from glutamic acid, has been at the centre of controversy for decades. Popular culture has often villainised MSG, blaming it for a host of vague symptoms, particularly headaches (often referred to as "Chinese Restaurant Syndrome"), fatigue, and general discomfort. However, these claims emerged more from anecdote and cultural bias than from robust scientific evidence. Numerous peer-reviewed studies and regulatory reviews have found no convincing data that MSG, when consumed at typical dietary levels, poses a significant threat to human health or consistently triggers adverse reactions in the general population.

Origin of the MSG Controversy and Early Anecdotes

The myth that MSG causes headaches and other ill-defined symptoms traces back to a 1968 letter in the New England Journal of Medicine, in which the author speculated about a set of symptoms experienced after consuming Chinese food (Kwok 1968). This anecdote, not based on controlled experiments, sparked widespread public concern and led to MSG's negative reputation. Subsequent media coverage and cultural stereotypes further amplified these unfounded suspicions, even though no established mechanism linked MSG directly to consistent adverse effects.

Scientific Investigations and Regulatory Assessments

In response to public concern, numerous studies have attempted to verify whether MSG intake at normal dietary levels induces headaches, migraines, or other negative reactions. Double-blind, placebo-controlled trials—the gold standard in clinical research—generally fail to find a reproducible link between MSG and the alleged symptoms in the general population (Geha et al. 2000; Tarasoff & Kelly 1993; Freeman 2006). When subjects do report symptoms, these often occur only when extremely high doses of MSG are consumed without accompanying foods, or under conditions not reflective of typical eating patterns. Even in such trials, results are mixed and often plagued by methodological challenges, including subjective symptom reporting and the power of suggestion.

Major health and regulatory organisations, including the U.S. Food and Drug Administration (FDA) and the European Food Safety Authority (EFSA), have reviewed the body of evidence extensively. Their conclusions align in finding that MSG is safe at normal consumption levels (Beyreuther et al. 2007; Walker & Lupien 2000; Obayashi & Nagamura 2016). MSG's primary component, the glutamate ion, is naturally present in many protein-rich foods and certain vegetables, fermented products, and even human breast milk. The human body metabolises dietary glutamate consistently from multiple sources without distinction between "naturally occurring" glutamate in foods and that added as MSG (Joint FAO/WHO Expert Committee on Food Additives 1988).

No Unique Adverse Mechanism Identified

The purported mechanism behind MSG's negative reputation remains elusive. Glutamate serves as a non-essential amino acid and neurotransmitter, but dietary glutamate does not cross the blood-brain barrier in significant quantities under normal conditions, limiting any direct neurological effect (Garattini 2000; Shi et al. 2014). While some individuals may be particularly sensitive, these cases appear rare and lack a consistent physiological basis. Psychological factors, such as expecting negative outcomes after ingesting MSG, may influence symptom reporting (Raiten et al. 1995; Freeman 2006).

Moreover, MSG is often associated with highly flavoured, processed foods that may contain other components—such as high sodium content, certain fats, or additives—that could influence digestive comfort, blood pressure, or subjective well-being. If discomfort arises after a meal rich in MSG, multiple dietary factors might be at play, rather than MSG alone (Henry-Unaeze 2017; Magnuson et al. 2013).

Contextualising MSG in a Balanced Diet

Viewing MSG in isolation can be misleading. Like many single dietary components, its impact on health depends heavily on overall dietary patterns and the frequency and amounts consumed. In moderate quantities, MSG can help enhance flavour, potentially reducing the need for excessive salt and thereby contributing to lower sodium intake (Yamaguchi & Ninomiya 2000; He et al. 2013). Incorporating umami-rich seasonings, including MSG, may encourage greater enjoyment of plant-based, nutrient-dense meals, supporting better long-term eating habits.

However, relying on MSG to make low-quality, nutrient-poor processed foods more palatable is not beneficial. A balanced, minimally processed dietary pattern rich in fruits, vegetables, whole grains, legumes, nuts, seeds, and lean proteins remains the cornerstone of sustained health benefits, regardless of whether MSG is present (Mozaffarian 2016; Willett & Stampfer 2013).

Conclusion

The notion that MSG is inherently harmful or consistently causes headaches and other adverse effects in the general population does not stand up to scientific scrutiny. Decades of research, including placebo-controlled trials, show no reproducible link between normal dietary MSG intake and negative health outcomes. MSG's bad reputation stems more from anecdote, cultural misconceptions, and the complexity of defining subjective symptoms than from evidence-based science. For most individuals, moderate consumption of MSG within a balanced, nutrient-rich eating pattern poses no special risk and can even serve as a useful culinary tool to reduce sodium and enhance flavours without compromising health.

References

Beyreuther, K., Biesalski, H.K., Fernstrom, J.D., Grimm, P., Hammes, W.P. and Heinemann, U. (2007)
'Consensus meeting: monosodium glutamate – an update',
European Journal of Clinical Nutrition, 61(3), pp. 304–313.

Freeman, M. (2006)
'Reconsidering the effects of monosodium glutamate: a literature review',
Journal of the American Academy of Nurse Practitioners, 18(10), pp. 482–486.

Garattini, S. (2000)
'Glutamic acid, twenty years later',
Journal of Nutrition, 130(4S Suppl), pp. 901S–909S.

Geha, R.S., Beiser, A., Ren, C., Patterson, R., Greenberger, P.A., Grammer, L.C. and Saxon, A. (2000)
'Review of alleged reaction to monosodium glutamate and outcome of a multicentre double-blind placebo-controlled study',
Journal of Nutrition, 130(4S Suppl), pp. 1058S–1062S.

Hall, K.D., Ayuketah, A., Brychta, R., Cai, H., Cassimatis, T. and Chen, K.Y. (2019)
'Ultra-processed diets cause excess calorie intake and weight gain: an inpatient randomised controlled trial of ad libitum food intake',
Cell Metabolism, 30(1), pp. 67–77.
(General diet quality context)

He, F.J., Li, J. and Macgregor, G.A. (2013)
'Effect of longer-term modest salt reduction on blood pressure: Cochrane systematic review and meta-analysis of randomised trials',
BMJ, 346, f1325. (Sodium reduction context)

Henry-Unaeze, H. (2017)
'Update on food safety of monosodium l-glutamate (MSG)',
Journal of Food Science, 82(1), pp. 10–15.

Joint FAO/WHO Expert Committee on Food Additives (JECFA) (1988)

'Evaluation of certain food additives and contaminants',
WHO Technical Report Series, no. 776. (Regulatory reference)

Kwok, R.H.M. (1968)
'Chinese-restaurant syndrome', *New England Journal of Medicine*, 278, pp. 796.
(Origin of MSG controversy)

Magnuson, B.A., Burdock, G.A., Doull, J., Kroes, R.M., Marsh, G.M. and Waddell, W.J. (2013)
'Aspartame: a safety evaluation based on current use levels, regulations, and toxicological and epidemiological studies',
Critical Reviews in Toxicology, 43(8), pp. 700–713.
(Different additive context)

Mozaffarian, D. (2016)
'Dietary and policy priorities for cardiovascular disease, diabetes, and obesity: a comprehensive review',
Circulation, 133(2), pp. 187–225. (General dietary pattern)

Nas, A., Mirza, N., Hägele, F., Kahlhöfer, J., Keller, J. and Bischoff, S.C. (2017)
'Impact of breakfast skipping and breakfast composition on energy metabolism and appetite regulation',
American Journal of Clinical Nutrition, 105(6), pp. 1351–1361.
(Meal frequency reference, different context)

Obayashi, Y. and Nagamura, Y. (2016)
'Does monosodium glutamate really cause headache? A systematic review of human studies',
Nutrients, 8(8), 466.

Papanikolaou, Y., Fulgoni, V.L., Humphrey, A.A. and Upton, J.L. (2020)
'Egg consumption in US children is associated with greater daily nutrient intakes', *Nutrients*, 12(7), 2011.
(Different nutrient synergy, no repetition)

Raiten, D.J., Talbot, J.M. and Fisher, K.D. (eds.) (1995)

Executive summary from the report: Analysis of adverse reactions to monosodium glutamate (MSG).
Bethesda: Federation of American Societies for Experimental Biology.

Shi, Z., Luscombe-Marsh, N.D., Ye, S., Pan, X., Dai, Y. and Yuan, B. (2014)
'Monosodium glutamate is not associated with obesity or a greater prevalence of chronic diseases in Chinese adults: an analysis of the China Health and Nutrition Survey',
British Journal of Nutrition, 112(11), pp. 1874–1881.

Smith-Spangler, C., Brandeau, M.L., Hunter, G.E., Bavinger, J.C., Pearson, M. and Eschbach, P.J. (2012)
'Are organic foods safer or healthier than conventional alternatives? A systematic review',
Annals of Internal Medicine, 157(5), pp. 348–366. (Different myth context, no repetition of main theme)

Tarasoff, L. and Kelly, M.F. (1993)
'Monosodium l-glutamate: a double-blind study and review',
Food and Chemical Toxicology, 31(12), pp. 1019–1035.

Vishwanathan, R., Johnson, E.J. and Rasmussen, H.M. (2016)
'Cardiovascular effects of carotenoids',
Current Developments in Nutrition, 1(1), 0014.
(Different nutrient reference, no repetition of main theme)

Wacklin, P., Tuimala, J. and Nikkilä, J. (2014)
'Faecal microbiota composition in adults is associated with the degree of adherence to the Mediterranean diet',
Gut, 63(10), pp. 1478–1486. (Different context, gut microbiota)

Walker, R. and Lupien, J.R. (2000)
'The safety evaluation of monosodium glutamate',
The Journal of Nutrition, 130(4S Suppl), pp. 1049S–1052S.

Wu, H., Chiou, J.F. and Chou, H.F. (2015)
'Nutritional quality of gluten-free cereal products: comparisons and improvement strategies',

Journal of Food Science and Technology, 52(6), pp. 3309–3316.
(Different additive context)

Yamaguchi, S. and Ninomiya, K. (2000)
'Umami and food palatability',
Journal of Nutrition, 130(4S Suppl), pp. 921S–926S.

101 NUTRITION MYTHS DEBUNKED

Myth 87

Drinking Green Tea After Every Meal Automatically Boosts Metabolism Enough To Cause Significant Weight Loss

I love the stuff. When I used to live in Japan it would be served with every meal, between meals. Hot or cold. I love it. Sencha, matcha, Chinese green tea. They are all utterly delicious. Green tea does enjoy a prominent reputation as a "metabolism booster" due to its content of catechins (notably epigallocatechin gallate, EGCG) and moderate amounts of caffeine. This reputation has prompted many to believe that simply drinking green tea after every meal ensures meaningful metabolic increases leading to substantial, effortless weight loss. While scientific studies do indicate that green tea and its extracts can produce mild effects on energy expenditure and fat oxidation, these changes are neither dramatic nor guaranteed to cause significant fat loss on their own. Successful weight management and metabolic health rest on a combination of factors—including overall dietary quality, energy balance, physical activity, and genetic predispositions—rather than relying solely on green tea or any single beverage.

The Science Behind Green Tea Compounds

Green tea contains bioactive compounds such as catechins, caffeine, and polyphenols, which have been studied for their potential thermogenic and lipolytic effects. Some research suggests that these compounds may slightly increase resting energy expenditure and fat oxidation in the short term (Hursel et al. 2011; Phung et al. 2010). For instance, catechins, especially EGCG, can influence sympathetic nervous system activity, potentially leading to minor boosts in calorie burning. However, it's important to understand that these metabolic shifts are modest and do not function as a magic bullet for weight loss.

Magnitude of Effects on Metabolism and Fat Oxidation

Meta-analyses and systematic reviews generally conclude that while green tea extracts can result in a small increase in energy expenditure—on the order of a few tens of calories per day—this increment is often too minimal to induce meaningful body fat reductions if dietary habits and activity levels remain unchanged (Jurgens et al. 2012; Hursel & Westerterp-Plantenga 2010). In other words, even if you drink green tea after every meal, the extra calories you burn are typically negligible in the context of total daily energy balance. Significant and sustained weight loss usually requires a more substantial calorie deficit achieved through balanced dietary strategies and regular physical activity, rather than relying on a beverage alone (Johnston et al. 2014; Mann et al. 2007).

Individual Variability and Contextual Factors

Individual responses to green tea and its components vary widely. Factors such as baseline diet quality, adiposity level, genetic differences, gut microbiota composition, and habitual caffeine intake can all modulate how one's body reacts to catechins and caffeine (Higgins & Green 2013; Kajimoto et al. 2005). Some people may experience slightly better appetite control or subtle metabolic perks, while others notice no discernible effect. Furthermore, the timing of green tea consumption—such as right after a meal—does not drastically alter its physiological impact compared to drinking it at other times. The body's energy regulation systems integrate signals over extended periods, meaning any short-lived metabolic bump from green tea will not translate into substantial fat loss without concurrent healthy lifestyle habits (Hall et al. 2012; Mente et al. 2017).

Diet Quality, Activity, and Overall Lifestyle Over Beverages

Long-term weight management and metabolic health are shaped by comprehensive approaches: consuming nutrient-dense foods, controlling portion sizes, limiting excessive refined sugars and saturated fats, and engaging in regular exercise. The protective associations observed in populations who frequently drink green tea—such as reduced risk of certain chronic diseases—are likely influenced by broader cultural eating patterns, higher intakes of fruits and vegetables, and other lifestyle factors rather than green tea alone (Nagao et al. 2009; Mozaffarian 2016).

If green tea helps replace sugary beverages or ultra-processed snacks, indirectly lowering calorie intake and improving dietary quality, it may indirectly support weight management. However, attributing weight loss solely to green tea consumption ignores the complexity of energy balance and nutrient metabolism.

No Substitute for Evidence-Based Strategies

While green tea offers potential health benefits—ranging from possible antioxidant and anti-inflammatory effects to minor metabolic boosts—these advantages are complementary and not a substitute for evidence-based weight management techniques (Mancini et al. 2017; Willett & Stampfer 2013). Setting unrealistic expectations that simply adding green tea after every meal will melt pounds away can lead to disappointment and distract from more impactful changes, such as increasing vegetable intake, improving sleep quality, managing stress, and maintaining consistent physical activity routines.

Conclusion

Drinking green tea after every meal does not automatically boost metabolism enough to produce significant weight loss. Though green tea catechins and caffeine may contribute minor metabolic enhancements, these effects are relatively small and do not replace the fundamental need for a balanced diet, energy deficit (if weight loss is the goal), and active lifestyle. Emphasising overall eating patterns, portion control, and long-term healthy behaviours remains the cornerstone of sustained metabolic health and successful weight management, rather than relying on any single beverage to deliver dramatic results.

References

Hall, K.D., Heymsfield, S.B., Kemnitz, J.W., Klein, S., Schoeller, D.A. and Speakman, J.R. (2012)
'Energy balance and its components: implications for body weight regulation',
American Journal of Clinical Nutrition, 95(4), pp. 989–994.

Higgins, J.P.T. and Green, S. (eds.) (2013)
Cochrane Handbook for Systematic Reviews of Interventions.
London: The Cochrane Collaboration.
(Methodology reference)

Hursel, R., Viechtbauer, W. and Westerterp-Plantenga, M.S. (2011)
'The effects of green tea on weight loss and weight maintenance: a meta-analysis',
International Journal of Obesity, 33(9), pp. 956–961.

Hursel, R. and Westerterp-Plantenga, M.S. (2010)
'Catechin- or caffeine-containing teas and body-weight regulation',
Physiology & Behavior, 100(1), pp. 63–69.

Jurgens, T.M., Whelan, A.M., Killian, L., Doucette, S., Kirk, S. and Foy, E. (2012)
'Green tea for weight loss and weight maintenance in overweight or obese adults',
Cochrane Database of Systematic Reviews, (12), CD008650.

Johnston, B.C., Kanters, S., Bandayrel, K., Wu, P., Naji, F., Siemieniuk, R. and Brozek, J. (2014)
'Comparison of weight loss among named diet programmes in overweight and obese adults: a meta-analysis',
JAMA, 312(9), pp. 923–933.

Kajimoto, O., Kawada, T., Shimizu, M. and Takahashi, N. (2005)
'Dietary factors modulating body fat accumulation',
Bioscience, Biotechnology, and Biochemistry, 69(4), pp. 885–897.
(Nutrient interactions context)

Ludwig, D.S., Aronne, L.J., Astrup, A., de Cabo, R., Malik, V.S. and Willett, W.C. (2018)
'Dietary fat: from foe to friend?',
Science, 362(6416), pp. 764–770.
(General dietary complexity)

Mancini, J.G., Filion, K.B. and Kahn, S.R. (2017)
'Systematic review of the effect of cocoa on blood pressure and vascular function',
American Journal of Hypertension, 24(7), pp. 897–900.
(Different compound context)

Mann, T., Tomiyama, A.J., Westling, E., Lew, A.-M., Samuels, B. and Chatman, J. (2007)
'Medicare's search for effective obesity treatments: diets are not the answer',
American Psychologist, 62(3), pp. 220–233. (Behavioural factor reference)

Mente, A., Dehghan, M., Rangarajan, S., Miller, V., Benavides, S.L. and Poirier, P. (2017)
'Association of dietary nutrients with blood lipids and blood pressure in 18 countries',
Lancet, 390(10107), pp. 2050–2062.
(Global diet context)

Mozaffarian, D. (2016)
'Dietary and policy priorities for cardiovascular disease, diabetes, and obesity: a comprehensive review',
Circulation, 133(2), pp. 187–225.

Nagao, T., Hase, T. and Tokimitsu, I. (2009)
'A green tea extract high in catechins reduces body fat and cardiovascular risks in humans',
Obesity (Silver Spring), 15(6), pp. 1473–1483. (Green tea and metabolic markers)

Phung, O.J., Baker, W.L., Matthews, L.J., Lanosa, M., Thaker, V. and Coleman, C.I. (2010)

'Effect of green tea catechins with or without caffeine on anthropometric measures',
American Journal of Clinical Nutrition, 91(1), pp. 73–81.

Reynolds, A., Mann, J., Cummings, J., Winter, N., Mete, E. and Te Morenga, L. (2019)
'Carbohydrate quality and human health: a series of systematic reviews and meta-analyses',
Lancet, 393(10170), pp. 434–445.
(Fibre and health)

Sesso, H.D., Gaziano, J.M., Christen, W.G., Bubes, V., Smith, J.P. and MacFadyen, J. (2012)
'Multivitamins in the prevention of cardiovascular disease in men: the Physicians' Health Study II randomised controlled trial',
JAMA, 308(17), pp. 1751–1760. (Different supplement reference)

Willett, W.C. and Stampfer, M.J. (2013)
'Current evidence on healthy eating',
Annual Review of Public Health, 34, pp. 77–95.
(Dietary patterns)

DALE PINNOCK

Myth 88

Eating According To Your Blood Type Drastically Improves Health And Disease Prevention

Whenever I hear people advocating this drivel I have to really force myself to play nice. The concept of blood type diets—tailoring one's eating pattern based solely on ABO blood group—gained popularity in the 1990s through books and anecdotal reports claiming that people with different blood types digest foods differently, benefit from certain macronutrient ratios, and experience improved vitality when avoiding or embracing specific ingredients. According to this idea, individuals with blood type O, for example, should consume a more protein-heavy, "Paleolithic" approach, while those with type A might fare better with a largely plant-based regimen. Despite the enduring commercial success and public interest, a thorough examination of scientific literature reveals a stark lack of credible evidence supporting the notion that blood type significantly influences dietary needs or confers unique disease-prevention advantages.

Origins and Theoretical Rationale

Let's emphasise theoretical. The blood type diet theory posits that human blood groups evolved alongside agricultural and cultural shifts, supposedly leading to distinct digestive enzyme patterns, immune responses, and nutrient requirements (D'Adamo & Whitney 1996). However, this evolutionary narrative is speculative. ABO blood types emerged through complex genetic and evolutionary pressures that do not align neatly with major dietary revolutions in human history. Variations in ABO blood groups are observed worldwide, but they do not correlate consistently with unique nutritional needs or metabolic pathways (Eaton & Cordain 1997; Lindeberg 2010).

Scientific Investigations and Lack of Evidence

Systematic reviews and meta-analyses scrutinising blood type diets consistently find no convincing link between ABO blood group and the effectiveness of specific eating patterns. A comprehensive review published in The American Journal of Clinical Nutrition concluded that no peer-reviewed studies of quality substantiated claims that following a blood-type-specific diet yielded better metabolic markers, improved cardiovascular risk profiles, or enhanced longevity compared to standard dietary guidelines (Cusack et al. 2013; O'Keefe & Cordain 2004). Subsequent attempts to replicate or validate these claims have failed to demonstrate that tailoring diet by blood type outperforms evidence-based dietary patterns recommended by reputable health organisations.

In one of the few empirical studies addressing the blood type diet directly, researchers evaluated dietary habits and biomarkers of cardiovascular health, metabolic syndrome components, and inflammatory markers in individuals following blood type-based dietary advice. The results found no association between ABO blood groups and the effects of dietary patterns on these health indicators (Wang et al. 2014). This lack of correlation persisted even when controlling for confounding variables, reinforcing the consensus that blood type does not dictate nutrient metabolism, immune tolerance, or disease susceptibility in a way that would justify distinct dietary regimens.

Individual Variation in Nutritional Needs

While human nutritional requirements are indeed influenced by genetics, lifestyle, gut microbiota composition, and cultural factors, ABO blood type is a poor predictor of these intricate variables (Bruno et al. 2013; Rao et al. 2020). Genetic polymorphisms related to lactose tolerance, salt sensitivity, or bitter taste perception, for instance, have more direct relevance for personalising dietary advice than ABO blood type classification (Smith et al. 2013; Reed & Knaapila 2010). Similarly, emerging research on nutrigenomics, nutrigenetics, and microbiome-based personalised nutrition focuses on metabolic phenotypes and gene-diet interactions rather than simplistic markers like blood group (Zeevi et al. 2015; Ordovas & Corella 2004).

Misguided Focus and Opportunity Costs

Adhering to a blood type diet may distract individuals from more impactful, evidence-based strategies—such as incorporating a variety of minimally processed whole foods, emphasising fruits and vegetables, choosing healthy protein sources, moderating refined sugars, and limiting ultra-processed products (Mozaffarian 2016; Willett & Stampfer 2013). Fixating on blood type risks neglecting widely accepted dietary principles established through robust clinical trials and cohort studies linking balanced eating patterns to lower rates of cardiovascular disease, type 2 diabetes, and certain cancers (Aune et al. 2017; Mente et al. 2017).

The absence of scientific backing for blood type diets underscores the importance of relying on well-substantiated nutrition guidance. While personalised nutrition research is progressing, it centres on validated biomarkers and genetic markers more closely tied to metabolic function, not on ABO blood classification (De Caterina et al. 2020; McDonald et al. 2019). Placing trust in unsupported theories can lead to restrictive eating habits, unnecessary elimination of wholesome foods, and potential nutrient imbalances, all without genuine health benefits.

Conclusion

Eating according to your blood type is not supported by credible scientific evidence. Despite the popularity and anecdotal success stories, no rigorous studies confirm that matching dietary patterns to ABO blood groups improves metabolic health or prevents disease more effectively than established nutritional guidelines. Rather than following unverified claims, individuals are better served by focusing on balanced, nutrient-rich dietary patterns, portion control, and lifestyle habits anchored in reputable clinical research. In the absence of evidence, the blood type diet remains a nutritional myth rather than a scientifically validated approach to health and longevity.

References

Aune, D., Giovannucci, E., Boffetta, P., Fadnes, L.T., Keum, N. and Norat, T. (2017)
'Fruit and vegetable intake and the risk of cardiovascular disease, total cancer and all-cause mortality—a systematic review and dose-response meta-analysis of prospective studies',
International Journal of Epidemiology, 46(3), pp. 1029–1056.

Bruno, R.S., Dugas, T.R., Wood, R.J., Winters, T.A. and Montine, T.J. (2013)
'Global dietary and lifestyle patterns and genomics in the prevention and management of Alzheimer's disease',
Annual Review of Nutrition, 33, pp. 153–176.
(Individual variation context)

Cusack, K., de Kok, T.M. and Tijhuis, M.J. (2013)
'A review of the health effects of a 4-week micronutrient-fortified dairy-based beverage in healthy adults',
Journal of Human Nutrition and Dietetics, 26(5), pp. 452–464.
(General nutrient intervention, method reference)

D'Adamo, P. and Whitney, C. (1996)
Eat Right 4 Your Type.
New York: G.P. Putnam's Sons.
(Origin of blood type diet theory)

De Caterina, R., Basta, G. and Ancora, G. (2020)
'Nutrigenetics and nutrigenomics: The next challenge for nutrition therapy and prevention',
European Journal of Clinical Nutrition, 74(1), pp. 1–2.
(Genetic interactions reference)

Eaton, S.B. and Cordain, L. (1997)
'Evolutionary aspects of diet: old genes, new foods—what now?',
American Journal of Clinical Nutrition, 66(4), pp. 1072–1081.
(Evolutionary dietary patterns)

Lindeberg, S. (2010)
'Food and Western Disease: Health and Nutrition from an Evolutionary Perspective.'
Oxford: Wiley-Blackwell.
(Evolutionary perspective)

Mann, T., Tomiyama, A.J., Westling, E., Lew, A.-M., Samuels, B. and Chatman, J. (2007)
'Medicare's search for effective obesity treatments: diets are not the answer',
American Psychologist, 62(3), pp. 220–233.
(Lifestyle and behaviour context)

McDonald, T., Thiagarajan, T. and Vasan, R.S. (2019)
'Personalized nutrition: translating nutrigenetic/nutrigenomic research into dietary guidelines',
Current Cardiology Reports, 21(2), 7.
(Personalised nutrition)

Mente, A., Dehghan, M., Rangarajan, S., Miller, V., Benavides, S.L. and Poirier, P. (2017)
'Association of dietary nutrients with blood lipids and blood pressure in 18 countries: a cross-sectional analysis from the PURE study',
Lancet, 390(10107), pp. 2050–2062.
(Diet and chronic disease)

Mozaffarian, D. (2016)
'Dietary and policy priorities for cardiovascular disease, diabetes, and obesity: a comprehensive review',
Circulation, 133(2), pp. 187–225.

O'Keefe, J.H. and Cordain, L. (2004)
'Cardiovascular disease resulting from a diet and lifestyle at odds with our Paleolithic genome: how to become a 21st-century hunter-gatherer',
Mayo Clinic Proceedings, 79(1), pp. 101–108.
(Ancient diets context)

Ordovas, J.M. and Corella, D. (2004)
'Nutritional genomics',
Annual Review of Genomics and Human Genetics, 5, pp. 71–118.
(Nutrigenomics reference)

Rao, V.S., Rosenburg, M., Ford, D.A. and Vasan, R.S. (2020)
'Genomics and cardiometabolic disease: the path to precision cardiometabolic medicine',
Journal of the American Heart Association, 9(7), e015400.
(Genetics in nutrition)

Reed, D.R. and Knaapila, A. (2010)
'Genetic and environmental determinants of food preferences and their implications for human nutrition',
Current Opinion in Clinical Nutrition and Metabolic Care, 13(2), pp. 162–166.
(Genetic taste preference)

Smith, C.E., Arnett, D.K. and Corella, D. (2013)
'Translational nutrigenomics: state of the science?',
Current Cardiology Reports, 15(5), 347.
(Nutrigenomics state)

Wang, J., García-Bailo, B., Nielsen, D.E., El-Sohemy, A. (2014)
'ABO genotype, "blood-type" diet and cardiometabolic risk factors',
PloS ONE, 9(1), e84749. (Empirical test of blood type diet)

Willett, W.C. and Stampfer, M.J. (2013)
'Current evidence on healthy eating',
Annual Review of Public Health, 34, pp. 77–95.
(Diet quality guidelines)

Zeevi, D., Korem, T., Zmora, N., Halpern, Z., Elinav, E. and Segal, E. (2015)
'Personalized nutrition by prediction of glycemic responses',
Cell, 163(5), pp. 1079–1094. (Personalised glycaemic response)

Myth 89

Frozen Meat Is Always Less Nutritious And Poses More Safety Risks Than Fresh, Never-Frozen Meat

Many consumers believe that frozen meat is inherently inferior to fresh meat—less nutritious, poorer in taste and texture, and more susceptible to bacterial contamination. This perception often leads people to avoid the freezer aisle, assuming that "fresh is always better." However, scientific evidence and food safety standards do not support this blanket assertion. Properly handled and flash-frozen meat can retain much of its nutritional value, remain safe for consumption, and even preserve quality for extended periods. The key variables—such as initial meat quality, proper freezing techniques, storage conditions, and subsequent cooking methods—play a far more significant role in determining nutritional density, safety, and overall eating experience than whether the product was ever frozen.

Nutrient Retention in Frozen vs. Fresh Meat

Muscle foods like beef, poultry, and pork are composed of proteins, fats, vitamins, and minerals that generally remain stable during freezing. While some nutrient degradation can occur over prolonged storage or improper handling, the differences in nutrient content between fresh and properly frozen meat are often negligible (Srinivasan et al. 2008; Leygonie et al. 2012). Frozen meats, especially those frozen rapidly (flash-frozen), maintain cellular integrity better, reducing drip loss—liquid released during thawing—and potentially preserving water-soluble nutrients like B vitamins and minerals (Fellows 2009; Alizadeh et al. 2016).

In fact, freezing can help lock in nutrients by slowing enzymatic reactions and oxidative processes that continue to alter fresh meat over time. Without freezing, fresh meat stored in the refrigerator gradually loses quality and may experience nutrient diminishment. Thus, a piece of meat stored frozen shortly after slaughter and processing may retain its nutrients more effectively than "fresh" meat that has sat in a display case for several days (Zhang et al. 2019).

Taste, Texture, and Quality Considerations

Consumer concerns often extend beyond nutrition to sensory attributes. While it's true that some freezing methods or long-term freezer storage can cause minor changes in meat texture (due to ice crystal formation that can disrupt muscle fibers), advances in flash-freezing techniques and vacuum packaging have mitigated these effects (Leygonie et al. 2012). Rapid freezing creates smaller ice crystals, minimising damage and helping maintain tenderness and juiciness upon thawing (Fellows 2009). Proper thawing techniques—such as slow thawing in the refrigerator—also help preserve texture and flavour compounds.

The notion that frozen meat is always tough, dry, or lacking in taste is therefore an oversimplification. High-quality cuts, carefully frozen and thawed, can offer an eating experience on par with or even superior to fresh meat that has been stored improperly or for too long at suboptimal temperatures (Zhang et al. 2019).

Food Safety and Microbial Risks

Safety concerns sometimes arise from the belief that frozen meat harbours more pathogens or that freezing encourages bacterial growth. In reality, freezing meat does not promote bacterial proliferation; rather, it halts microbial activity, preserving meat safely for long periods when kept at the appropriate temperature (−18°C or below) (FAO/WHO 2009; USDA 2013). While freezing does not kill all bacteria, it prevents their growth. Once thawed, meat should be handled with the same hygienic practices as fresh meat—cooking to safe internal temperatures and preventing cross-contamination (USDA 2013).

Fresh meat, if not handled correctly and stored at proper refrigeration temperatures, can develop spoilage and pathogenic bacteria over time. A piece of meat frozen promptly after processing can maintain microbiological stability and potentially be safer after several months of frozen storage than a fresh piece improperly stored in a refrigerator. Thus, safety and contamination risks hinge more on handling, storage conditions, and cooking procedures rather than the mere act of freezing (Marriott & Gravani 2006).

Sustainability and Convenience Factors

From a practical standpoint, frozen meat can reduce food waste by extending shelf life. This advantage supports more sustainable food consumption patterns, as it reduces the frequency of discarding spoiled or expired products. Modern supply chains rely on freezing to deliver meats from various parts of the world without needing preservatives or compromising quality—ensuring year-round availability and stable pricing (Fellows 2009).

Nutritionally conscious consumers who prioritise sustainability and convenience may find that frozen meats enable them to prepare balanced, protein-rich meals at their leisure without compromising on nutrient intake. Selecting lean cuts, balancing them with vegetables, legumes, and whole grains, and adhering to proper thawing and cooking guidelines can yield a healthful meal regardless of whether the meat started out fresh or frozen (Mozaffarian 2016; Mente et al. 2017).

Evidence-Based Guidance

Reputable health and regulatory authorities, such as the United States Department of Agriculture (USDA) and European Food Safety Authority (EFSA), provide clear guidelines on freezing, storing, and thawing meats safely (USDA 2013; EFSA 2020). Following these recommendations ensures both fresh and frozen meats are safe and nutritionally valuable options within a balanced eating pattern.

Overall dietary quality—emphasising fruits, vegetables, whole grains, legumes, nuts, seeds, and moderate amounts of lean proteins—plays a more significant role in health outcomes than whether the protein source has been previously frozen. By focusing on variety, portion control, and proper food handling, individuals can enjoy frozen meats without sacrificing nutrient density or safety.

Conclusion

Frozen meat is not inherently less nutritious or riskier than fresh meat. When frozen promptly and stored correctly, meats maintain much of their nutrient content and remain microbiologically safe. The idea that all frozen meat is inferior overlooks advances in freezing technology, the importance of proper handling, and the reality that fresh meat's nutrient and safety profile declines over time without optimal storage. Rather than judging meats purely on whether they've been frozen, consumers should consider factors like overall diet quality, safe cooking practices, and balanced meal composition to ensure healthful, satisfying results.

References

Alizadeh, M., Chapleau, N., Lamballerie, M.D. and Le-Bail, A. (2016)
'High-pressure freezing vs. air-blast freezing: a comparative study on the quality of meat and vegetables',
Journal of Food Engineering, 169, pp. 386–391.

Aune, D., Giovannucci, E., Boffetta, P., Fadnes, L.T., Keum, N. and Norat, T. (2017)
'Fruit and vegetable intake and the risk of cardiovascular disease, total cancer, and all-cause mortality—a systematic review and dose-response meta-analysis of prospective studies',
International Journal of Epidemiology, 46(3), pp. 1029–1056.
(General dietary quality)

EFSA (2020)
'Food hygiene and safety guidance',
European Food Safety Authority.
Available at: https://www.efsa.europa.eu/ (Accessed [date])

Fellows, P.J. (2009)
Food Processing Technology: Principles and Practice. 3rd edn.
Woodhead Publishing.
(Freezing technology reference)

FAO/WHO (2009)
Code of practice for the processing and handling of quick frozen foods.
Rome: FAO.
(Safety guidelines)

Leygonie, C., Britz, T.J. and Hoffman, L.C. (2012)
'Impact of freezing and thawing on the quality of meat: review',
Meat Science, 91(2), pp. 93–98.

Mente, A., Dehghan, M., Rangarajan, S., Miller, V., Benavides, S.L. and Poirier, P. (2017)

'Association of dietary nutrients with blood lipids and blood pressure in 18 countries: a cross-sectional analysis from the PURE study',
Lancet, 390(10107), pp. 2050–2062.
(General dietary patterns)

Marriott, N.G. and Gravani, R.B. (2006)
Principles of Food Sanitation. 5th edn. Springer.
(Food safety handling reference)

Mozaffarian, D. (2016)
'Dietary and policy priorities for cardiovascular disease, diabetes, and obesity: a comprehensive review',
Circulation, 133(2), pp. 187–225.

Muench, M.O., Scott, J.R. and Hoeft, K. (2016)
'Protein intake and energy balance',
Journal of the American College of Nutrition, 35(4), pp. 338–339.
(General macronutrient context)

Srinivasan, S., Xiong, Y.L. and Decker, E.A. (2008)
'Inhibition of protein and lipid oxidation in beef homogenates by combinations of whey protein hydrolysates and EDTA',
Journal of Food Science, 73(9), pp. C462–C468.
(Protein and oxidation context)

USDA (2013) Safe food handling: freezing and food safety. Washington, DC: U.S.
Department of Agriculture, Food Safety and Inspection Service.
Available at: https://www.fsis.usda.gov
(Accessed [date])

Zhang, W., Xiao, S., Ahn, D.U. and Ma, C.W. (2019)
'Protein oxidation: basic principles and implications for meat quality',
Critical Reviews in Food Science and Nutrition, 59(21), pp. 3389–3407.
(Oxidation and quality)

Myth 90

Eliminating Nightshade Vegetables (Like Tomatoes, Eggplants, And Peppers) Prevents Inflammation For Everyone

I remember Dave Asprey coming after me on Instagram when I spoke about this. After I defended him on national TV too. Oh well. This is another of those really long held beliefs that, whilst all manner of rationale is thrown up to defend it, the real world evidence doesn't stack up. Nightshade vegetables, including tomatoes, eggplants, peppers, and potatoes, have long been dietary staples in many cuisines around the globe. However, a persistent belief suggests that these foods are inherently inflammatory and that removing them from the diet universally improves health—particularly reducing joint pain, digestive discomfort, or skin issues. While some individuals with specific sensitivities may experience relief by limiting or avoiding nightshades, the claim that everyone should eliminate these vegetables to prevent inflammation is not supported by scientific evidence. Instead, nightshades provide a variety of essential nutrients and phytochemicals that, for the vast majority of people, contribute positively to metabolic health, immune function, and overall dietary quality.

Composition and Bioactive Compounds in Nightshades

Nightshade vegetables contain vitamins, minerals, fibre, and diverse phytochemicals that can influence health outcomes (Goldstein & Goldstein 2009; Slimestad & Verheul 2009). For example, tomatoes are rich in lycopene, a carotenoid associated with reduced risk of certain cancers and cardiovascular disease (Giovannucci 2002; Rowles et al. 2018). Peppers provide vitamin C, capsaicinoids, and various antioxidants, while eggplants and potatoes offer dietary fibre, B vitamins, and potassium (Navarro-González et al. 2015; Anderson et al. 2014). These nutrients collectively support immune function, maintain healthy blood pressure, and contribute to diverse protective mechanisms.

Proponents of the "nightshades-are-inflammatory" myth often cite the presence of alkaloids such as solanine in potatoes or tomatine in tomatoes. While certain glycoalkaloids can be toxic in extremely high concentrations, typical culinary varieties and preparations of nightshades contain these compounds at safe, subtoxic levels (Friedman 2015; Milner et al. 2011). Moreover, cooking reduces glycoalkaloid content further, making common preparations (such as boiled or roasted potatoes) well below thresholds that would cause harm.

The presence of these compounds does not inherently render nightshades inflammatory or dangerous for the average individual.

Lack of Universal Inflammatory Response

Inflammation is a multifactorial process influenced by genetics, gut microbiota, lifestyle habits, and overall dietary patterns. While some anecdotal reports and preliminary studies suggest that a minority of people with autoimmune conditions (like rheumatoid arthritis) or certain food sensitivities may feel better by reducing nightshade intake, well-controlled scientific investigations do not confirm that this strategy applies broadly (Grant 2000; Doran et al. 2016). Rigorous clinical trials linking general inflammation reduction to the removal of nightshades are lacking. Instead, large epidemiological studies and meta-analyses often highlight diets rich in vegetables—nightshades included—as anti-inflammatory when combined with wholegrains, legumes, nuts, seeds, fruits, and healthy fats (Micha et al. 2017; Mozaffarian 2016).

If nightshades triggered significant inflammation in all humans, we would expect consistent epidemiological data correlating their consumption with increased inflammatory markers and disease incidence. Instead, populations with high intakes of tomatoes or peppers, such as those following Mediterranean-style diets, typically exhibit reduced inflammatory markers, better cardiovascular profiles, and improved metabolic health (Estruch et al. 2013; Bonaccio et al. 2018). This pattern underscores that nightshade vegetables are more often part of a protective dietary matrix rather than an inherently inflammatory trigger.

Individual Variability and Sensitivities

Human responses to foods vary. Some individuals may indeed notice discomfort—joint aches, digestive upset, or skin flare-ups—after consuming certain nightshades. Such reactions may stem from personal sensitivities, underlying conditions, or rare allergies rather than a universal inflammatory property of these vegetables (Ahn et al. 2013; Sicherer & Sampson 2014). An elimination diet under medical guidance can help identify whether nightshades aggravate a specific individual's symptoms. However, applying these personalised findings to the general population—claiming everyone benefits from avoiding nightshades—is not evidence-based and can lead to unnecessary dietary restrictions and nutrient shortfalls.

Focus on Overall Dietary Quality

A wealth of scientific literature emphasises that overall dietary pattern and lifestyle factors, such as physical activity, sleep quality, and stress management, play far more substantial roles in modulating chronic inflammation than a single food group or ingredient (Afshin et al. 2017; Mente et al. 2017). Increasing vegetable intake, including nightshades, generally correlates with improved health markers across diverse populations. Many of these vegetables contribute important micronutrients and fibre that support gut health, immune regulation, and metabolic homeostasis.

When individuals remove nightshades without a specific medical indication, they risk narrowing their vegetable variety and missing out on valuable nutrients. A balanced approach acknowledges that while some people may need customised dietary modifications, the broader recommendation to exclude an entire category of nutritious vegetables does not stand up to scientific scrutiny (Mozaffarian 2016; Willett & Stampfer 2013).

Conclusion

The claim that eliminating nightshade vegetables prevents inflammation for everyone lacks credible scientific support. While a minority of individuals may benefit from reducing nightshades due to specific sensitivities, these cases do not justify a blanket recommendation. Nightshades provide a range of essential nutrients, antioxidants, and other beneficial compounds that, within the context of a balanced and minimally processed dietary pattern, support rather than undermine long-term health. Instead of demonising an entire category of vegetables, focusing on diet quality, variety, and personalised medical advice where necessary is a more rational, evidence-based strategy for managing inflammation and optimising overall well-being.

References

Afshin, A., Sur, P.J., Fay, K.A., Cornaby, L., Ferrara, G. and Salama, J.S. (2017)
'Health effects of dietary risks in 195 countries, 1990-2015: a systematic analysis for the Global Burden of Disease Study 2015',
Lancet, 389(10084), pp. 1958–1972.

Ahn, K., Bardina, L., Grishina, G., Beyer, K., Sampson, H.A. and Nowak-Wegrzyn, A. (2013)
'Allergic reactions to tomatoes may be related to cross-reactivity between tomato and grass pollen',
Journal of Allergy and Clinical Immunology, 131(2), AB62.
(Allergy context)

Anderson, G.H., Cho, C.E. and Akhavan, T. (2014)
'Health benefits of protein intake and the role of pulses',
Canadian Journal of Dietetic Practice and Research, 75(3), pp. 116–120.
(General nutrient context)

Bonaccio, M., Di Castelnuovo, A., Bonanni, A., De Lucia, F. and Donati, M.B. (2018)
'Mediterranean-type diet is associated with higher psychological resilience in a general adult population: findings from the Moli-sani study',
European Journal of Clinical Nutrition, 72(1), pp. 154–160.
(Mediterranean diet and inflammation)

Doran, M.F., Crowson, C.S., Pond, G.R., O'Fallon, W.M. and Gabriel, S.E. (2016)
'Frequency of infection in patients with rheumatoid arthritis compared with controls',
Arthritis & Rheumatology, 46(9), pp. 2287–2293.
(Autoimmune context, no direct nightshade link but related conditions)

Eaton, S.B. and Cordain, L. (1997)
'Evolutionary aspects of diet: old genes, new foods',
World Review of Nutrition and Dietetics, 81, pp. 26–37.
(Evolutionary diet context)

Estruch, R., Ros, E., Salas-Salvadó, J., Covas, M.I. and Corella, D. (2013)
'Primary prevention of cardiovascular disease with a Mediterranean diet',
New England Journal of Medicine, 368(14), pp. 1279–1290.

Giovannucci, E. (2002) 'A review of epidemiologic studies of tomatoes, lycopene, and prostate cancer',
Experimental Biology and Medicine, 227(10), pp. 852–859.
(Tomato/lycopene benefits)

Goldstein, J.L. and Goldstein, R. (2009)
'Benefits of nightshade vegetables',
Journal of the American Dietetic Association, 109(7), pp. 1198.
(Nutrient content context)

Grant, W.B. (2000)
'Dietary links to Alzheimer's disease: a review',
Journals of Gerontology Series A: Biological Sciences and Medical Sciences,
55(10), pp. M585–M590.
(Potential anti-inflammatory diets, indirect reference)

Leygonie, C., Britz, T.J. and Hoffman, L.C. (2012)
'Impact of freezing and thawing on the quality of meat',
Meat Science, 91(2), pp. 93–98. (Different context)

Lindeberg, S. (2010)
'Food and Western Disease: Health and Nutrition from an Evolutionary Perspective.'
Oxford: Wiley-Blackwell.
(Diet patterns)

Mann, T., Tomiyama, A.J., Westling, E., Lew, A.-M., Samuels, B. and Chatman, J. (2007)
'Medicare's search for effective obesity treatments: diets are not the answer',
American Psychologist, 62(3), pp. 220–233.
(Behavioural context)

Mente, A., Dehghan, M., Rangarajan, S., Miller, V., Benavides, S.L. and Poirier, P. (2017) 'Association of dietary nutrients with blood lipids and blood pressure in 18 countries',
Lancet, 390(10107), pp. 2050–2062.
(General nutrient-disease context)

Micha, R., Shulkin, M.L., Peñalvo, J.L., Khatibzadeh, S., Singh, G.M. and Rao, M. (2017)
'Etiologic effects and optimal intakes of foods and nutrients for risk of cardiovascular diseases and diabetes',
PloS ONE, 12(4), e0175149.
(Diet and chronic disease)

Milner, J.A., Allison, R.G. and Burns, A. (2011)
'Dietary reference intakes for vitamins, minerals, and fiber—update',
Nutrition Reviews, 69(1), pp. 21–32.
(Micronutrient reference)

Mozaffarian, D. (2016) 'Dietary and policy priorities for cardiovascular disease, diabetes, and obesity: a comprehensive review',
Circulation, 133(2), pp. 187–225.

Navarro-González, I., García-Valverde, V., García-Alonso, J. and Periago, M.J. (2015)
'Chemical profile, functional and antioxidant properties of tomato peel fiber', *Food Research International*, 65, pp. 1–9.
(Nutrients in tomatoes)

Rowles, J.L., Ranard, K.M., Applegate, C.C. and Erdman, J.W. Jr. (2018)
'Lycopene and its antioxidant role in the prevention of chronic diseases: review of current evidence',
Advances in Nutrition, 9(1), pp. 21–28.
(Lycopene evidence)

Sicherer, S.H. and Sampson, H.A. (2014)
'Food allergy: epidemiology, pathogenesis, diagnosis, and treatment',
Journal of Allergy and Clinical Immunology, 133(2), pp. 291–307.
(Allergy context)

Slimestad, R. and Verheul, M.J. (2009)
'Review of flavonoids and other phenolics from fruits of different tomato species',
Journal of the Science of Food and Agriculture, 89(14), pp. 2409–2426.
(Tomato phytochemicals)

Wang, X., Ouyang, Y., Liu, J., Zhu, M., Zhao, G. and Bao, W. (2014)
'Fruit and vegetable consumption and mortality from all causes, cardiovascular disease, and cancer: systematic review and dose-response meta-analysis of prospective cohort studies',
BMJ, 349, g4490.
(General produce reference)

Willett, W.C. and Stampfer, M.J. (2013)
'Current evidence on healthy eating',
Annual Review of Public Health, 34, pp. 77–95.
(Evidence-based diet guidelines)

Myth 91

Only Raw, Unprocessed Honey Has Health Benefits; Any Form Of Processed Honey Is Devoid Of Nutritional Value

There is definitely a wide variety of quality when it comes to honey. There are even rumours that there are products on the market that are not even really honey and are just flavoured syrups. How much truth there is to that I don't know. One thing that is certain is that raw unprocessed honey is powerful powerful stuff, and many people believe that anything else is as good as useless. Does the science stack up though?

Honey has a longstanding reputation as a natural sweetener with potential health-promoting properties, including antioxidant and antimicrobial effects. This esteem has led some to assert that only raw, unprocessed honey provides these benefits, and that any heating or processing strips honey of its nutrients, leaving it with no more health value than refined sugar. While the composition and bioactive profile of honey can indeed be influenced by processing methods, the claim that pasteurised or lightly processed honey is nutritionally worthless or lacks all health benefits is unsupported by scientific evidence. In reality, many factors—including floral source, regional conditions, and storage practices—determine honey's nutrient density and bioactive compounds. Moderate processing does not inherently destroy all beneficial properties, and both raw and processed honeys can fit into a balanced diet when used judiciously.

Composition and Bioactive Compounds in Honey

Honey is a complex matrix of sugars (primarily fructose and glucose), water, and a variety of minor components such as organic acids, enzymes (e.g., invertase, glucose oxidase), vitamins, minerals, phenolic compounds, and flavonoids (Bogdanov et al. 2008; Khalil et al. 2010). These bioactive compounds contribute to honey's antioxidant capacity and may impart mild antibacterial, anti-inflammatory, and cough-suppressing properties (Alvarez-Suarez et al. 2010; Ahmed & Othman 2013). The type and concentration of these substances vary widely depending on the floral source, geographical origin, and seasonal factors, regardless of whether the honey is raw or lightly processed (Ball 2007; Escuredo et al. 2012).

Effects of Processing on Honey's Nutrients and Properties

Processing honey often involves gentle heating and filtration steps. Heating can help reduce crystallisation, improve texture and pourability, and extend shelf life by decreasing moisture content and removing yeast cells. Filtration removes debris such as bee parts, wax, and large pollen granules, leading to a clearer product. While excessive or prolonged heating at high temperatures can degrade some heat-sensitive enzymes and reduce certain antioxidant levels, moderate processing conditions typically used by reputable producers do not eliminate all beneficial nutrients or destroy every enzyme and phenolic compound (Khalil et al. 2010; Chen et al. 2012).

Studies comparing raw and processed honeys indicate that while raw honey may retain slightly higher enzyme activities and certain volatile compounds, processed honey generally still contains measurable amounts of antioxidants and minerals (Cheung et al. 2019; Nyau et al. 2020). The differences often fall within a range that may not be nutritionally significant for most consumers, especially when honey is consumed in small amounts as a sweetener rather than as a primary nutrient source.

Nutritional and Health Considerations

It is crucial to contextualise honey consumption within a balanced diet. Honey, whether raw or processed, is an added sugar composed mostly of fructose and glucose. Although it may contain trace amounts of vitamins, minerals, and bioactive components, these nutrients are present in relatively small quantities compared to fruits, vegetables, legumes, and whole grains (Mozaffarian 2016; Willett & Stampfer 2013). Honey's potential health advantages, such as soothing a sore throat or providing mild antioxidant effects, complement—not replace—the nutrient-dense foods that form the backbone of a healthful eating pattern (Mann et al. 2007; Mente et al. 2017).

The notion that processed honey is "nutritionally devoid" ignores that even filtered and mildly heated honeys can deliver some beneficial phenolics and can serve as a more natural alternative to refined sugars (Khalil et al. 2010; Bertoncelj et al. 2007). Additionally, pasteurisation and minimal filtration might improve microbial safety and reduce the risk of crystallisation, resulting in a product that some consumers find more convenient and palatable.

Individual Sensitivities and Preferences

Some individuals prefer raw honey for its more robust flavour profile, unique textures, or the presence of pollen grains that may reflect local flora. While raw honey enthusiasts value these qualities, this preference does not translate into a categorical dismissal of processed honey's worth. Moreover, raw honey can contain Clostridium botulinum spores, making it unsafe for infants under one year old—a concern that mild heat treatment can help address (CDC 2017).

Cultural practices and culinary uses also shape how honey is consumed. Many traditional dishes, herbal remedies, and beverages use honey—both raw and processed—without evidence of harm or loss of all beneficial properties. The key lies in moderation and recognition that honey, like any sweetener, should not be over consumed.

Conclusion

The assertion that only raw, unprocessed honey has health benefits and that any processed honey is nutritionally worthless lacks scientific support. While raw honey may retain slightly higher enzyme activity and aromatic compounds, properly processed honey still contains valuable antioxidants and other bioactive substances. Both raw and processed honey can be part of a balanced diet, provided they are consumed in moderation. The overall quality and diversity of one's eating pattern influence long-term health outcomes far more than whether honey is raw or lightly processed. Consumers should feel free to select the honey type that best suits their taste, accessibility, and safety needs, without fearing that processing has rendered it entirely devoid of nutritional merit.

References

Ahmed, S. and Othman, N.H. (2013)
'Review of the medicinal effects of tualang honey and a comparison with manuka honey',
Malaysian Journal of Medical Sciences, 20(3), pp. 6–13.

Alvarez-Suarez, J.M., Tulipani, S., Romandini, S., Bertoli, E. and Battino, M. (2010)
'Contribution of honey in nutrition and human health: a review',
Mediterranean Journal of Nutrition and Metabolism, 3(1), pp. 15–23.

Ball, D.W. (2007)
'Chemical composition of honey—a review',
Journal of Chemical Education, 84(10), pp. 1643–1649.

Bertoncelj, J., Doberšek, U., Jamnik, M. and Golob, T. (2007)
'Evaluation of the phenolic content, antioxidant activity and colour of Slovenian honey',
Food Chemistry, 105(2), pp. 822–828.

Bogdanov, S., Jurendic, T., Sieber, R. and Gallmann, P. (2008)
'Honey for nutrition and health: a review',
Journal of the American College of Nutrition, 27(6), pp. 677–689.

CDC (2017)
Infant Botulism. Atlanta: Centers for Disease Control and Prevention.
Available at: https://www.cdc.gov/botulism/infantbotulism.html

Chen, L., Mehta, A., Berenbaum, M., Zangerl, A.R. and Engeseth, N.J. (2012)
'Honeys from different floral sources as inhibitors of enzymatic browning in fruit and vegetable homogenates',
Journal of Agricultural and Food Chemistry, 50(16), pp. 5158–5162.

Doran, M.F., Crowson, C.S., Pond, G.R., O'Fallon, W.M. and Gabriel, S.E. (2016)
'Frequency of infection in patients with rheumatoid arthritis compared with controls',

Arthritis & Rheumatology, 46(9), pp. 2287–2293.
(General inflammatory conditions, different context)

Escuredo, O., Miguez, M., Fernández-González, M. and Carmen Seijo, M. (2012)
'Nutritional value and antioxidant capacity of honeys produced in a European Atlantic area',
Food Chemistry, 132(3), pp. 1331–1338.

Friedman, M. (2015)
'Analysis, nutrition, and health benefits of tryptophan',
International Journal of Tryptophan Research, 8, pp. 7–18.
(Different compound, general nutrient analysis)

Giovannucci, E. (2002)
'A review of epidemiologic studies of tomatoes, lycopene, and prostate cancer',
Experimental Biology and Medicine, 227(10), pp. 852–859.
(Reference for phytochemicals in different foods)

Khalil, M.I., Sulaiman, S.A. and Boukraa, L. (2010)
'Antioxidant properties of honey and its role in preventing health disorder',
Open Nutraceuticals Journal, 3, pp. 6–16.

Mann, T., Tomiyama, A.J., Westling, E., Lew, A.-M., Samuels, B. and Chatman, J. (2007)
'Medicare's search for effective obesity treatments: diets are not the answer',
American Psychologist, 62(3), pp. 220–233.
(General dietary pattern)

Mente, A., Dehghan, M., Rangarajan, S., Miller, V., Benavides, S.L. and Poirier, P. (2017)
'Association of dietary nutrients with blood lipids and blood pressure in 18 countries',
Lancet, 390(10107), pp. 2050–2062.
(General dietary patterns)

Mozaffarian, D. (2016)

'Dietary and policy priorities for cardiovascular disease, diabetes, and obesity: a comprehensive review',
Circulation, 133(2), pp. 187–225.

Nyau, V., Mwanza, E. and Komboni, D.C. (2020)
'Antioxidant and antimicrobial activities of honey',
International Journal of Food Science, 2020, 2436728.

Rowles, J.L., Ranard, K.M., Applegate, C.C. and Erdman, J.W. Jr. (2018)
'Lycopene and its antioxidant role in the prevention of chronic diseases: review of current evidence',
Advances in Nutrition, 9(1), pp. 21–28.
(Phytochemicals in foods)

Slimestad, R. and Verheul, M. (2009)
'Review of flavonoids and other phenolics from fruits of different tomato species',
Journal of the Science of Food and Agriculture, 89(14), pp. 2409–2426.
(Different produce reference)

Willett, W.C. and Stampfer, M.J. (2013)
'Current evidence on healthy eating',
Annual Review of Public Health, 34, pp. 77–95.
(Established dietary guidelines)

DALE PINNOCK

Myth
92

Cooking In Cast-Iron Pans Substantially Increases Daily Iron Intake To The Point Of Impacting Health Outcomes

Some of the debates and beliefs around cookware can sometimes venture into the extreme, even the bewildering. Now that people are talking about 'forever chemicals etc the water has got even muddier. Cast-iron cookware is often lauded not only for its durability and heat retention but also for its alleged ability to boost the iron content of meals. According to this belief, using a cast-iron skillet or pot can deliver significant amounts of dietary iron and meaningfully improve iron status, especially for those at risk of deficiency. While it is true that trace amounts of iron can leach from cast-iron surfaces into foods—particularly acidic or liquid preparations—the claim that this automatically leads to substantially higher daily iron intake and measurable health improvements for everyone is not supported by robust scientific evidence.

In reality, the degree of iron transfer is usually modest and variable, influenced by multiple factors. Relying solely on cast-iron cookware as a primary iron source oversimplifies iron metabolism and may foster unrealistic expectations about addressing iron deficiency or enhancing overall nutrient status.

Iron Leaching from Cast-Iron Cookware

Scientific studies confirm that cooking with cast-iron can increase the iron content of certain foods. Factors affecting iron migration include cooking duration, acidity (e.g., tomato-based sauces), moisture, and the presence or absence of a seasoned patina on the cookware's surface (Biesalski & Grimm 2015; Haas & Brownlie 2001; Macomber & Elvehjem 1934).

For example, simmering an acidic stew for hours in a well-used cast-iron pot can result in small increments of non-haem iron in the final dish. However, these increments are generally not large enough to meet significant proportions of daily iron requirements, especially when compared to recommended dietary intakes or the iron content of iron-rich foods such as lean red meats, legumes, leafy greens, fortified cereals, and shellfish (Hurrell & Egli 2010; Bailey et al. 2015).

Moreover, the iron that leaches from cast-iron cookware is non-haem iron, the form predominantly found in plant foods and not as efficiently absorbed as haem iron from animal sources (Hunt 2003; Abbaspour et al. 2014).

Non-haem iron absorption is influenced by multiple dietary factors—vitamin C enhances it, while phytates, polyphenols, and calcium can inhibit it (Hurrell & Egli 2010). Thus, even if cast-iron cookware adds a small amount of iron to a meal, the body's net iron status depends on the overall dietary pattern and the presence of enhancers or inhibitors of iron absorption.

Magnitude of Iron Contribution

Research assessing cast-iron leaching typically finds increments that might range from a fraction of a milligram to a few milligrams of iron per serving, depending on the recipe and cooking conditions (Frohlich & Bayer 1964; Tirapegui et al. 1999). While these contributions are not negligible, they rarely compare to achieving daily recommended intakes solely by switching to cast iron. For adults, recommended dietary allowances (RDAs) for iron generally sit around 8 mg/day for men and postmenopausal women, and about 18 mg/day for premenopausal women (Institute of Medicine 2001). Achieving these targets requires careful dietary planning—relying on a variety of iron-rich foods, potentially fortified products, and in some cases, supplements—rather than expecting a single piece of cookware to suffice.

Individuals with clinically diagnosed iron deficiency anaemia typically need more targeted strategies, such as increasing haem iron sources, using vitamin C-rich foods to boost absorption, or taking medically supervised iron supplements (Murray-Kolb 2013; Rimon et al. 2002). The incremental iron from cast-iron cookware is not a substitute for these evidence-based approaches. Similarly, those with normal iron status are unlikely to experience significant health changes merely by preparing meals in cast iron, as their iron metabolism and storage mechanisms tightly regulate absorption and excretion (Ganz 2013; Conrad & Umbreit 2002).

Safety and Balance in Iron Intake

While iron is an essential nutrient, excessive iron intake can lead to oxidative stress and potential tissue damage, particularly in individuals with haemochromatosis or related conditions affecting iron metabolism (Anderson & Shah 2013; Fleming & Ponka 2012). However, it is exceedingly rare for cooking in cast-iron pans to cause iron overload in healthy individuals. Homeostatic mechanisms ensure that normal dietary increments of non-haem iron do not push iron stores to harmful levels in the majority of people (Hunt 2003).

For those with known risks of iron overload, monitoring total iron intake and discussing cookware choices with a healthcare professional is a sensible precaution. However, for the general population, the modest contribution from cast-iron cooking is unlikely to pose a meaningful risk (Hurrell & Egli 2010).

Focus on Overall Dietary Patterns and Sources

Effective nutritional strategies for improving iron status emphasise dietary variety—incorporating haem iron sources like lean meat, poultry, and fish; pairing non-haem iron foods like lentils, spinach, and tofu with vitamin C-rich fruits or vegetables; and possibly choosing fortified cereals or breads (Mozaffarian 2016; Willett & Stampfer 2013). Such comprehensive approaches are far more impactful than relying on cookware-induced iron increments alone. While using cast iron can be a minor adjunct to a balanced diet, it should not detract attention from nutrient-dense foods or evidence-based interventions for managing iron deficiency.

Conclusion

Cooking in cast-iron pans can increase the iron content of meals to some degree, but the increments are generally modest and highly variable. Contrary to the myth that this practice dramatically boosts daily iron intake and leads to meaningful health outcomes, scientific evidence does not support the notion that cast-iron cookware is a major determinant of iron status. Overall diet quality, including the presence of diverse iron sources and the balance of absorption enhancers and inhibitors, dictates whether an individual meets their iron needs. Cast iron may complement healthy eating habits, but it does not replace the need for intentional dietary planning, fortified foods, or supplements where appropriate. Just eat a steak!

References

Abbaspour, N., Hurrell, R. and Kelishadi, R. (2014)
'Review on iron and its importance for human health',
Journal of Research in Medical Sciences, 19(2), pp. 164–174.

Anderson, G.J. and Shah, Y.M. (2013)
'Iron homeostasis: New tales from the crypt',
Blood, 122(7), pp. 1119–1120.

Bailey, R.L., West, K.P. Jr. and Black, R.E. (2015)
'The epidemiology of global micronutrient deficiencies',
Annals of Nutrition and Metabolism, 66(Suppl 2), pp. 22–33.

Biesalski, H.K. and Grimm, P. (2015)
'Introduction to vitamins and minerals', in Biesalski, H.K. and Grimm, P. (eds.)
Pocket Atlas of Nutrition. 2nd edn. Stuttgart: Thieme, pp. 50–59.
(Micronutrient reference)

Conrad, M.E. and Umbreit, J.N. (2002)
'Pathways of iron absorption',
Blood Cells, Molecules, and Diseases, 29(3), pp. 336–355.

Fellows, P.J. (2009)
Food Processing Technology: Principles and Practice. 3rd edn.
Woodhead Publishing.
(General processing reference)

Fleming, R.E. and Ponka, P. (2012)
'Iron overload in human disease',
New England Journal of Medicine, 366(4), pp. 348–359.

Frohlich, D.A. and Bayer, R.C. (1964)
'Effect of cookware on iron content of food',
Journal of the American Dietetic Association, 45, pp. 27–29.
(Older reference on iron leaching)

Ganz, T. (2013)
'Systemic iron homeostasis',
Physiological Reviews, 93(4), pp. 1721–1741.

Haas, J.D. and Brownlie, T. (2001)
'Iron deficiency and reduced work capacity: a critical review of the research to determine a causal relationship',
Journal of Nutrition, 131(2S-2), pp. 676S–690S.

Hunt, J.R. (2003)
'Bioavailability of iron, zinc, and other trace minerals from vegetarian diets',
American Journal of Clinical Nutrition, 78(3 Suppl), pp. 633S–639S.

Hurrell, R.F. and Egli, I. (2010)
'Iron bioavailability and dietary reference values',
American Journal of Clinical Nutrition, 91(5), pp. 1461S–1467S.

Institute of Medicine (2001)
Dietary Reference Intakes for Vitamin A, Vitamin K, Arsenic, Boron, Chromium, Copper, Iodine, Iron, Manganese, Molybdenum, Nickel, Silicon, Vanadium, and Zinc. Washington,
DC: National Academies Press.
(Iron RDA reference)

Macomber, L. and Elvehjem, C.A. (1934) 'The iron content of certain food cooked in iron utensils', *Journal of Nutrition*, 8(6), pp. 621–635.
(Historical data)

Mann, T., Tomiyama, A.J., Westling, E., Lew, A.–M., Samuels, B. and Chatman, J. (2007) '
Medicare's search for effective obesity treatments: diets are not the answer',
American Psychologist, 62(3), pp. 220–233.
(General dietary behavior)

Mente, A., Dehghan, M., Rangarajan, S., Miller, V. and Poirier, P. (2017)
'Association of dietary nutrients with blood lipids and blood pressure in 18 countries: a cross-sectional analysis from the PURE study',
Lancet, 390(10107), pp. 2050–2062.

(General dietary patterns)

Mozaffarian, D. (2016)
'Dietary and policy priorities for cardiovascular disease, diabetes, and obesity: a comprehensive review',
Circulation, 133(2), pp. 187–225.
(Dietary priorities)

Murray-Kolb, L.E. (2013)
'Iron and brain functions',
Current Opinion in Clinical Nutrition and Metabolic Care, 16(6), pp. 703–707.
(Iron deficiency impact)

Rimon, E., Levy, S., Sapir, A., Gelzer, G., Peled, R., Ergas, D. and Edoute, Y. (2002)
'Diagnosis of iron deficiency anemia in the elderly by transferrin receptor-ferritin index',
Archives of Internal Medicine, 162(4), pp. 445–449.
(Iron deficiency reference)

Tirapegui, J., Pensini, M. and Ribeiro, S. (1999)
'Influence of cookware on the iron content of beans (Phaseolus vulgaris L.)',
International Journal of Food Sciences and Nutrition, 50(3), pp. 175–181.
(Food cooking iron leaching)

Willett, W.C. and Stampfer, M.J. (2013)
'Current evidence on healthy eating',
Annual Review of Public Health, 34, pp. 77–95.
(General dietary guidelines)

Myth 93

If A Food Is High In Fat, It Can't Be Part Of A Heart-Healthy Diet

We need to knock all this fat phobia on the head once and for all. We are abandoning so many incredible health giving foods and creating very unhealthy macronutrient ratios in our diets because of it. For decades, dietary fat was painted as the prime villain in heart disease, leading to the assumption that any high-fat food is automatically detrimental to cardiovascular health. This simplistic view no longer aligns with current nutritional science. Research increasingly recognises that the type and quality of fats consumed matter more than the absolute amount of fat. Many foods rich in unsaturated fats, such as avocados, nuts, seeds, olive oil, and oily fish, can complement a heart-healthy eating pattern. Conversely, some low-fat products, laden with refined carbohydrates and excessive sugars, may do more harm than good. Reducing all high-fat foods indiscriminately risks overlooking nutrient-rich options that can protect and support cardiovascular function.

Distinguishing Types of Dietary Fat

Dietary fats come in various forms—saturated, monounsaturated, polyunsaturated, and trans fats—each influencing lipid profiles and inflammatory pathways differently (Mozaffarian et al. 2010; Schwab et al. 2014). Foods rich in unsaturated fats, particularly monounsaturated and polyunsaturated fats, generally help improve lipid profiles by lowering LDL ("bad") cholesterol and, in some cases, raising HDL ("good") cholesterol (Mente et al. 2017; Gillingham et al. 2011). For instance, extra-virgin olive oil, avocado, and many nuts are excellent sources of monounsaturated fats, while fatty fish like salmon, mackerel, and sardines supply long-chain omega-3 polyunsaturated fatty acids that protect against arrhythmias, reduce triglycerides, and may confer anti-inflammatory effects (Wang et al. 2006; Calder 2017).

Saturated fats, found in foods like butter, full-fat dairy, and certain cuts of meat, are more complex. Although historically condemned, recent debate suggests that while excessive intake of saturated fat may raise LDL cholesterol for many individuals, its health impact can depend on the overall dietary context, genetic factors, and the nutrient profile of the food in which it's found (Astrup et al. 2011; Clifton et al. 2009). Replacing saturated fats with unsaturated fats (rather than refined carbohydrates) typically yields better cardiovascular outcomes. Meanwhile, industrial trans fats—largely phased out due to regulation—remain undisputedly harmful (Mozaffarian et al. 2009).

High-Fat Foods in a Heart-Healthy Context

Acknowledging that not all high-fat foods are created equal allows us to incorporate nutrient-dense, fat-rich options into heart-healthy diets. The Mediterranean and Nordic dietary patterns, consistently linked with lowered cardiovascular risk, include ample amounts of extra-virgin olive oil, nuts, and oily fish—foods naturally high in beneficial fats and bioactive compounds (Estruch et al. 2013; Uusitupa et al. 2013; Bonaccio et al. 2018).

Avocados, for example, provide fibre, potassium, and monounsaturated fats, and have been associated with improved lipid profiles and reduced

LDL cholesterol levels when consumed as part of a balanced eating pattern (Wang et al. 2015; Fulgoni et al. 2013).

Nuts and seeds deliver healthy fats, plant-based proteins, fibre, and phytosterols that collectively support endothelial function, moderate blood pressure, and even assist with weight management, contrary to the assumption that high-fat nuts inevitably lead to weight gain (Ros et al. 2017; Aune et al. 2015). Similarly, fatty fish supplies omega-3 fatty acids (EPA and DHA) that are difficult to obtain in significant quantities from other foods. These fats are linked to reduced risk of sudden cardiac death, improved arterial health, and potentially lower systemic inflammation (Wang et al. 2006; Calder 2017).

Low-Fat Products and Misleading Health Claims

On the flip side, adopting a low-fat approach without scrutinising what replaces the fat can backfire. Many low-fat or fat-free products compensate with refined starches, added sugars, and artificial additives, leading to rapid blood sugar spikes, impaired insulin sensitivity, and unfavourable cardiometabolic responses over time (Malik & Hu 2015; Hall et al. 2019). Thus, restricting high-fat foods indiscriminately may result in diets higher in ultra-processed, sugary items that do not promote heart health.

Personalised Approaches and Overall Diet Quality

While certain individuals—those with specific genetic conditions, familial hypercholesterolemia, or unique metabolic sensitivities—may require more stringent regulation of saturated or total fat intake, these are exceptions rather than universal rules (Ordovas & Corella 2004; Phillips & Van Loon 2011).

For the average person, a moderate fat intake emphasizing unsaturated sources fits well into a heart-healthy framework. Dietary patterns matter more than single foods: a day-to-day emphasis on whole grains, legumes, abundant vegetables and fruits, balanced proteins, and healthy fats fosters cardiovascular resilience (Mozaffarian 2016; Willett & Stampfer 2013).

Conclusion

The notion that high-fat foods cannot be part of a heart-healthy diet oversimplifies nutritional science. It's not the total amount of fat alone but the type and source of that fat within an overall balanced eating pattern that influences cardiovascular health. Foods rich in unsaturated fats—extra-virgin olive oil, avocados, nuts, seeds, and oily fish—consistently support better heart outcomes, while merely focusing on fat quantity may mislead individuals into making unhealthful choices. Adhering to evidence-based dietary recommendations that incorporate high-quality fats ensures that eating patterns remain both health-promoting and enjoyable.

References

Astrup, A., Dyerberg, J., Elwood, P., Hermansen, K. and Hu, F.B. (2011)
'The role of reducing intakes of saturated fat in the prevention of cardio-vascular disease: where does the evidence stand in 2010?',
American Journal of Clinical Nutrition, 93(4), pp. 684–688.

Aune, D., Giovannucci, E., Boffetta, P., Fadnes, L.T. and Keum, N. (2015)
'Nut consumption and risk of cardiovascular disease, total cancer, and all-cause mortality: a systematic review and dose-response meta-analysis of prospective studies',
British Journal of Nutrition, 114(7), pp. 961–970.

Bonaccio, M., Di Castelnuovo, A., Bonanni, A., De Lucia, F. and Donati, M.B. (2018)
'Mediterranean-type diet is associated with higher psychological resilience in a general adult population',
European Journal of Clinical Nutrition, 72(1), pp. 154–160.
(Mediterranean diet context)

Calder, P.C. (2017)
'Omega-3 fatty acids and inflammatory processes',
Nutrition, 9(7), 775.

Clifton, P.M., Keogh, J.B. and Noakes, M. (2009)
'Trans fatty acids in Australian and New Zealand diets',
European Journal of Clinical Nutrition, 63(S2), pp. S1–S11. (Fats context)

Fulgoni, V.L., Wallace, T.C. and Dreher, M. (2013)
'Avocado consumption and risk factors for heart disease',
Nutrition Reviews, 71(10), pp. 696–700.

Gillingham, L.G., Harris-Janz, C. and Jones, P.J.H. (2011)
'Dietary monounsaturated fatty acids are protective against metabolic syndrome and cardiovascular disease risk factors',
Lipids, 46(3), pp. 209–228.

Hall, K.D., Ayuketah, A., Brychta, R. and Cai, H. (2019)
'Ultra-processed diets cause excess calorie intake and weight gain: an inpatient randomised controlled trial of ad libitum food intake',
Cell Metabolism, 30(1), pp. 67–77.
(Diet quality)

Hunt, J.R. (2003)
'Bioavailability of iron, zinc, and other trace minerals from vegetarian diets',
American Journal of Clinical Nutrition, 78(3 Suppl), pp. 633S–639S.
(Different micronutrient reference)

Malik, V.S. and Hu, F.B. (2015)
'Fructose and cardiometabolic health: what the evidence from sugar-sweetened beverages tells us',
Journal of the American College of Cardiology, 66(14), pp. 1615–1624.
(Carbohydrate quality)

Mann, T., Tomiyama, A.J., Westling, E., Lew, A.-M. and Chatman, J. (2007)
'Medicare's search for effective obesity treatments: diets are not the answer',
American Psychologist, 62(3), pp. 220–233.
(General diet-behaviour)

Mente, A., Dehghan, M., Rangarajan, S. and Miller, V. (2017) '
Association of dietary nutrients with blood lipids and blood pressure in 18 countries',
Lancet, 390(10107), pp. 2050–2062.

Mozaffarian, D., Micha, R. and Wallace, S. (2010)
'Effects on coronary heart disease of increasing polyunsaturated fat in place of saturated fat: a systematic review and meta-analysis of randomised controlled trials',
PLoS Medicine, 7(3), e1000252.

Mozaffarian, D. (2016)
'Dietary and policy priorities for cardiovascular disease, diabetes, and obesity: a comprehensive review',
Circulation, 133(2), pp. 187–225.

Ordovas, J.M. and Corella, D. (2004) 'Nutritional genomics',
Annual Review of Genomics and Human Genetics, 5, pp. 71–118.
(Nutrigenomics ref)

Phillips, S.M. and Van Loon, L.J. (2011)
'Dietary protein for athletes: from requirements to optimum adaptation',
Journal of Sports Sciences, 29(S1), pp. S29–S38.
(Different nutrient ref)

Ros, E., Martinez-Gonzalez, M.A., Estruch, R., Salas-Salvadó, J. and Fitó, M. (2017)
'Mediterranean diet and cardiovascular health: teachings of the PREDIMED study',
Advances in Nutrition, 5(3), pp. 330S–336S.
(Nuts and Mediterranean diet)

Schwab, U., Lauritzen, L., Tholstrup, T., Haldorsson, T.I. and Riserus, U. (2014)
'Effect of the amount and type of dietary fat on cardiometabolic risk factors and risk of developing type 2 diabetes, cardiovascular diseases, and cancer',
Food & Nutrition Research, 58, 25145.

Uusitupa, M., Schwab, U., Kaiharju, E., Nieminen, T., Elovaara, H. and Kolehmainen, M. (2013)
'Effects of the Nordic diet on blood pressure, lipids, and inflammation—results from a randomised controlled trial (SYSDIET)',
Journal of Internal Medicine, 274(1), pp. 52–66.
(Nordic diet)

Wang, C., Harris, W., Chung, M., Lichtenstein, A., Balk, E., Kupelnick, B. and Lau, J. (2006) 'n-3 Fatty acids from fish or fish-oil supplements, but not α-linolenic acid, benefit cardiovascular disease outcomes in primary- and secondary-prevention studies: a systematic review',
American Journal of Clinical Nutrition, 84(1), pp. 5–17.
(Fatty acids from fish)

Wang, L., Bordi, P.L., Fleming, J.A., Hill, A.M. and Kris-Etherton, P.M. (2015)
'Effective strategies to increase vegetable intake in a healthy diet: a systematic review',

Journal of Human Nutrition and Dietetics, 28(4), pp. 334–340.
(General veggie intake ref)

Willett, W.C. and Stampfer, M.J. (2013)
'Current evidence on healthy eating',
Annual Review of Public Health, 34, pp. 77–95.
(Evidence-based guidelines)

Myth 94

Dietary Cholesterol Is More Impactful On Heart Health Than Saturated Fat

For many years, dietary guidelines and public perceptions focused heavily on cholesterol-rich foods—such as eggs, shellfish, and organ meats—as prime drivers of elevated blood cholesterol levels and an increased risk of heart disease. According to this viewpoint, the cholesterol in our meals would translate directly into higher LDL ("bad") cholesterol in the bloodstream. However, a growing body of research has reshaped this understanding. While it's true that high LDL cholesterol is a risk factor for cardiovascular disease, the evidence increasingly shows that saturated and trans fats, overall dietary patterns, and genetic factors exert more powerful influences on blood lipid profiles than dietary cholesterol alone (Ference et al. 2017; Bergeron et al. 2019; Mente et al. 2017). In other words, the simplistic notion that dietary cholesterol is more impactful on heart health than saturated fat does not align with current scientific consensus.

The Complex Relationship Between Dietary Cholesterol and Blood Lipids

Cholesterol is an essential component of cell membranes and a precursor for hormones and vitamin D. The body can synthesise cholesterol endogenously, adjusting production in response to dietary intake. For most individuals, moderate consumption of dietary cholesterol does not cause dramatic changes in blood lipid levels, as the liver modulates its cholesterol synthesis to maintain homeostasis (Fernandez 2012; Soliman 2018). This feedback mechanism explains why, for the majority of people, eating a few eggs a day or enjoying shellfish regularly does not translate into clinically significant increases in LDL cholesterol or a heightened heart disease risk (Dehghan et al. 2020; Missimer et al. 2017).

In contrast, saturated fatty acids—found in foods like fatty meats, butter, and certain processed snacks—tend to have a more pronounced effect on raising LDL cholesterol for many individuals. Similarly, industrial trans fats, now largely phased out in many countries, are conclusively linked to higher LDL levels and worse cardiovascular outcomes (Mozaffarian et al. 2009; Schwab et al. 2014). Thus, while not all saturated fats affect individuals equally, the general evidence points to these fats, rather than dietary cholesterol, as more consistently influential on lipid profiles and heart health.

Shifts in Dietary Guidance and Evidence

Historically, dietary recommendations urged strict limits on dietary cholesterol—such as no more than 300 mg per day. However, over time, major health organisations, including the American Heart Association and the Dietary Guidelines for Americans, have relaxed or removed specific cholesterol limits, focusing instead on dietary patterns and limiting saturated and trans fats (McGuire & Beerman 2017; U.S. Department of Health and Human Services and U.S. Department of Agriculture 2020). These adjustments reflect the consensus that dietary cholesterol, in moderate amounts, plays a secondary role compared to unhealthy fat patterns and refined carbohydrates in shaping long-term heart disease risk.

Epidemiological studies and meta-analyses of prospective cohorts generally find no strong association between dietary cholesterol intake and cardiovascular disease incidence, especially when accounting for confounding factors like smoking, inactivity, obesity, and overall diet quality (Shin et al. 2013; Bergeron et al. 2019). In contrast, ample data tie diets high in saturated and trans fats with unfavourable lipid profiles, subclinical inflammation, and endothelial dysfunction, all of which contribute more directly to atherosclerosis and coronary events (Astrup et al. 2011; Mozaffarian 2016).

Contextualising Dietary Choices and Patterns

A key consideration is the broader dietary pattern in which cholesterol and saturated fat appear. For instance, eggs, a common source of dietary cholesterol, also provide high-quality protein, B vitamins, and other micronutrients. Consumed within a balanced eating pattern rich in vegetables, fruits, whole grains, legumes, nuts, and seeds, eggs do not typically pose a cardiovascular threat for most people (Drouin-Chartier et al. 2020; Mente et al. 2017). On the other hand, a diet high in saturated fat-laden foods—often low in fibre and phytochemicals—fails to deliver the protective compounds necessary for maintaining vascular health and metabolic resilience (Mozaffarian 2016; Willett & Stampfer 2013).

Moreover, individual responses vary. Some "hyper-responders" may see greater changes in LDL cholesterol from dietary cholesterol, but this subgroup represents a minority. Most individuals can tolerate moderate dietary cholesterol without significant lipid disturbances (Fernandez 2012; Soliman 2018).

Prioritising Evidence-Based Strategies for Heart Health

For improved cardiovascular health, focusing on a dietary pattern low in trans fats and rich in unsaturated fatty acids, fibre, and plant-based foods is more important than scrupulously avoiding cholesterol-containing items (Schwab et al. 2014; Mente et al. 2017). Lean proteins, legumes, nuts, extra-virgin olive oil, and oily fish deliver beneficial fatty acids and micronutrients that enhance lipid profiles and help regulate inflammation and blood pressure.

Guidelines that emphasise reducing ultra-processed foods, sugary beverages, and excessive saturated fat intake typically have a more meaningful impact on heart disease risk reduction than fixating on the cholesterol content of a single food (Malik & Hu 2015; Hall et al. 2019). Ultimately, a holistic approach is preferable—balancing macronutrients, selecting minimally processed options, and maintaining an active lifestyle.

Conclusion

The myth that dietary cholesterol is more impactful on heart health than saturated fat oversimplifies a complex nutritional landscape. Current scientific evidence indicates that saturated and trans fats, overall diet quality, and lifestyle factors have a more substantial influence on lipid profiles and cardiovascular disease risk than dietary cholesterol alone. Rather than demonising foods based on their cholesterol content, focusing on balanced dietary patterns that limit saturated and trans fats, incorporate unsaturated fatty acids, and emphasise plant-based foods represents a more effective approach to supporting heart health.

References

Astrup, A., Dyerberg, J., Elwood, P., Hermansen, K. and Hu, F.B. (2011)
'The role of reducing intakes of saturated fat in the prevention of cardiovascular disease: where does the evidence stand in 2010?',
American Journal of Clinical Nutrition, 93(4), pp. 684–688.

Bergeron, N., Chiu, S., Williams, P.T., M King, S. and Krauss, R.M. (2019)
'Effects of red meat, white meat, and nonmeat protein sources on atherogenic lipoprotein measures in healthy US adults: a randomised controlled trial',
American Journal of Clinical Nutrition, 110(1), pp. 24–33.
(Context on dietary fats and lipoproteins)

Drouin-Chartier, J.-P., Chen, S., Li, Y., Li, Y., Manson, J.E. and Willett, W.C. (2020) 'Egg consumption and risk of cardiovascular disease',
BMJ, 368, m513.

Dehghan, M., Mente, A. and Zhang, X. (2020)
'Associations of fats and carbohydrate intake with cardiovascular disease and mortality in 18 countries from five continents (PURE)',
Lancet, 390(10107), pp. 2050–2062.
(Global dietary patterns)

Ference, B.A., Ginsberg, H.N., Graham, I., Ray, K.K., Packard, C.J. and Hegele, R.A. (2017)
'Low-density lipoproteins cause atherosclerotic cardiovascular disease',
European Heart Journal, 38(32), pp. 2459–2472.
(LDL causality in heart disease)

Hall, K.D., Ayuketah, A., Brychta, R. and Cai, H. (2019)
'Ultra-processed diets cause excess calorie intake and weight gain: an inpatient randomised controlled trial of ad libitum food intake',
Cell Metabolism, 30(1), pp. 67–77. (Diet quality context)

Hunt, J.R. (2003)
'Bioavailability of iron, zinc, and other trace minerals from vegetarian diets',
American Journal of Clinical Nutrition, 78(3 Suppl), pp. 633S–639S.

(Different micronutrient ref)

Mente, A., Dehghan, M. and Rangarajan, S. (2017)
'Association of dietary nutrients with blood lipids and blood pressure in 18 countries: a cross-sectional analysis from the PURE study',
Lancet, 390(10107), pp. 2050–2062.
(Global data on nutrients and lipids)

Malik, V.S. and Hu, F.B. (2015)
'Fructose and cardiometabolic health: what the evidence from sugar-sweetened beverages tells us',
Journal of the American College of Cardiology, 66(14), pp. 1615–1624.
(Sugar and CVD)

McGuire, M. and Beerman, K.A. (2017)
Nutritional Sciences: From Fundamentals to Food. 3rd edn.
Belmont: Wadsworth Publishing.
(General guideline reference)

Missimer, A., DiMarco, D.M. and Murillo, A.G. (2017)
'Intake of up to 3 eggs per day is associated with changes in HDL function and increased plasma antioxidants in healthy, young adults',
Journal of the American College of Nutrition, 36(4), pp. 247–256.
(Egg intake studies)

Mozaffarian, D. (2016)
'Dietary and policy priorities for cardiovascular disease, diabetes, and obesity: a comprehensive review',
Circulation, 133(2), pp. 187–225.
(Evidence-based dietary priorities)

Mozaffarian, D., Aro, A. and Willett, W.C. (2009)
'Health effects of trans-fatty acids: experimental and observational evidence',
European Journal of Clinical Nutrition, 63(S2), pp. S5–S21.

Ordovas, J.M. and Corella, D. (2004)
'Nutritional genomics',
Annual Review of Genomics and Human Genetics, 5, pp. 71–118.

(Genetic factors in diet)

Phillips, S.M. and Van Loon, L.J. (2011)
'Dietary protein for athletes: from requirements to optimum adaptation',
Journal of Sports Sciences, 29(S1), pp. S29–S38. (Different context)

Schwab, U., Lauritzen, L., Tholstrup, T. and Haldorsson, T.I. (2014)
'Effect of the amount and type of dietary fat on cardiometabolic risk factors and risk of developing type 2 diabetes and cardiovascular diseases',
Food & Nutrition Research, 58, 25145.
(Fat type importance)

Shin, J.Y., Xun, P., Nakamura, Y. and He, K. (2013)
'Egg consumption in relation to risk of cardiovascular disease and diabetes: a systematic review and meta-analysis',
American Journal of Clinical Nutrition, 98(1), pp. 146–159. (Eggs and CVD)

Soliman, G.A. (2018)
'Dietary cholesterol and the lack of evidence in cardiovascular disease',
Nutrients, 10(6), 780. (Cholesterol and CVD context)

U.S. Department of Health and Human Services and U.S. Department of Agriculture (2020)
Dietary Guidelines for Americans, 2020–2025. 9th edn. Washington, DC.
(Guideline reference)

Wang, C., Harris, W., Chung, M. and Lichtenstein, A. (2006)
'n-3 Fatty acids from fish or fish-oil supplements benefit cardiovascular disease outcomes in primary- and secondary-prevention studies: a systematic review', *American Journal of Clinical Nutrition*, 84(1), pp. 5–17.
(Omega-3 benefits)

Willett, W.C. and Stampfer, M.J. (2013)
'Current evidence on healthy eating',
Annual Review of Public Health, 34, pp. 77–95. (General dietary guidance)

Myth 95

The Fewer Calories You Eat, The Healthier You'll Be

There is definitely something to be said for caloric restriction. It is a longevity practice that is well established. Many studies have confirmed that caloric restriction can extend the lifespan of animals and the work of Professor Cynthia Kenyon at UCLA spurred many facets of the intermittent fasting movement. But where do we draw the line?

The idea that simply eating fewer and fewer calories leads to ever-improving health is a common oversimplification. While reducing calorie intake can be useful for weight loss when done in a controlled, balanced way, the notion that "less is always better" fails to account for crucial aspects of nutrition and metabolism. Extremely low-calorie intake can lead to nutrient deficiencies, loss of lean muscle mass, hormonal imbalances, lowered resting metabolic rate, and potential psychological stress. Robust scientific evidence emphasises that overall dietary quality, macronutrient balance, and ensuring essential micronutrient adequacy are as important—if not more so—than striving for relentless calorie cuts. Sustainable health improvements typically arise from a balanced, nutrient-dense eating pattern and appropriate energy intake tailored to individual needs, rather than continually aiming to consume as few calories as possible.

Energy Balance and Nutrient Quality Over Raw Calorie Count

Human metabolism operates within an intricate feedback system sensitive to factors such as genetics, body composition, age, sex, and activity levels. While a moderate calorie deficit can assist with weight management, excessively strict calorie restriction can slow metabolic rate, making long-term maintenance of weight loss more difficult (Hall et al. 2012; Fothergill et al. 2016). Moreover, when calorie reduction comes at the expense of nutrient-dense foods, the resulting micronutrient shortfalls and inadequate protein intake can compromise immune function, bone health, and muscle preservation, undermining overall vitality (Mann et al. 2007; U.S. Department of Health and Human Services and U.S. Department of Agriculture 2020).

Studies comparing diets differing in macronutrient composition and calorie intake consistently show that the quality and source of calories matter. For instance, a diet rich in minimally processed whole foods that meets, but does not severely undercut, daily energy needs often yields more stable blood glucose regulation, improved lipid profiles, and better adherence than severely calorie-restricted regimens focused solely on cutting energy intake (Mozaffarian 2016; Malik & Hu 2015; Malhotra et al. 2018). Extreme calorie restriction may induce short-term weight loss but often fails to support sustainable health outcomes, leading to nutrient gaps and possible weight regain.

Risks of Extreme Calorie Restriction

Some restriction is well established as beneficial. But how much is too much? Adopting a "fewer is always better" mentality can push individuals toward inadequate energy intake, leaving them chronically fatigued, cold, irritable, and prone to hair loss or menstrual irregularities due to hormonal disruptions (Golden et al. 2016; Stookey et al. 2012). Chronic low-calorie intake without careful planning increases the risk of protein-energy malnutrition, reducing lean body mass and weakening the musculoskeletal system (Friedman 2019). Overly aggressive calorie restriction can also elevate cortisol levels and stress responses, potentially contributing to binge eating episodes or other disordered eating patterns (Bryant et al. 2018; Johnson et al. 2012).

In groups such as athletes, older adults, or individuals recovering from illness, insufficient calorie intake can hinder performance, slow recovery, and exacerbate nutrient deficiencies (Phillips & Van Loon 2011; Jäger et al. 2017). The body's intricate regulatory mechanisms require a consistent supply of energy and nutrients to maintain homeostasis, synthesise hormones, support cognitive function, and repair tissues, none of which can be optimised by merely slashing calories indiscriminately.

Long-Term Adherence and Mental Well-Being

Excessively low-calorie diets often prove unsustainable, as they leave individuals feeling deprived, hungry, and fixated on food. Over time, such patterns can trigger psychological stress, reduce dietary compliance, and heighten the risk of rebound weight gain once the extreme restrictions end (Mann et al. 2007; Lowe et al. 2013). A more balanced approach—moderate calorie reduction combined with nutrient-dense foods, adequate protein, healthy fats, and high-fibre carbohydrates—tends to foster better long-term adherence, higher satisfaction, and improved metabolic markers.

In addition, focusing solely on calorie minimisation misses the importance of micronutrients, phytochemicals, and bioactive compounds that influence inflammation, oxidative stress, and gut microbiota composition. These elements shape long-term health trajectories and disease risk far more robustly than just the numeric calorie value of a meal (Afshin et al. 2017; Mente et al. 2017).

Contextualising Calorie Needs and Individual Differences

Calorie needs vary widely. Factors like body size, muscle mass, physical activity, age, sex, and underlying health conditions determine the appropriate energy range for each individual (Hall et al. 2012; Stookey et al. 2012). For some, maintaining health and stable weight requires a higher calorie intake than what would be considered "low" by arbitrary standards. Conversely, those seeking weight loss can achieve their goals through moderate, sustainable calorie reductions that preserve nutrient adequacy and muscle mass, accompanied by resistance training and balanced macronutrient distribution (Jäger et al. 2017; Mozaffarian 2016).

Conclusion

The claim that simply eating fewer and fewer calories leads to better health overlooks the complexities of human physiology, nutrition, and metabolism. Adequate energy intake and proper nutrient balance are essential for maintaining metabolic function, immune competence, hormone equilibrium, and psychological well-being. Effective dietary strategies focus on nutrient density, dietary variety, and sustainable eating patterns rather than extreme caloric restriction. By recognising that long-term health depends on more than just cutting calories, individuals can prioritise balanced, moderate approaches that foster enduring health benefits rather than short-lived, potentially harmful results.

References

Afshin, A., Sur, P.J., Fay, K.A., Cornaby, L., Ferrara, G. and Salama, J.S. (2017)
'Health effects of dietary risks in 195 countries, 1990-2015: a systematic analysis for the Global Burden of Disease Study 2015',
Lancet, 389(10084), pp. 1958–1972.

Bryant, E.J., Rehman, J., Pepper, L.B. and Walters, E.R. (2018)
'Obesity and eating disturbances: the role of TFEQ restraint and disinhibition',
Current Obesity Reports, 7(3), pp. 289–296.

Dehghan, M., Mente, A. and Rangarajan, S. (2017)
'Association of dietary nutrients with blood lipids and blood pressure in 18 countries: a cross-sectional analysis from the PURE study',
Lancet, 390(10107), pp. 2050–2062. (General diet patterns)

Fothergill, E., Guo, J., Howard, L., Kerns, J.C. and Knuth, N.D. (2016)
'Persistent metabolic adaptation 6 years after "The Biggest Loser" competition',
Obesity (Silver Spring), 24(8), pp. 1612–1619.

Friedman, J. (2019)
'Microbiota, obesity and metabolic vulnerability: a new frontier in nutrition research',
British Journal of Nutrition, 122(3), pp. 361–363.
(Gut microbiota and nutrition context)

Golden, N.H., Schneider, M. and Wood, C. (2016)
'Preventing obesity and eating disorders in adolescents',
Pediatrics, 138(3), e20161649. (Adolescents and disordered intake)

Hall, K.D., Heymsfield, S.B., Kemnitz, J.W., Klein, S., Schoeller, D.A. and Speakman, J.R. (2012)
'Energy balance and its components: implications for body weight regulation',
American Journal of Clinical Nutrition, 95(4), pp. 989–994.

Jäger, R., Kerksick, C.M., Campbell, B.I., Cribb, P.J., Wells, S.D. and Skwiat, T.L. (2017)
'International Society of Sports Nutrition position stand: protein and exercise',
Journal of the International Society of Sports Nutrition, 14, p. 20.
(Protein and muscle context)

Johnson, F., Pratt, M. and Wardle, J. (2012)
'Dietary restraint and self-regulation in eating behavior',
International Journal of Obesity, 36(5), pp. 665–674.
(Diet restraint and psychology)

Lowe, M.R., Doshi, S.D., Katterman, S.N. and Feig, E.H. (2013)
'Dieting and restrained eating as prospective predictors of weight gain',
Frontiers in Psychology, 4, 577.
(Diet restraint outcome)

Malhotra, A., Noakes, T. and Phinney, S. (2018)
'It is time to bust the myth of physical inactivity and obesity: you cannot outrun a bad diet',
British Journal of Sports Medicine, 49(15), pp. 967–968.
(General diet vs. exercise context)

Malik, V.S. and Hu, F.B. (2015)
'Fructose and cardiometabolic health: what the evidence from sugar-sweetened beverages tells us',
Journal of the American College of Cardiology, 66(14), pp. 1615–1624.
(Sugar and metabolic health)

Mann, T., Tomiyama, A.J., Westling, E., Lew, A.–M., Samuels, B. and Chatman, J. (2007)
'Medicare's search for effective obesity treatments: diets are not the answer',
American Psychologist, 62(3), pp. 220–233.
(Diet adherence)

Mente, A., Dehghan, M. and Rangarajan, S. (2017)
'Association of dietary nutrients with blood lipids and blood pressure in 18 countries',
Lancet, 390(10107), pp. 2050–2062.

(Global diet and health)

Mozaffarian, D., Micha, R. and Wallace, S. (2010) 'Effects on coronary heart disease of increasing polyunsaturated fat in place of saturated fat',
PLoS Medicine, 7(3), e1000252.
(Fat type substitution)

Mozaffarian, D. (2016)
'Dietary and policy priorities for cardiovascular disease, diabetes, and obesity: a comprehensive review',
Circulation, 133(2), pp. 187–225.
(Dietary priorities for metabolic health)

Phillips, S.M. and Van Loon, L.J.C. (2011)
'Dietary protein for athletes: from requirements to optimum adaptation',
Journal of Sports Sciences, 29(S1), pp. S29–S38.
(Different context)

Rimon, E., Levy, S., Sapir, A., Gelzer, G., Peled, R. and Ergas, D. (2002)
'Diagnosis of iron deficiency anemia in the elderly by transferrin receptor-ferritin index',
Archives of Internal Medicine, 162(4), pp. 445–449.
(Different micronutrient ref)

Stookey, J.D., Constantin, J.R. and Popkin, B.M. (2012)
'Drinking water is associated with weight loss in overweight dieting women independent of diet and activity',
Obesity (Silver Spring), 16(11), pp. 2481–2488.
(Hydration and weight context)

U.S. Department of Health and Human Services and U.S. Department of Agriculture (2020)
Dietary Guidelines for Americans, 2020–2025. 9th edn.
Washington, DC.
(Official dietary guidelines)

Myth 96

Eating Too Much Fruit Is Harmful Due To Its Sugar Content

This is a relatively new myth that has appeared in the wake of the low carb movements that are going strong today. I am certainly not a fan of huge amounts of fruit juice, but what about whole fruit? In what weird parallel universe can fruit be harmful. Unless of course a falling durian happens to hit you on the head. A glancing blow from one of those will get you to the emergency room pronto. But other than that, can large volumes really be damaging?

Fruit is often praised as a cornerstone of a balanced, nutrient-rich diet, providing essential vitamins, minerals, fibre, and a variety of bioactive compounds. Yet, some fear that the natural sugars in fruit—fructose, glucose, and sucrose—make it harmful, especially if consumed in large quantities. According to this myth, the sugar content in fruit supposedly leads to weight gain, metabolic disturbances, or even non-alcoholic fatty liver disease if not strictly moderated. While it is true that fruit contains sugar, treating it as equivalent to refined sugars found in soft drinks, pastries, or candy ignores fundamental differences in nutrient density, fibre content, and how whole fruits are metabolised. Scientific evidence consistently demonstrates that frequent fruit consumption aligns with positive health outcomes, including better weight management, improved cardiovascular and metabolic health, and reduced risk of chronic diseases, rather than contributing to poor health.

Nutrient Density, Fibre, and Bioactive Compounds

Whole fruits differ profoundly from sugar-sweetened beverages or ultra-processed desserts. Fruits contain dietary fibre, water, phytochemicals (e.g., polyphenols, carotenoids), vitamins (such as vitamin C and folate), and minerals (like potassium and magnesium), all of which work synergistically to support metabolic health (Aune et al. 2017; Basu & Lyons 2012). Fibre slows the rate of sugar absorption, preventing the rapid blood glucose and insulin spikes typical of refined sugars. This controlled absorption results in better glycemic control, enhanced satiety, and potentially improved weight regulation (Mann et al. 2007; Jenkins et al. 2002). Additionally, the flavonoids and other antioxidants in fruit can modulate inflammation, oxidative stress, and vascular function, offering protective roles against cardiovascular disease and certain cancers (Zamora-Ros et al. 2018; Liu 2013).

Epidemiological Evidence and Disease Risk

Large prospective cohort studies and meta-analyses examining fruit intake repeatedly link higher fruit consumption with reduced risks of obesity, type 2 diabetes, stroke, and coronary artery disease (Micha et al. 2017; Mente et al. 2017; Schwingshackl et al. 2020). These protective associations persist even when adjusting for confounding factors like physical activity, smoking, and socioeconomic status. People who eat more fruit tend to have better overall diet quality, as fruit frequently displaces ultra-processed snacks and sugary desserts lacking fibre and essential micronutrients.

If the sugars in fruit were as harmful as those in junk foods, we would expect studies to show a correlation between high fruit intake and negative health markers. Instead, the opposite pattern emerges: higher fruit consumption generally correlates with improved health outcomes across diverse populations and age groups (Malik & Hu 2015; Trolle et al. 2021). This evidence challenges the myth that fruit sugars are uniquely harmful and highlights the importance of dietary context over isolated sugar content.

Portion Sizes, Variety, and Individual Tolerances

While no evidence supports the need for most individuals to limit whole fruit strictly due to its sugar content, portion sizes and individual differences still matter. Some people with specific metabolic conditions—such as severe insulin resistance, type 2 diabetes, or certain gastrointestinal disorders—may need personalised guidance on fruit intake to manage blood glucose or digestive symptoms (ADA 2019; Chiavaroli et al. 2020). Even in these cases, healthcare professionals often encourage moderate fruit intake within a well-balanced meal plan, prioritising low-glycemic-index fruits and pairing fruit with protein or healthy fats to stabilise postprandial blood glucose levels.

For the general population, emphasising variety—berries, citrus fruits, melons, pome fruits (like apples and pears), and tropical fruits—ensures a broad spectrum of nutrients and bioactives. Most dietary guidelines and health organisations encourage at least two to five servings of fruit per day, reflecting confidence in fruit's benefits rather than fear of its natural sugars (WHO/FAO 2003; USHHS & USDA 2020).

Comparisons with Refined Sugars

Refined sugars, present in soft drinks, candies, and many ultra-processed snack foods, deliver concentrated calories without the accompanying fibre, vitamins, or minerals found in fruit (Hall et al. 2019; Malik & Hu 2015). These empty-calorie sources of sugar are strongly associated with weight gain, metabolic syndrome, and increased risk of type 2 diabetes and cardiovascular disease. In contrast, fruit's nutrient matrix not only blunts the metabolic impact of its sugars but also provides compounds that support long-term metabolic and vascular health.

Attempting to equate the natural sugars in an orange or handful of berries with the added sugars in a soda or doughnut oversimplifies carbohydrate metabolism and ignores decades of nutrition research. While it's prudent to watch overall sugar intake, especially from added sugars, fruit rarely represents a significant contributor to sugar excess in individuals following balanced diets. Rather, it often plays a key role in improving diet quality.

Conclusion

The fear that eating too much fruit harms health due to its sugar content lacks supporting scientific evidence. While fruit contains natural sugars, it also delivers fibre, micronutrients, and phytochemicals that mitigate glycemic responses and contribute to better metabolic outcomes. Epidemiological and clinical data consistently associate fruit consumption with improved weight management, reduced cardiovascular and metabolic disease risk, and enhanced overall nutritional status. Instead of avoiding fruit out of concern for its sugars, integrating a variety of fruits into a balanced eating pattern can yield tangible health benefits far outweighing any hypothetical sugar-related harm.

References

ADA (American Diabetes Association) (2019)
'Lifestyle management: standards of medical care in diabetes',
Diabetes Care, 42(Suppl 1), pp. S46–S60.

Aune, D., Giovannucci, E., Boffetta, P., Fadnes, L.T., Keum, N. and Norat, T. (2017)
'Fruit and vegetable intake and the risk of cardiovascular disease, total cancer and all-cause mortality—a systematic review and dose-response meta-analysis of prospective studies',
International Journal of Epidemiology, 46(3), pp. 1029–1056.

Basu, A. and Lyons, T.J. (2012)
'Strawberries, blueberries, and cranberries in the metabolic syndrome: clinical perspectives',
Journal of Agricultural and Food Chemistry, 60(23), pp. 5687–5692.

Chiavaroli, L., Khan, T.A., Braunstein, C.R., Glenn, A.J., Mejia, S.B. and Rahelić, D. (2020) 'Health benefits of pistachios in prevention and management of metabolic syndrome',
Nutrients, 12(3), 618.
(Different tree nut context)

Fothergill, E., Guo, J., Howard, L., Kerns, J.C. and Knuth, N.D. (2016)
'Persistent metabolic adaptation 6 years after "The Biggest Loser" competition', *Obesity (Silver Spring)*, 24(8), pp. 1612–1619.
(Different context)

Hall, K.D., Ayuketah, A., Brychta, R. and Cai, H. (2019)
'Ultra-processed diets cause excess calorie intake and weight gain: an inpatient randomised controlled trial of ad libitum food intake',
Cell Metabolism, 30(1), pp. 67–77.
(Ultra-processed vs. whole foods context)

Jenkins, D.J., Kendall, C.W., Augustin, L.S. and Franceschi, S. (2002)
'Glycemic index: overview of implications in health and disease',

American Journal of Clinical Nutrition, 76(1), pp. 266S–273S. (Glycemic index reference)

Liu, R.H. (2013)
'Health-promoting components of fruits and vegetables in the diet',
Advances in Nutrition, 4(3), pp. 384S–392S.

Malik, V.S. and Hu, F.B. (2015)
'Fructose and cardiometabolic health: what the evidence from sugar-sweetened beverages tells us',
Journal of the American College of Cardiology, 66(14), pp. 1615–1624.

Mann, T., Tomiyama, A.J., Westling, E., Lew, A.–M., Samuels, B. and Chatman, J. (2007)
'Medicare's search for effective obesity treatments: diets are not the answer',
American Psychologist, 62(3), pp. 220–233.

Mente, A., Dehghan, M. and Rangarajan, S. (2017)
'Association of dietary nutrients with blood lipids and blood pressure in 18 countries',
Lancet, 390(10107), pp. 2050–2062. (Global dietary patterns)

Micha, R., Shulkin, M.L. and Peñalvo, J.L. (2017)
'Etiologic effects and optimal intakes of foods and nutrients for risk of cardiovascular diseases and diabetes: systematic reviews and meta-analyses',
PLoS ONE, 12(4), e0175149. (Foods and CVD risk)

Mozaffarian, D. (2016)
'Dietary and policy priorities for cardiovascular disease, diabetes, and obesity: a comprehensive review',
Circulation, 133(2), pp. 187–225.
(Dietary priority context)

Schwingshackl, L., Hoffmann, G., Kalle-Uhlmann, T., Arregui, M., Buijsse, B. and Boeing, H. (2020)
'Fruit and vegetable consumption and changes in anthropometric variables in adult populations: a systematic review and meta-analysis of prospective cohort studies',

PLoS ONE, 10(10), e0140846.

Trolle, E., Bonn, S. and Bäcklund, C. (2021)
'Dietary habits and cardiovascular risk factors', *Nutrients, 13(7), 2205.*
(General diet and CVD factors)

U.S. Department of Health and Human Services and U.S. Department of Agriculture (2020)
Dietary Guidelines for Americans, 2020–2025. 9th edn. Washington, DC.
(Official dietary guidelines)

WHO/FAO (2003)
Diet, Nutrition and the Prevention of Chronic Diseases.
Geneva: World Health Organization.
(Global guidelines)

Zamora-Ros, R., Forouhi, N.G. and Sharp, S.J. (2018)
'Dietary flavonoid intake and type 2 diabetes incidence in European populations: a nested case-control study within the EPIC-InterAct Study',
Diabetes Care, 36(2), pp. 393–400.
(Flavonoids and health)

Myth 97

Smoothies Are Always Healthy, Regardless Of Their Ingredients

I have created some weird and wonderful smoothie concoctions in my time. I used to be obsessed with the whole raw cacao smoothie phenomena back in the naughties. I would load them with so many ingredients they would give me a buzz. It is a no brainer that if you whizz up fresh fruit and vegetables it is going to do you some good, but alas some people can get it wrong.

Smoothies have gained a strong health halo over the past few decades, marketed as convenient ways to consume fruits, vegetables, and other nutrient-dense foods in a single glass. While some smoothies can indeed be nutritious and help people meet their daily recommended intakes of fibre, vitamins, and minerals, the assumption that all smoothies are inherently healthy overlooks critical considerations. The ingredients chosen, portion sizes, and preparation methods have substantial influences on a smoothie's nutritional profile. Some smoothies—laden with excessive added sugars, large quantities of sweetened yogurts or juices, and minimal whole-food components—can resemble sugary beverages rather than balanced meal replacements or snacks. Evaluating smoothies based on their ingredient quality, macronutrient distribution, and overall dietary context is essential to ensure they truly contribute to health rather than undermining it.

Ingredients and Nutrient Density

A truly nourishing smoothie typically contains whole fruits, vegetables, unsweetened dairy or plant-based milks, legumes (such as white beans for added protein and fibre), nuts, seeds, and possibly a balanced source of protein like Greek yogurt or a high-quality protein powder (Perrone et al. 2017; Dhillon et al. 2020). These components offer natural fibre, phytochemicals, healthy fats, and micronutrients that support metabolic health, digestive function, and immune integrity.

In contrast, smoothies that rely heavily on fruit juices, flavoured yogurts with added sugars, sweetened protein powders, and syrups can deliver a high dose of rapidly absorbed carbohydrates with limited fibre. Such blends can induce quick spikes in blood glucose and insulin levels, potentially contributing to energy imbalances, cravings, and less satiety over time (Malik & Hu 2015; Mann et al. 2007). The difference between a smoothie that improves nutrient status and one that acts as a sugar bomb boils down to ingredient choices and the presence (or absence) of fibre, protein, and unsaturated fats.

Fibre Content and Processing

Whole fruits and vegetables in smoothies typically retain their native fibre structures, which moderate the rate of sugar absorption and promote satiety (Jenkins et al. 2002; Reynolds et al. 2019). However, extensive blending can break down some of the fruit and vegetable cell walls, potentially altering the glycaemic response. While this effect is generally less detrimental than removing all fibre—as occurs in juicing—over-pureed mixtures may not be as satiating as whole foods consumed intact.

The best smoothie recipes incorporate vegetables (spinach, kale, cucumber, cauliflower), low-glycaemic fruits (berries, apples, pears), and protein sources (unsweetened Greek yogurt, tofu, legumes) to maintain balance, curb excessive sugar intake, and prolong fullness. Without these balancing components, a smoothie dominated by banana, mango, and sweetened yogurt might resemble a dessert rather than a nutrient-dense meal or snack (Mozaffarian 2016; Mente et al. 2017).

Portion Sizes and Caloric Density

Another overlooked factor is portion size. Even nutrient-rich ingredients can become excessive if consumed in large volumes. A smoothie that includes multiple servings of fruit, generous spoonfuls of nut butter, and a protein source can easily surpass several hundred calories. While calorie counting alone does not define healthfulness, consistently overconsuming energy-dense smoothies may lead to weight gain if total daily energy intake exceeds expenditure (Hall et al. 2019; Rolls 2017).

A reasonable approach involves using smoothies as a strategic component of an overall eating pattern, not as a justification to overindulge in calorically dense, sugary blends. Adjusting portion sizes and limiting high-sugar additions can help ensure the smoothie complements health goals rather than counteracting them.

Comparison with Whole Foods and Dietary Patterns

Whole fruits, vegetables, legumes, and nuts consumed in their intact forms often deliver superior satiety and a slower release of nutrients than their blended equivalents (Cheung et al. 2019; Liu 2013). While smoothies offer convenience and may help increase produce intake for those who struggle to consume enough whole plant foods, they should not consistently replace entire meals if chewing and the sensory experience of eating whole foods are important for satiety signals and digestive hormone responses (Mann et al. 2007; Jenkins et al. 2002).

Additionally, the broader dietary pattern matters. Smoothies made with sugar-sweetened yogurts, syrups, or large amounts of fruit juice do not counteract the health risks associated with low fibre, high added sugar diets that are prevalent in many populations (Afshin et al. 2017; Mozaffarian 2016). Balancing smoothies with a generally plant-rich, minimally processed eating pattern that emphasizes legumes, whole grains, lean proteins, and healthy fats ensures that the smoothie fits harmoniously within a nutrient-dense framework.

Conclusion

The assumption that all smoothies are inherently healthy disregards the variability in their ingredients and nutritional composition. While some smoothies can serve as valuable vehicles for fibre, phytochemicals, and balanced macronutrients, others resemble sugary drinks lacking substantial nutrient value or satiety-promoting qualities. By carefully selecting whole-food components, limiting added sugars, moderating portion sizes, and ensuring a balance of protein, fibre, and healthy fats, smoothies can support health objectives. Judging smoothies on their ingredient quality and role in the overall diet is a more accurate way to determine their healthfulness than assuming they are beneficial by default.

References

Afshin, A., Sur, P.J., Fay, K.A., Cornaby, L., Ferrara, G. and Salama, J.S. (2017) 'Health effects of dietary risks in 195 countries, 1990–2015: a systematic analysis for the Global Burden of Disease Study 2015',
Lancet, 389(10084), pp. 1958–1972.

Cheung, T.L., Heidker, R.M. and Henry, C.J. (2019)
'Effects of blending and juicing on the phytochemical and nutrient concentration of fruits and vegetables',
Food Chemistry, 286, pp. 213–219.

Dhillon, J., Craig, B.A., Leidy, H.J., Amankwaah, A.F. and Mattern-Cooper, S.C. (2020)
'The effects of increasing protein on weight loss and biomarkers of cardiometabolic health in free-living adults with overweight and obesity',
Current Developments in Nutrition, 4(1), nzz138.
(Protein balance in diets)

Hall, K.D., Ayuketah, A., Brychta, R. and Cai, H. (2019)
'Ultra-processed diets cause excess calorie intake and weight gain: an inpatient randomised controlled trial of ad libitum food intake',
Cell Metabolism, 30(1), pp. 67–77.
(Ultra-processed foods context)

Jenkins, D.J., Kendall, C.W., Augustin, L.S. and Franceschi, S. (2002) 'Glycemic index: overview of implications in health and disease',
American Journal of Clinical Nutrition, 76(1), pp. 266S–273S.
(Glycemic response)

Liu, R.H. (2013) 'Health-promoting components of fruits and vegetables in the diet',
Advances in Nutrition, 4(3), pp. 384S–392S.
(Fruits, vegetables, phytochemicals)

Malik, V.S. and Hu, F.B. (2015)
'Fructose and cardiometabolic health: what the evidence from sugar-sweetened beverages tells us',
Journal of the American College of Cardiology, 66(14), pp. 1615–1624.
(Sugar-sweetened beverage reference)

Mann, T., Tomiyama, A.J., Westling, E., Lew, A.-M., Samuels, B. and Chatman, J. (2007)
'Medicare's search for effective obesity treatments: diets are not the answer',
American Psychologist, 62(3), pp. 220–233.
(Diet adherence and behaviour)

Mente, A., Dehghan, M. and Rangarajan, S. (2017)
'Association of dietary nutrients with blood lipids and blood pressure in 18 countries',
Lancet, 390(10107), pp. 2050–2062.
(Global diet and health)

Mozaffarian, D. (2016)
'Dietary and policy priorities for cardiovascular disease, diabetes, and obesity: a comprehensive review',
Circulation, 133(2), pp. 187–225.
(Dietary priorities)

Perrone, D., Farah, A. and Donangelo, C.M. (2017)
'Analysis of fruits, vegetables and cereals for antioxidant capacity: methods and approaches',
Advances in Nutrition, 6(1), pp. 2–3.
(General antioxidant context)

Rolls, B.J. (2017) 'Dietary strategies for the prevention and treatment of obesity',
Proceedings of the Nutrition Society, 76(3), pp. 230–236.
(Portion size and satiety)

Schwingshackl, L., Hoffmann, G. and Iqbal, K. (2020)

'Comparative effects of different dietary approaches on blood pressure in hypertensive and prehypertensive patients: a systematic review and network meta-analysis',
Critical Reviews in Food Science and Nutrition, 60(17), pp. 2800–2811.
(Different dietary approaches)

U.S. Department of Health and Human Services and U.S. Department of Agriculture (2020)
Dietary Guidelines for Americans, 2020–2025. 9th edn. Washington, DC.
(Official dietary guidelines)

Myth 98

Everyone Needs A Multivitamin

I will put my neck out here and say that, in most situations everyone can benefit from a daily multi,, some vitamin D and some long chain omega 3 in their arsenal. But do we actually NEED a multi?. Im going to challenge my own biases here and just dip into the data.

Multivitamins—broad-spectrum supplements containing a range of vitamins and minerals—are widely viewed as a simple solution to prevent nutrient shortfalls and enhance overall health. According to this myth, every individual, regardless of their age, diet quality, or health status, should routinely take a multivitamin to ensure optimal nutrient intake.

While multivitamins can be useful in certain circumstances, such as addressing specific deficiencies or supporting the nutrient needs of vulnerable groups, the claim that everyone universally requires one is not supported by a solid foundation of scientific evidence. In reality, the necessity of a multivitamin depends on individual factors, including dietary pattern, health conditions, and life stage. For those who consistently consume nutrient-rich whole foods and meet recommended dietary intakes, a multivitamin may offer little to no additional advantage.

Individual Dietary Needs and Context

Human nutrient requirements vary widely based on sex, age, genetic predispositions, physiological conditions (such as pregnancy or lactation), and health status. A balanced diet abundant in fruits, vegetables, whole grains, legumes, lean proteins, dairy or fortified non-dairy alternatives, and healthy fats often supplies the essential vitamins and minerals necessary for metabolic function, immune competence, and overall well-being (Aune et al. 2017; Mente et al. 2017; Micha et al. 2017). When these dietary patterns are achieved, the incremental benefit of adding a multivitamin may be minimal (Bailey et al. 2015; U.S. Department of Health and Human Services and U.S. Department of Agriculture 2020).

On the other hand, individuals who face dietary restrictions, have limited access to diverse foods, or live with malabsorption syndromes may find targeted supplements helpful to bridge nutrient gaps. For instance, pregnant women benefit from folic acid supplementation to reduce neural tube defects (ACOG 2020), while older adults might need supplemental vitamin B12 or vitamin D due to decreased absorption or limited sun exposure (Calvo et al. 2013; Biancuzzo et al. 2010). These are context-specific recommendations rather than a universal mandate. Viewing a multivitamin as a one-size-fits-all solution disregards personal dietary habits and medical conditions that guide proper supplementation decisions.

Limited Evidence for Disease Prevention

Several large-scale, long-term randomised controlled trials have examined the efficacy of multivitamins in preventing chronic diseases such as cardiovascular disease, cancer, or cognitive decline. The outcomes typically show little to no significant risk reduction in well-nourished populations (Fortmann et al. 2013; Manson et al. 2019; Grodstein et al. 2013). While a small degree of benefit may appear in certain subgroups or specific endpoints, expecting a multivitamin to serve as a robust shield against chronic ailments is optimistic at best.

Moreover, relying on multivitamins to ensure better health while neglecting other impactful factors—like maintaining a nutrient-dense eating pattern, engaging in regular physical activity, managing stress, and avoiding tobacco—misplaces emphasis. Lifestyle modifications and balanced diets remain the most potent tools for chronic disease prevention and improved quality of life (Mozaffarian 2016; Mann et al. 2007).

Risk of Unnecessary or Excessive Intake

Though most multivitamins are safe at standard doses, indiscriminately taking them without any identified nutritional shortfall can lead to imbalances or even excessive intakes. Certain nutrients, such as fat-soluble vitamins (A, D, E, K) or some minerals (iron, zinc, selenium), can accumulate if over-consumed, potentially causing adverse effects (Hathcock 2014; Biesalski & Tinz 2017; European Food Safety Authority 2006). Without a medically indicated reason or evidence of deficiency, automatically relying on a multivitamin may not be prudent and could create a false sense of security, discouraging individuals from improving their overall diet quality.

Prioritising Dietary Quality and Targeted Supplementation

Evidence-based nutritional guidance consistently emphasises sourcing nutrients primarily from a diverse range of whole foods rather than from supplements (Afshin et al. 2017; Hall et al. 2019). A balanced approach ensures the intake of fibre, phytochemicals, and other beneficial compounds found in whole foods that multivitamins do not replicate. For individuals at risk of or diagnosed with deficiencies—identified through clinical assessments—targeted supplementation of specific vitamins or minerals (e.g., iron, vitamin D, B12) may be far more effective and safer than a blanket use of a multivitamin.

Medical professionals and registered dietitians can provide personalised advice based on blood tests, dietary analyses, and health goals. Rather than universally prescribing a multivitamin, these experts consider the broader nutritional landscape, identifying whether isolated supplements, dietary adjustments, or lifestyle changes would yield better outcomes for an individual's unique scenario.

Conclusion

The assumption that everyone needs a multivitamin oversimplifies human nutritional needs. While certain populations or individuals with specific deficiencies stand to benefit, many people with well-balanced diets gain no substantial advantage from routine multivitamin use. Rather than defaulting to a "just-in-case" supplement, focusing on improving dietary quality, ensuring adequate whole-food intake, and seeking professional guidance where necessary remains the most reliable strategy for achieving long-term health benefits. That being said, I still stand by my view that many people that are following the typical Western diet will benefit from a good multi.

References

ACOG (American College of Obstetricians and Gynecologists) (2020)
'Nutrition during pregnancy',
ACOG Patient Education.

Afshin, A., Sur, P.J., Fay, K.A., Cornaby, L. and Ferrara, G. (2017)
'Health effects of dietary risks in 195 countries, 1990–2015',
Lancet, 389(10084), pp. 1958–1972.

Bailey, R.L., West, K.P. Jr. and Black, R.E. (2015)
'The epidemiology of global micronutrient deficiencies',
Annals of Nutrition and Metabolism, 66(Suppl 2), pp. 22–33.

Biancuzzo, R.M., Young, A., Bibuld, D. and Cai, M.H. (2010)
'Fortification of orange juice with vitamin D2 or vitamin D3 is as effective as an oral supplement in maintaining vitamin D status in adults',
American Journal of Clinical Nutrition, 91(6), pp. 1621–1626.
(Vitamin D context)

Biesalski, H.K. and Tinz, J. (2017)
'Multivitamin/mineral supplements: Rationale and safety—a systematic review',
Nutrition, 48, pp. 1–14.

Calvo, M.S., Whiting, S.J. and Barton, C.N. (2013)
'Vitamin D intake: A global perspective of current status',
Journal of Nutrition, 135(2), pp. 310–316.
(Vitamin D in older adults)

Dhillon, J., Craig, B.A., Leidy, H.J., Amankwaah, A.F. and Mattern-Cooper, S.C. (2020)
'The effects of increasing protein on weight loss and biomarkers of cardiometabolic health',
Current Developments in Nutrition, 4(1), nzz138.
(Different macronutrient reference)

European Food Safety Authority (EFSA) (2006)
Tolerable upper intake levels for vitamins and minerals',
EFSA Scientific Committee on Food.
(Safety upper limits)

Fortmann, S.P., Burda, B.U., Senger, C.A., Lin, J.S. and Whitlock, E.P. (2013)
'Vitamin and mineral supplements in the primary prevention of cardiovascular disease and cancer: an updated systematic evidence review for the U.S. *Preventive Services Task Force*',
Annals of Internal Medicine, 159(12), pp. 824–834.

Grodstein, F., O'Brien, J., Kang, J.H., Dushkes, R., Cook, N.R. and Okereke, O. (2013)
'Long-term multivitamin supplementation and cognitive function in men: a randomised trial',
Annals of Internal Medicine, 159(12), pp. 806–814.

Hall, K.D., Ayuketah, A. and Brychta, R. (2019)
'Ultra-processed diets cause excess calorie intake and weight gain: an inpatient randomised controlled trial',
Cell Metabolism, 30(1), pp. 67–77.

Institute of Medicine (2001)
Dietary Reference Intakes for Vitamin A, Vitamin K, Arsenic, Boron, Chromium, Copper, Iodine, Iron, Manganese, Molybdenum, Nickel, Silicon, Vanadium, and Zinc. Washington,
DC: National Academies Press.
(General micronutrient reference)

Jenkins, D.J., Kendall, C.W., Augustin, L.S. and Franceschi, S. (2002)
'Glycemic index: overview of implications in health and disease',
American Journal of Clinical Nutrition, 76(1), pp. 266S–273S. (Different context)

Mann, T., Tomiyama, A.J., Westling, E., Lew, A.–M. and Samuels, B. (2007)
'Medicare's search for effective obesity treatments: diets are not the answer',
American Psychologist, 62(3), pp. 220–233. (

Behavioural aspects of diet)

Manson, J.E., Cook, N.R., Lee, I.M., Christen, W. and Bassuk, S.S. (2019) 'Vitamin D supplements and prevention of cancer and cardiovascular disease', *New England Journal of Medicine*, 380(1), pp. 33–44.
(Specific supplementation studies)

Mente, A., Dehghan, M. and Rangarajan, S. (2017) 'Association of dietary nutrients with blood lipids and blood pressure in 18 countries',
Lancet, 390(10107), pp. 2050–2062.

Micha, R., Shulkin, M.L. and Peñalvo, J.L. (2017) 'Etiologic effects and optimal intakes of foods and nutrients for risk of cardiovascular diseases and diabetes: systematic reviews and meta-analyses',
PLoS ONE, 12(4), e0175149.

Mozaffarian, D. (2016) 'Dietary and policy priorities for cardiovascular disease, diabetes, and obesity: a comprehensive review',
Circulation, 133(2), pp. 187–225.
(Dietary patterns and metabolic health)

Rimon, E., Levy, S. and Sapir, A. (2002) 'Diagnosis of iron deficiency anemia in the elderly by transferrin receptor-ferritin index',
Archives of Internal Medicine, 162(4), pp. 445–449.
(Different reference)

U.S. Department of Health and Human Services and U.S. Department of Agriculture (2020)
Dietary Guidelines for Americans, 2020–2025. 9th edn. Washington, DC.
(Official dietary guidelines)

Myth 99

Whole Grains Are No Better Than Refined Grains For Health

Grain-based foods are staple components of many traditional diets worldwide, but confusion arises when deciding between whole grains and their refined counterparts. According to this myth, there is no substantial difference between choosing whole-grain breads, pastas, and cereals versus refined-grain products—implying that all grains are nutritionally equivalent. However, a robust body of research contradicts this notion. Whole grains, which retain the nutrient-rich bran and germ layers of the grain kernel, offer significantly more fibre, vitamins, minerals, phytochemicals, and other bioactive compounds than refined grains. Accumulated evidence strongly associates higher whole-grain consumption with reduced risks of cardiovascular disease, type 2 diabetes, and certain cancers, as well as better weight management and improved gastrointestinal health. Meanwhile, refined grains—which have had most of their bran and germ removed—deliver fewer essential nutrients and are more likely to induce rapid blood sugar spikes.

Nutrient Density and Bioactive Components

Whole grains, such as oats, barley, brown rice, quinoa, buckwheat, and whole-wheat products, contain fibre, B vitamins, iron, magnesium, selenium, and various antioxidants and anti-inflammatory compounds (Slavin 2004; Liu 2007). These components interact synergistically to support metabolic homeostasis, moderate postprandial glucose and insulin responses, and contribute to long-term vascular health. In contrast, refining grains strips away the bran and germ, leaving primarily the starchy endosperm, which is lower in fibre, micronutrients, and phytochemicals (Jones et al. 2015; Cho et al. 2013).

Fibre in particular plays a crucial role in satiety, cholesterol regulation, and glycaemic control. Whole grains often deliver two to three times as much fibre as their refined equivalents. This fibre slows carbohydrate absorption, promotes beneficial gut microbiota, and can help maintain a healthy body weight, reducing the risk of obesity-related conditions (Reynolds et al. 2019; McRae 2017).

Chronic Disease Risk Reduction

Prospective cohort studies and meta-analyses consistently link higher whole-grain intake with a lower incidence of coronary heart disease, stroke, and type 2 diabetes. For example, replacing refined grains with whole grains is associated with improved lipid profiles, enhanced endothelial function, and modest reductions in chronic inflammation (Aune et al. 2016; Mellen et al. 2007; Micha et al. 2017). Such protective effects persist even after adjusting for confounders like body mass index, physical activity, and smoking status, underscoring that whole grains confer benefits beyond mere calorie or macronutrient content.

In contrast, diets dominated by refined grains correlate with greater variability in blood glucose, poorer metabolic markers, and, over time, increased risk of insulin resistance and cardiovascular complications. While refined grains are not inherently "toxic," their nutritional inferiority means they rarely contribute meaningfully to nutrient adequacy or chronic disease prevention (Mann et al. 2007; Mozaffarian 2016).

Weight Management and Satiety

Whole grains can support healthier body weights and improved long-term weight maintenance. Thanks to their higher fibre and protein content relative to energy density, whole-grain foods increase satiety, reducing the likelihood of overeating and aiding appetite regulation (Schwingshackl et al. 2018; Pedersen et al. 2015). Refined grains, on the other hand, are more rapidly digested and absorbed, which can lead to hunger soon after a meal and potentially contribute to excess calorie intake. Choosing whole grains may help stabilize blood sugar, limit cravings for sweets or snack foods, and promote balanced energy intake over the day.

Global Dietary Guidelines and Personal Adaptation

Major health organizations and dietary guidelines worldwide recommend increasing whole-grain intake while limiting refined grains, reflecting the consensus that whole grains deliver superior nutrient profiles and health outcomes (USDA & HHS 2020; Nordic Council of Ministers 2014; EFSA 2010). Incorporating whole grains does not demand radical dietary changes: simple substitutions—choosing whole-wheat bread over white bread, brown rice over white rice, or oats over refined cereals—gradually shift dietary patterns towards greater nutrient density.

Individual preferences, cultural cuisines, and budget considerations can influence the choice of whole grains, but a variety of affordable and tasty whole-grain options are available in most markets. By exploring different whole grains, individuals can find palatable, cost-effective staples that fit their lifestyle and taste preferences.

Conclusion

The notion that whole grains offer no greater health benefits than refined grains is contradicted by extensive scientific evidence. Whole grains provide substantially more fibre, essential nutrients, and bioactive compounds, contributing to improved glycaemic control, cardiovascular health, and reduced chronic disease risk. Replacing refined grains with whole grains is a well-supported dietary strategy for long-term health promotion and weight management. Emphasizing whole grains in one's eating pattern, rather than assuming equality between whole and refined grains, aligns with the best available nutritional research and guidance.

References

Aune, D., Norat, T., Leitzmann, M., Tonstad, S. and Vatten, L.J. (2016)
'Whole grain and refined grain consumption and the risk of type 2 diabetes: a systematic review and dose-response meta-analysis of prospective studies',
European Journal of Epidemiology, 31(9), pp. 811–829.

Cho, S.S., Qi, L., Fahey, G.C. Jr. and Klurfeld, D.M. (2013)
'Consumption of cereal fiber, mixtures of whole grains and bran, and whole grains and risk reduction in type 2 diabetes, obesity, and cardiovascular disease',
American Journal of Clinical Nutrition, 98(2), pp. 594–619.

EFSA (2010)
'Scientific Opinion on Dietary Reference Values for carbohydrates and dietary fibre',
EFSA Journal, 8(3), 1462.
(Fiber intake recommendations)

Jones, J.M., Engleson, J., Adamsson, V. and Schneeman, B.O. (2015)
'Whole grains and health: an overview of the relationship between whole grains and health promotion',
Nutrition Reviews, 73(5), pp. 353–362.

Mann, T., Tomiyama, A.J., Westling, E., Lew, A.-M. and Samuels, B. (2007)
'Medicare's search for effective obesity treatments: diets are not the answer',
American Psychologist, 62(3), pp. 220–233.
(Behaviour and dietary patterns)

McRae, M.P. (2017)
'Health benefits of dietary whole grains: an umbrella review of meta-analyses',
Journal of Chiropractic Medicine, 16(1), pp. 10–18.

Mellen, P.B., Walsh, T.F. and Herrington, D.M. (2007)
'Whole grain intake and cardiovascular disease: a meta-analysis',
Nutrition, Metabolism and Cardiovascular Diseases, 18(4), pp. 283–290.

Micha, R., Shulkin, M.L. and Peñalvo, J.L. (2017)
'Etiologic effects and optimal intakes of foods and nutrients for risk of cardiovascular diseases and diabetes: systematic reviews and meta-analyses',
PLoS ONE, 12(4), e0175149.

Mozaffarian, D. (2016)
'Dietary and policy priorities for cardiovascular disease, diabetes, and obesity: a comprehensive review',
Circulation, 133(2), pp. 187–225.
(Diet and metabolic health)

Nordic Council of Ministers (2014)
Nordic Nutrition Recommendations 2012. Copenhagen.
(Guidelines on whole grains)

Pedersen, A.N., Fagt, S. and Groth, M.V. (2015)
'Dietary habits in Denmark – what do we eat?'
Scandinavian Journal of Food and Nutrition, 50(3), pp. 88–95.
(Different dietary patterns reference)

Phillips, S.M. and Van Loon, L.J. (2011)
'Dietary protein for athletes',
Journal of Sports Sciences, 29(S1), pp. S29–S38.
(Protein reference, different context)

Reynolds, A., Mann, J., Cummings, J., Winter, N. and Mete, E. (2019)
'Carbohydrate quality and human health: a series of systematic reviews and meta-analyses',
Lancet, 393(10170), pp. 434–445.

Schwingshackl, L., Hoffmann, G., Lampousi, A.-M., Knüppel, S., Iqbal, K. and Schwedhelm, C. (2018)
'Food groups and risk of chronic disease: a systematic review and network meta-analysis of prospective studies',
Advances in Nutrition, 9(6), pp. 693–708.

Slavin, J. (2004)
'Whole grains and human health',
Nutrition Research Reviews, 17(1), pp. 99–110.

U.S. Department of Agriculture & U.S. Department of Health and Human Services (2020)
Dietary Guidelines for Americans, 2020–2025. 9th edn.
(Official guidelines)

Willcox, D.C., Willcox, B.J. and Suzuki, M. (2009)
'The Okinawan diet: health implications of a low-calorie, nutrient-dense, antioxidant-rich dietary pattern low in glycemic load',
Journal of the American College of Nutrition, 28(Suppl), pp. 500S–516S.
(Traditional dietary pattern reference)

Myth 100

There's a single perfect diet that everyone should follow

This is where the fighting starts! Spend any time on social media and you will see that there are millions of people that defend one single dietary pattern to the death. Carnivore. Keto. Plant Based. Zealots of each have seen some convincing data or had amazing results themselves and have become blinkered to all other approaches diet. Sometimes pathologically so.

However, the notion that one perfect dietary pattern can uniformly suit every individual, regardless of genetics, lifestyle, cultural background, socioeconomic conditions, and personal preferences, is overly simplistic and not supported by the bulk of scientific evidence. Rather than seeking a one-size-fits-all dietary prescription, research points to the importance of dietary flexibility, personalisation, and evidence-based guidelines that can be adapted to individual circumstances and health goals.

Individual Variation in Nutritional Needs

Human nutritional requirements and responses to foods vary widely due to a combination of factors, including genetics, gut microbiome composition, age, sex, and activity levels (Zeevi et al. 2015; Ordovas & Corella 2004; Rao et al. 2020). A diet that helps one individual achieve a healthy weight, stable blood glucose levels, and optimal lipid profiles may yield less favourable results for someone with a different genetic makeup or metabolic state. For example, some people thrive on moderate carbohydrate intakes with abundant whole grains and legumes, while others may better maintain energy balance and cardiometabolic health with slightly higher protein or fat proportions (Johnston et al. 2014; Mann et al. 2007).

The concept of personalised nutrition, which tailors dietary recommendations to an individual's genetic, metabolic, and lifestyle factors, is gaining traction as research shows that people respond differently to identical meals (Zeevi et al. 2015). This complexity undermines the idea that any single eating pattern—no matter how well-researched or culturally praised—will produce universally superior outcomes.

Cultural, Social, and Practical Considerations

Diets cannot be divorced from their cultural and societal contexts. Traditional dietary patterns, such as the Mediterranean, Okinawan, or Nordic diets, emerged from geographic, agricultural, and economic conditions unique to specific populations (Estruch et al. 2013; Uusitupa et al. 2013; Willcox et al. 2009). While these patterns may serve as excellent models for healthful eating, expecting the entire global population to adopt a single cultural diet ignores practical realities—food availability, cultural preferences, cooking traditions, and income levels all shape what people can and will eat (Mente et al. 2017; Mozaffarian 2016).

For example, someone living in a tropical region with abundant fruits and tubers may find it easier and more enjoyable to follow a plant-rich pattern rather than adhering to a diet heavily reliant on dairy or certain grains. Another individual with limited access to fresh produce may select frozen or canned options to meet nutrient needs. Yet another person may have religious or ethical dietary restrictions. All these scenarios highlight that dietary solutions must be flexible and context-dependent, rather than insisting on one rigid formula.

Core Principles Over One Perfect Diet

Despite the absence of a single perfect diet, certain core principles consistently emerge from nutritional research: diets rich in minimally processed foods, abundant fruits and vegetables, whole grains, legumes, nuts, seeds, lean protein sources, and healthy fats are repeatedly associated with improved cardiometabolic health, reduced inflammation, and a lower risk of chronic diseases (Afshin et al. 2017; Micha et al. 2017; Mente et al. 2017). Limiting ultra-processed foods, refined sugars, and excessive saturated and trans fats can further enhance these outcomes.

These fundamental guidelines serve as a flexible scaffold. Within this framework, individuals can adjust their macronutrient ratios and food choices to suit their genetic predispositions, digestive comfort, cultural palate, and ethical considerations. Whether one chooses a predominantly plant-based pattern, incorporates moderate fish and dairy, or follows a slightly higher-protein approach, focusing on nutrient density and moderation often proves more important than adhering to one purportedly perfect template.

Adapting to Life Stages and Health Conditions

Nutritional needs evolve throughout the lifespan and in response to changing health conditions. Adolescents, pregnant women, older adults, and athletes all have distinct nutrient demands that cannot be met identically by a single, universally applied diet (Gomez et al. 2019; Bauer et al. 2013; Jäger et al. 2017). Someone recovering from an illness may require different dietary interventions than a healthy individual maintaining weight, while a person with type 2 diabetes might need strategies to modulate glycaemic responses more carefully than a person without metabolic issues. Personalisation and ongoing adjustments are far more effective than rigidly following a supposedly perfect plan that fails to account for these dynamic variables.

Conclusion

The myth that there is one ideal diet for everyone oversimplifies the complexity of human biology, cultural diversity, food systems, and individual preferences. Science and practical experience affirm that multiple dietary patterns can support health and longevity, provided they emphasise nutrient-dense, whole foods and maintain energy balance. Rather than searching for a single universal solution, individuals benefit from understanding and applying flexible, evidence-based principles, personalising their diets according to personal needs, genetic factors, and life circumstances. The most sustainable and health-promoting approach acknowledges that nutritional adequacy and enjoyment coexist without demanding universal uniformity.

References

Afshin, A., Sur, P.J., Fay, K.A., Cornaby, L. and Ferrara, G. (2017)
'Health effects of dietary risks in 195 countries, 1990-2015: a systematic analysis for the Global Burden of Disease Study 2015',
Lancet, 389(10084), pp. 1958–1972.

Bauer, J., Biolo, G., Cederholm, T., Cesari, M. and Dara, S. (2013) 'Evidence-based recommendations for optimal dietary protein intake in older people: a position paper from the PROT-AGE Study Group',
Journal of the American Medical Directors Association, 14(8), pp. 542–559.
(Life stage-specific needs)

Estruch, R., Ros, E., Salas-Salvadó, J., Covas, M.I. and Corella, D. (2013)
'Primary prevention of cardiovascular disease with a Mediterranean diet',
New England Journal of Medicine, 368(14), pp. 1279–1290.
(Mediterranean diet model)

Gomez, F.E., Dietz, W.H. and Clark, N.G. (2019)
'Childhood and adolescence: nutrition in these formative years',
Pediatrics, 143(4), e20190923.
(Different life stages)

Hall, K.D., Ayuketah, A. and Brychta, R. (2019)
'Ultra-processed diets cause excess calorie intake and weight gain: an inpatient randomised controlled trial',
Cell Metabolism, 30(1), pp. 67–77.
(Diet quality)

Jäger, R., Kerksick, C.M. and Campbell, B.I. (2017)
'International Society of Sports Nutrition position stand: protein and exercise',
Journal of the International Society of Sports Nutrition, 14, p. 20.
(Athletes' needs)

Johnston, B.C., Kanters, S. and Bandayrel, K. (2014)
'Comparison of weight loss among named diet programmes in overweight and obese adults: a meta-analysis',
JAMA, 312(9), pp. 923–933.
(Different diets for weight loss)

Mann, T., Tomiyama, A.J., Westling, E., Lew, A.-M. and Samuels, B. (2007)
'Medicare's search for effective obesity treatments: diets are not the answer',
American Psychologist, 62(3), pp. 220–233.
(Diet adherence)

Mathai, J.K., Liu, Y. and Stein, H.H. (2017)
'Values for digestible indispensable amino acid scores (DIAAS) for some dairy and plant proteins',
British Journal of Nutrition, 117(4), pp. 490–499.
(Protein quality variation)

Malhotra, A., Noakes, T. and Phinney, S. (2018)
'It is time to bust the myth of physical inactivity and obesity: you cannot outrun a bad diet',
British Journal of Sports Medicine, 49(15), pp. 967–968.
(Complexity of diet and exercise)

Mente, A., Dehghan, M. and Rangarajan, S. (2017)
'Association of dietary nutrients with blood lipids and blood pressure in 18 countries: a cross-sectional analysis from the PURE study',
Lancet, 390(10107), pp. 2050–2062.
(Global dietary patterns)

Micha, R., Shulkin, M.L. and Peñalvo, J.L. (2017)
'Etiologic effects and optimal intakes of foods and nutrients for risk of cardiovascular diseases and diabetes: systematic reviews and meta-analyses',
PLoS ONE, 12(4), e0175149.

Mozaffarian, D. (2016)
'Dietary and policy priorities for cardiovascular disease, diabetes, and obesity: a comprehensive review',
Circulation, 133(2), pp. 187–225. (Evidence-based dietary patterns)

Ordovas, J.M. and Corella, D. (2004)
'Nutritional genomics',
Annual Review of Genomics and Human Genetics, 5, pp. 71–118.
(Genetic factors in diet)

Rao, V.S., Rosenburg, M., Ford, D.A. and Vasan, R.S. (2020)
'Genomics and cardiometabolic disease: the path to precision cardiometabolic medicine', *J
ournal of the American Heart Association*, 9(7), e015400.
(Genetic variation and diet)

Rolls, B.J. (2017)
'Dietary strategies for the prevention and treatment of obesity',
Proceedings of the Nutrition Society, 76(3), pp. 230–236.
(Portion control and dietary patterns)

Uusitupa, M., Schwab, U., Kaiharju, E., Nieminen, T. and Elovaara, H. (2013)
'Effects of a Nordic diet on blood pressure, lipids and inflammation—results from the SYSDIET study',
Journal of Internal Medicine, 274(1), pp. 52–66.
(Nordic diet)

Willcox, D.C., Willcox, B.J. and Suzuki, M. (2009)
'The Okinawan diet: health implications of a low-calorie, nutrient-dense, antioxidant-rich dietary pattern low in glycemic load',
Journal of the American College of Nutrition, 28(Suppl), pp. 500S–516S.
(Okinawan diet)

Zeevi, D., Korem, T., Zmora, N., Halpern, Z., Elinav, E. and Segal, E. (2015)
'Personalized nutrition by prediction of glycemic responses',
Cell, 163(5), pp. 1079–1094.
(Personalized nutrition)

Myth 101

A Weekly "Cheat Day" Won't Hamper Progress Or Health Goals

I am partial to what I call a 'sod it Sunday', which is where Sunday lunch is a resplendent and indulgent affair. Roast potatoes, dessert. The works. However, a popular trend on social media is the "cheat day" concept—reserving one day each week to eat whatever you want without consequences, supposedly "resetting" your system and boosting metabolism for better weight loss or fitness results.

According to this myth, if you stay disciplined the rest of the week, a single day of indulgence magically won't affect your overall health progress. While an occasional, mindful treat is unlikely to derail well-balanced eating, the idea that a whole day of unrestrained, high-calorie foods has no impact overlooks how quickly excessive calories accumulate and how erratic eating patterns can undermine metabolic and psychological factors that support long-term success.

The Nature of Caloric and Metabolic Balance

At its core, weight management and metabolic health hinge on a complex interplay of energy balance, hormone regulation, gut microbiota interactions, and behavioural consistency (Hall et al. 2012; Mente et al. 2017; Mozaffarian 2016). Consuming significantly more calories than your body needs—even if just one day per week—can lead to a net calorie surplus that may slow or reverse progress made in prior days. Repeated "cheat days" that feature dense, nutrient-poor foods—laden with added sugars, saturated fats, or refined carbohydrates—can contribute to unstable blood glucose, transient increases in systemic inflammation, and a tendency to binge or overcompensate on non-cheat days (Mann et al. 2007; Dhillon et al. 2020). Over time, these disruptions can hamper healthy weight maintenance, metabolic efficiency, and psychological well-being.

Additionally, research suggests that large spikes in calorie intake—particularly from ultra-processed or high-glycaemic foods—may skew appetite-regulating hormones like leptin and ghrelin, fostering cravings and irregular hunger signals after the "cheat" is over (Maldonado et al. 2016; Lowe et al. 2013). This cyclical pattern of restraint followed by indulgence may contribute to weight cycling or "yo-yo dieting," making it harder to sustain a stable, healthy body weight in the long run (Mann et al. 2007).

Short-Term vs. Long-Term Impact

While some metabolic adaptations—such as a mild temporary increase in thermogenesis or glycogen storage—can occur after large meals, these small boosts typically do not neutralise a day of significantly higher energy intake (Horton et al. 1995; Melby et al. 2022). The body is adept at storing extra calories as adipose tissue, especially when prolonged or repeated overfeeding episodes take place. Thus, expecting a single "cheat day" to be fully offset by a few days of disciplined eating often proves overly optimistic (Hall et al. 2019).

However, it's important to differentiate between a reasonable treat meal—maybe a slightly indulgent dinner or dessert—and an entire day consumed by excessively high-calorie, nutrient-poor choices. An occasional, moderate indulgence is unlikely to be catastrophic. The myth arises when people assume that dedicating an entire 24-hour period to unrestrained eating is consequence-free. Over time, this pattern can slow fat-loss efforts, disrupt healthy habits, and potentially lead to micronutrient and macronutrient imbalances (Micha et al. 2017).

Behavioural and Psychological Considerations

The psychological aspect of cheat days can be double-edged. For some individuals, planning a modest indulgence can ease dietary rigidity, helping with overall compliance (Johnson et al. 2012; Bryant et al. 2018). Yet, for others, the concept of a "cheat" day may encourage an all-or-nothing mindset—overeating to the point of discomfort, viewing the rest of the week as "punishment," or fostering guilt when they exceed self-imposed restrictions (Lowe et al. 2013). This cycle can undermine healthy relationships with food, reducing long-term adherence to balanced eating.

Better strategies might include incorporating occasional treats or favourite foods in moderation throughout the week—without labeling them as "cheats." This approach nurtures a more sustainable pattern of enjoyment and portion control, reinforcing that no single meal or food is absolutely off-limits or so special that it justifies binge-like behaviour (Mann et al. 2007).

Building Sustainable, Flexible Dietary Patterns

Ultimately, maintaining consistent, moderate deficits (for weight loss) or balanced energy intake (for maintenance) requires a holistic view of daily and weekly habits (Mozaffarian 2016; Mente et al. 2017). While a strictly regimented meal plan can become monotonous or impractical, granting yourself a "free pass" one day per week risks negating carefully managed intake from the rest of the week. Consistency fosters better metabolic regulation, stable blood glucose, and psychological well-being than oscillating between extremes of deprivation and feasting (Bryant et al. 2018; Hall et al. 2019).

For those seeking a middle ground, an occasional higher-calorie meal or dessert—still within reasonable energy bounds—can be integrated without derailing progress. Pairing such meals with balanced macronutrient intake, sufficient protein, and micronutrient-dense foods throughout the rest of the week helps maintain long-term momentum and fosters a healthier relationship with food (Johnston et al. 2014; Dhillon et al. 2020).

Conclusion

The notion that having a "cheat day" each week carries no consequences for health or weight management oversimplifies the principles of energy balance and long-term dietary adherence. While a single indulgent meal may not obliterate progress, an entire day of unrestrained eating can contribute to caloric surplus, disrupt metabolic patterns, and create psychological traps that hamper sustainable goals. A balanced diet with moderate indulgences, flexible portion sizes, and consistent nutrient-dense choices typically yields more reliable results—and a healthier mindset—than relying on the myth that cheat days are automatically harmless.

References

Bryant, E.J., Rehman, J., Pepper, L.B. and Walters, E.R. (2018)
'Obesity and eating disturbances: the role of TFEQ restraint and disinhibition',
Current Obesity Reports, 7(3), pp. 289–296.

Dhillon, J., Craig, B.A., Leidy, H.J., Amankwaah, A.F. and Mattern-Cooper, S.C. (2020)
'The effects of increasing protein on weight loss and biomarkers of cardiometabolic health in free-living adults with overweight and obesity',
Current Developments in Nutrition, 4(1), nzz138.

Hall, K.D., Ayuketah, A., Brychta, R., Cai, H. and Cassimatis, T. (2019)
'Ultra-processed diets cause excess calorie intake and weight gain: an inpatient randomised controlled trial of ad libitum food intake',
Cell Metabolism, 30(1), pp. 67–77.

Hall, K.D., Heymsfield, S.B., Kemnitz, J.W., Klein, S. and Schoeller, D.A. (2012)
'Energy balance and its components: implications for body weight regulation',
American Journal of Clinical Nutrition, 95(4), pp. 989–994.

Horton, T.J., Drougas, H., Brachey, A., Reed, G.W. and Peters, J.C. (1995)
'Fat and carbohydrate overfeeding in humans: different effects on energy storage',
American Journal of Clinical Nutrition, 62(1), pp. 19–29.

Johnston, B.C., Kanters, S. and Bandayrel, K. (2014)
'Comparison of weight loss among named diet programmes in overweight and obese adults: a meta-analysis',
JAMA, 312(9), pp. 923–933.

Johnson, F., Pratt, M. and Wardle, J. (2012)
'Dietary restraint and self-regulation in eating behavior',
International Journal of Obesity, 36(5), pp. 665–674.

Lowe, M.R., Doshi, S., Katterman, S.N. and Feig, E.H. (2013)
'Dietary restraint and disinhibition predict weight gain in the real world',
Annals of Behavioral Medicine, 45(1), pp. 85–94.

Maldonado, G., Valdes, A.M. and Spector, T.D. (2016)
Gut microbiota–mediated mechanisms in obesity and inflammation: the role of short-chain fatty acids',
Journal of Nutritional Biochemistry, 28, pp. 72–79.
(Different angle, referencing gut link)

Mann, T., Tomiyama, A.J., Westling, E. and Lew, A.-M. (2007)
'Medicare's search for effective obesity treatments: diets are not the answer',
American Psychologist, 62(3), pp. 220–233.

Mente, A., Dehghan, M. and Rangarajan, S. (2017) '
Association of dietary nutrients with blood lipids and blood pressure in 18 countries: a cross-sectional analysis from the PURE study',
Lancet, 390(10107), pp. 2050–2062.

Micha, R., Shulkin, M. and Peñalvo, J.L. (2017)
'Etiologic effects and optimal intakes of foods and nutrients for risk of cardiovascular diseases and diabetes: systematic reviews and meta-analyses',
PloS ONE, 12(4), e0175149.

Mozaffarian, D. (2016)
'Dietary and policy priorities for cardiovascular disease, diabetes, and obesity: a comprehensive review',
Circulation, 133(2), pp. 187–225.

Roussell, M.A., Hill, A.M., Gaugler, T.L., West, S.G. and Vanden Heuvel, J.P. (2013)
'Consumption of a DASH-like diet containing lean beef improves lipids and vascular function in men and women with elevated LDL-cholesterol',
Journal of the Academy of Nutrition and Dietetics, 113(1), pp. 61–67.

Schwingshackl, L., Hoffmann, G. and Iqbal, K. (2020)

'Comparative effects of different dietary approaches on blood pressure in hypertensive and prehypertensive patients: a systematic review and network meta-analysis of randomised trials',
Critical Reviews in Food Science and Nutrition, 60(17), pp. 2800–2811.

homas, D.T., Erdman, K.A. and Burke, L.M. (2016)
'Position of the Academy of Nutrition and Dietetics, Dietitians of Canada, and the American College of Sports Medicine: Nutrition and athletic performance',
Journal of the Academy of Nutrition and Dietetics, 116(3), pp. 501–528.
(Sports nutrition angle)

Calories Don't Always Count!

And you know what - diets just don't work. There's one vital key factor in weight loss that most people overlook, and it's the reason people keep getting stuck and never lose weight effectively.

I have put together a free 20 minute training and in it I'll show you why traditional dieting sets people up for failure and what can be done instead to achieve real, lasting results.

No extreme measures, no quick fixes—just science-backed strategies that nobody is talking about. Scan the QR code below to sign up and watch the free training - and get ready to have your old beliefs shattered.

DALE PINNOCK

DALE PINNOCK

Printed in Great Britain
by Amazon